Mental Health Promotion, Prevention, and Intervention With Children and Youth: *A Guiding Framework for Occupational Therapy*

Edited by Susan Bazyk, PhD, OTR/L, FAOTA

Wendy – Welcome to this project. Here's to mental health! Sue

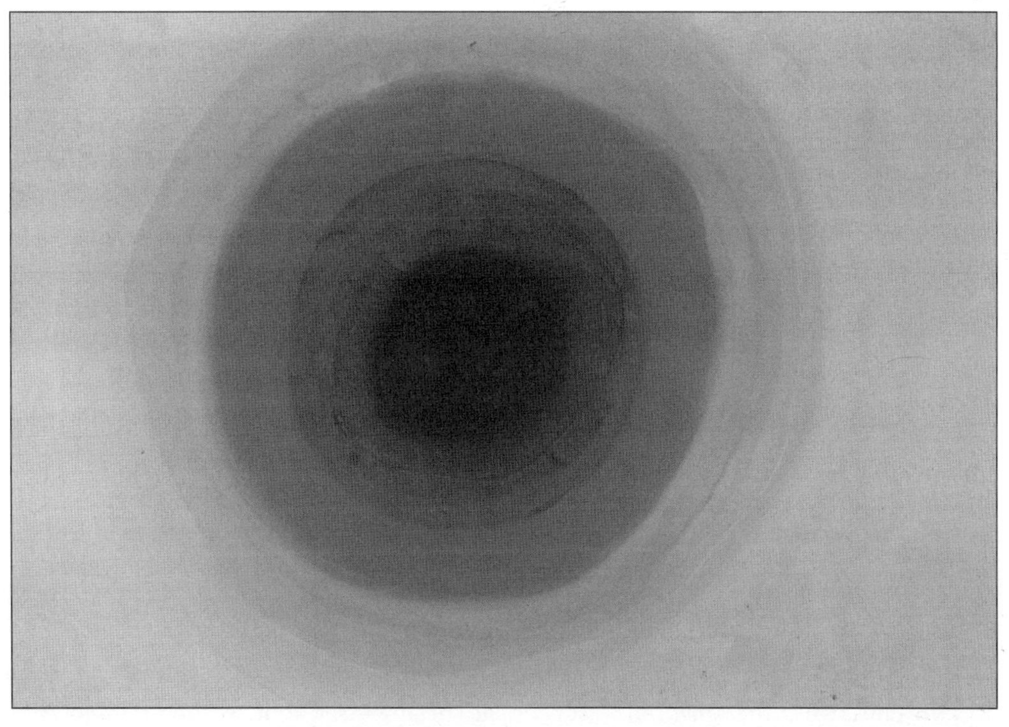

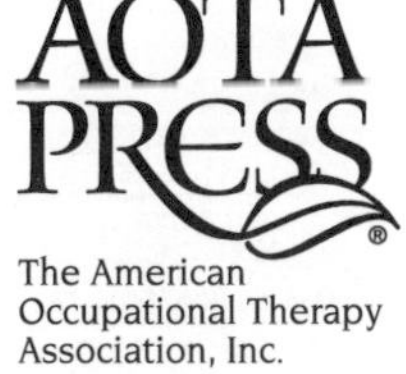

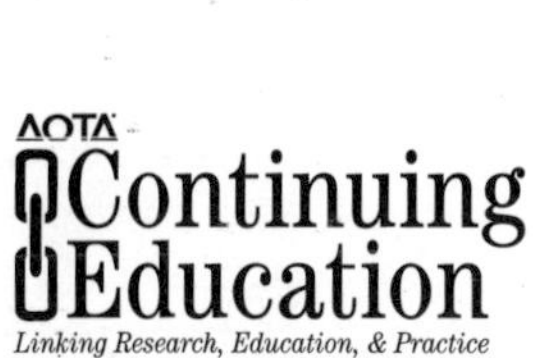

Centennial Vision
We envision that occupational therapy is a powerful, widely recognized, science-driven, and evidence-based profession with a globally connected and diverse workforce meeting society's occupational needs.

Vision Statement
The American Occupational Therapy Association advances occupational therapy as the pre-eminent profession in promoting the health, productivity, and quality of life of individuals and society through the therapeutic application of occupation.

Mission Statement
The American Occupational Therapy Association advances the quality, availability, use, and support of occupational therapy through standard-setting, advocacy, education, and research on behalf of its members and the public.

AOTA Staff
Frederick P. Somers, *Executive Director*
Christopher M. Bluhm, *Chief Operating Officer*
Maureen Freda Peterson, *Chief Professional Affairs Officer*

Chris Davis, *Director, AOTA Press*
Sarah D. Hertfelder, *Continuing Education Program Manager*
Caroline Polk, *Project Manager*
Cynthia Stock, *Electronic Quill Publishing Services, Compositor*

Beth Ledford, *Director, Marketing*
Emily Zhang, *Technology Marketing Specialist*
Jennifer Folden, *Marketing Specialist*

The American Occupational Therapy Association, Inc.
4720 Montgomery Lane
Bethesda, MD 20814
Phone: 301-652-AOTA (2682)
TDD: 800-377-8555
Fax: 301-652-7711
www.aota.org

Library of Congress Control Number: 2010918171
ISBN-13: 978-1-56900-274-3

About the Cover
The cover art is by Seth Chwast, who was born in 1983 and diagnosed with autism at an early age. An informal ambassador for autism, Chwast has spread hope by telling his story of finding his passion in art. He has exhibited in the United States and around the world. Visit www.SethChwastArt.com to see images of his art and learn more about his work.

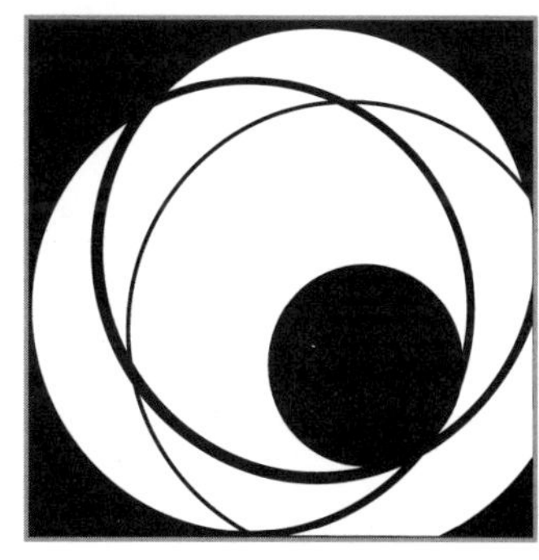

Contents

Dedication

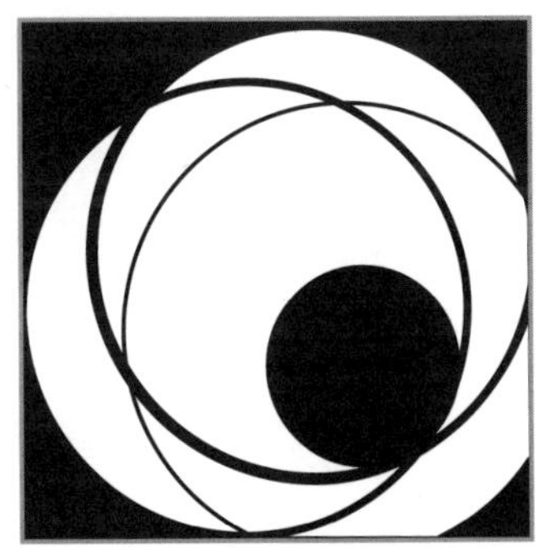

This book is dedicated to my parents.
To my mother, Lillian, who instilled in me a
thirst for knowledge and the value of caring
for others and who led me to occupational therapy;
and to my father, Leo, for teaching me the
value of persistence and hard work.

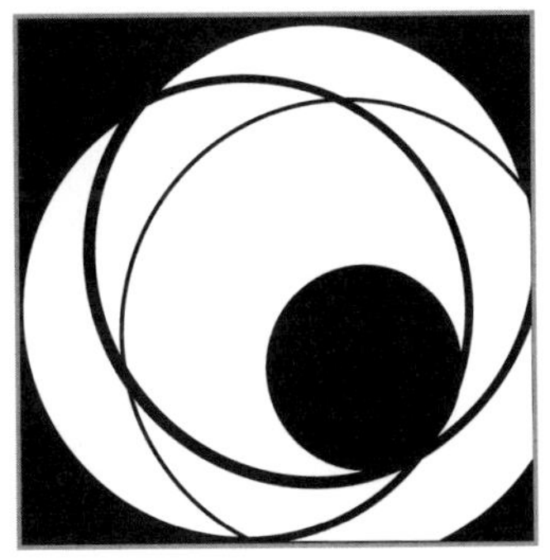

Acknowledgments

I would like to thank Barbara Hanft, Leslie Jackson, and Sandra Schefkind for inviting me to participate in a variety of national American Occupational Therapy Association activities over the past 20 years and for encouraging me to publish work related to the well-being of children and families. Such experiences have fueled my interest in children's mental health and confidence in sharing my voice. I am also deeply grateful to my family—John, Andrew, and Audrey—for their ongoing patience and support during the creation of this book.

A special acknowledgment is made to Andrea B. Sherwin, PhD, OTR/L, the co-author of Chapter 12. Dr. Sherwin served as an assistant professor in the Department of Occupational Therapy and Occupational Science at Towson University until her death in September 2010. Her family, colleagues, and friends honor her for her keen and inquisitive intellect, her commitment to family advocacy initiatives, and her deep passion for the profession of occupational therapy. She energized others by her undaunting spirit and her ability to appreciate the richness of life in the moment.

I also thank the following contributors for their practice examples and other materials that illustrate the concepts described in this volume:

- Chapter 3
  - *Robin M. Kirschenbaum, OTD, OTR/L*
  - *Susan Gara Mastromonaco, OTR/L*
- Chapter 5
  - *Waiming Cheung, MS, OTR*
  - *Ridvan Foxhall, OTS*
  - *Christina Francesconi, OTS*
  - *Bettina Franco, OTS*
  - *Carola Gomes, OTS*
  - *Kristina Mele, OTS*
  - *Glenn Yedowitz, MS, OTR*
- Chapter 10
  - *Claudette Fette, OTR*
  - *Diane Ventura, OTR/L.*

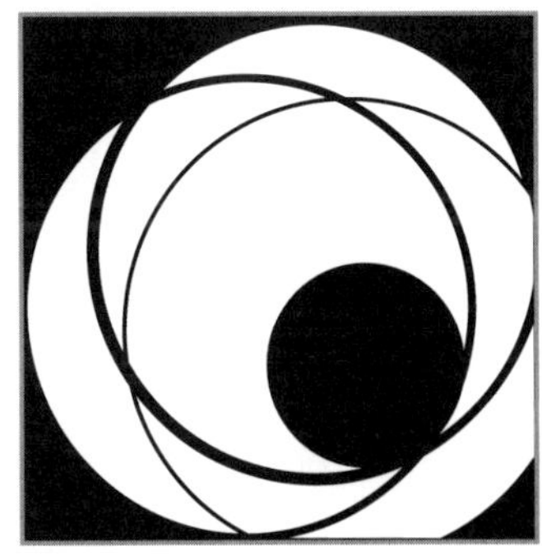

About the Editor

Susan Bazyk, PhD, OTR/L, FAOTA, is professor in the occupational therapy program at Cleveland State University, where she has taught for the past 26 years. She is also director of the graduate certificate program in school-based practice.

Bazyk earned a BS in occupational therapy from the Ohio State University, an MS in health science from the University of Florida, and a PhD in human services from Capella University. Throughout her career, she has specialized in occupational therapy practice with children and youth in home-, school-, and community-based settings. Her research and publications have contributed to several areas of practice, including parent–professional collaboration, understanding food refusal, occupation-based programming, and addressing the mental health needs of children.

Recently, Bazyk's scholarship has been guided by a commitment to exploring the needs of underserved populations—specifically, low-income urban youth. In an effort to meet real community needs and make occupational therapy accessible to underserved groups, she has developed a preventive occupational therapy program, the Occupational Therapy Groups for HOPE (*H*ealthy *O*ccupations for *P*ositive *E*motions). Offered by graduate occupational therapy students as a service learning initiative since 2003, the HOPE groups are embedded in an after-school program to address the structured leisure and social–emotional needs of low-income urban youth.

Bazyk has also been committed to the continued education of occupational therapy practitioners through publications (articles, book chapters, American Occupational Therapy Association [AOTA] documents) and presentations at local, state, and national occupational therapy conferences. Recent efforts have focused on occupational therapy's role in children's mental health. For example, she has authored a chapter on school mental health for the 3rd edition of *Occupational Therapy Services for Children and Youth Under IDEA* (AOTA Press, 2007). In addition, she has been an active member of the AOTA School Mental Health Task Group since 2006 under the leadership of Sandra Schefkind, pediatric coordinator at AOTA. One of the outcomes of this group has been the publication of an FAQ (2008) and Webinar (2009) on occupational therapy's role in school mental health.

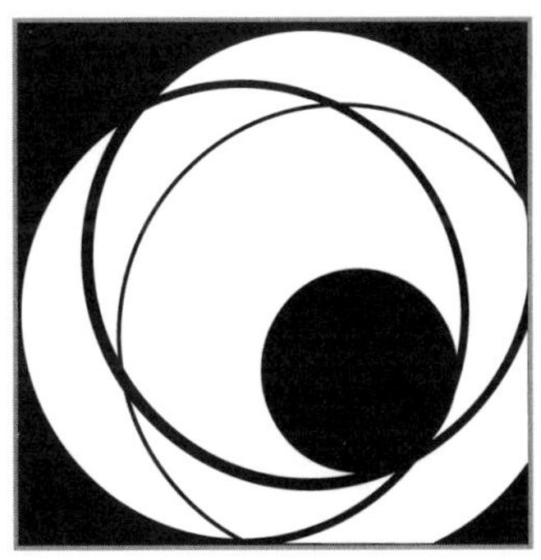

About the Authors

Karin Barnes, PhD, OTR, received a BS in occupational therapy and an MS in special education from the University of Kansas and a PhD in special education from the University of Texas at Austin. She is chair and associate professor of the Department of Occupational Therapy at the University of Texas Health Science Center, San Antonio. Her teaching and research areas are in school-based occupational therapy, team collaboration, occupational therapy interventions for students with emotional disturbance, and activity participation of children with burns.

Beata Batorowicz, MSc, OT Reg(Ont), has an MSc in occupational therapy from the University of Western Ontario and is a doctoral student in the rehabilitation science program at McMaster University. She is a Vanier Graduate Scholar and Strategic Training Fellow in Rehabilitation Research with the Canadian Institutes of Health Research and a fellow at the internationally renowned CanChild Centre for Childhood Disability Research at McMaster University.

Batorowicz has practiced as an occupational therapist for 11 years, providing community-based services and working with children who have little or no functional speech. She was previously a clinical services leader of augmentative and alternative communication, seating and mobility, and adaptive technology services at the Thames Valley Children's Centre in London, Ontario, and a lecturer in the School of Occupational Therapy at the University of Western Ontario. She has been actively involved in development of partnerships to promote inclusion of children with disabilities in after-school community programs. She has many peer-reviewed publications and presentations at international conferences. Her research interests include social inclusion and participation of children with disabilities, especially children who have complex needs and do not have a voice; psychosocial experiences of those children and their families; and environmental factors related to children's participation and their emotional well-being.

Alison Beck, PhD, OTR, is an associate professor in the Department of Occupational Therapy at the University of Texas Health Science Center, San Antonio. She earned a diploma in occupational therapy from St. Andrew's School of Occupational Therapy, Northampton, England; an MA in education from Incarnate Word College, San Antonio; and a PhD in educational administration from the University of Texas at Austin. She also holds a postgraduate certificate in play therapy and play diagnosis from the Institute of Child and Family Psychiatry, Ipswich, England. Beck's clinical practice has been in adolescent and adult psychiatric units and in urban and rural school systems. Her research includes issues and effective practices in the provision of occupational therapy services for students with severe emotional disturbance.

Sharon Brandenburger Shasby, EdD, OTR/L, FAOTA, received a BS in occupational therapy from the University of Florida, an MEd in clinical counseling from The Citadel, and an EdD in early childhood curriculum and instruction from the University of South Carolina. She is professor in the Department of Occupational Therapy at Eastern Kentucky University. Additionally, she has an appointment to the graduate faculty at the University of Kentucky, where she teaches in the interdisciplinary Rehabilitation Sciences Doctoral Program.

Brandenburger Shasby has extensive experience in providing related services to students with special needs in educational settings for more than 15 years. She has coordinated occupational and physical therapy services for large school systems in both urban and rural settings, and she has designed and taught school-based practice courses emphasizing best practice and functional outcomes to graduate students for 17 years. Her publications and presentations focus on school-based practice. Brandenburger Shasby has sustained a record of service to her professional national and state associations and holds the honor of being a Fellow of the American Occupational Therapy Association (AOTA). She has served for the past 2 years as a member of the AOTA task force defining the role of occupational therapy when working with students addressing mental health concerns.

Lisa Crabtree, PhD, OTR/L, earned a doctoral degree from Nova Southeastern University, a master's degree in special education from Syracuse University, and a bachelor's degree in occupational therapy from Utica College of Syracuse University. She has practiced for more than 30 years as an occupational therapist in school systems and community settings and is assistant professor in occupational therapy and occupational science at Towson University. Her research, teaching, and practice work has focused on the social participation and mental health of children, youth, and adults on the autism spectrum. She was appointed by the governor to the Maryland Commission on Autism, an advisory group designed to develop policy and programs for the state. As director of the Center for Adults With Autism, she develops educational, research, and outreach programs to meet the needs of transitioning youth and young adults on the autism spectrum. She educates and supervises graduate and undergraduate students from a variety of disciplines to support youth and young adults on the autism spectrum; conducts applied research on best practices with this population; and disseminates knowledge through local, national, and international conferences.

Janet V. DeLany, DEd, OTR/L, FAOTA, earned a doctoral degree in adult education from the Pennsylvania State University, a master's degree in health administration from the University of Notre Dame, a postbaccalaureate certificate degree in occupational therapy from the University of Pennsylvania, and a bachelor of arts in psychology from Immaculata University. She has practiced as an occupational therapist for 30 years with a focus on children and adolescents. For the past 20 years, DeLany has also been an occupational therapy educator, teaching at the associate, baccalaureate, master's, and doctoral levels. Currently, she is professor and director of the Doctor of Science in Occupational Science program at Towson University and directs the university's interdisciplinary postbaccalaureate certificate program in autism studies.

DeLany is chair of the AOTA Commission on Practice and a contributor to the *Occupational Therapy Practice Framework: Domain and Process* (2nd ed.). Her research interests include understanding the leadership and learning of women in health care professions, occupational challenges of teenage mothers, and autism. She is coauthor of a textbook on occupational therapy practice for children and adolescents.

Donna Downing, MS, OTR/L, is clinical faculty member in the Department of Occupational Therapy at the University of New Hampshire, where she earned her undergraduate and postgraduate degrees in occupational therapy. For more than 20 years, she has specialized in the field of psychiatry, working in long-term, acute care, and community settings. In December 2000, she became the clinical team leader of the Portland Identification and Early Referral (PIER) Program, a treatment research project working with youth between ages 12 and 25 who show early signs of a psychotic illness. PIER includes the family and client in every step of the assessment and treatment process. As part of the PIER Program, she introduced a smaller research study to gather data about the use of the Adolescent/Adult Sensory Profile and the Allen Cognitive Level Screen with adolescents.

From 2006 to 2010, Downing served as director of clinical training for the Early Detection and Intervention for the Prevention of Psychosis Program (EDIPPP), which is replicating PIER in five sites across the United States. Her role in EDIPPP was to guide clinical interventions and monitor fidelity to the PIER Model for all five sites. She has presented the role and work of EDIPPP occupational therapy practitioners at the 2009 AOTA Annual Conference & Expo and at the 2009 Annual Conference on Advancing School Mental Health.

Gillian A. King, PhD, has a doctorate in social psychology from the University of Western Ontario and is senior scientist with Bloorview Research Institute in Toronto. She has four appointments at the University of Western Ontario (in the Faculty of Education, School of Nursing, and Departments of Family Medicine and Psychology) and is associate clinical professor in the School of Rehabilitation Science at McMaster University.

King has authored or coauthored more than 100 articles in professional journals, has been an investigator on more than 40 grants, and has been an author on more than 180 peer-reviewed presentations. Her research interests are in the area of psychosocial aspects of childhood disability and health, including the participation and social inclusion of children with disabilities; family resilience; resilience in adolescents with mental health difficulties; delivery of health, social, and education services; and experiences of immigrant and refugee families raising children with disabling conditions. King recently held a Senior Research Fellowship from the Ontario Mental Health Foundation and received the John Whittaker Memorial Award for innovation in research.

Laurette Olson, PhD, OTR/L, is professor in the Graduate Program in Occupational Therapy, School of Health Professions and Natural Science, at Mercy College in Dobbs Ferry, New York. She earned her bachelor's degree in psychology at Fairfield University and her master's degree and doctorate in occupational therapy from New York University. She has been teaching group process and courses related to child and adolescent mental health for the past 15 years. Over the past 30 years, Olson has worked with children and adolescents in mental health and school-based settings. She has also developed and supervised group programs and has presented and written extensively about this work. Her book *Activity Groups in Family-Centered Treatment* was published in 2006. Olson is a member of the AOTA School Mental Health Work Group.

Theresa M. Petrenchik, PhD, OTR/L, earned a doctoral degree in occupational therapy from Nova Southeastern University; a postdoctoral research fellowship diploma from McMaster University in Hamilton, Ontario; and a bachelor of science in occupational therapy from Florida International University. She is assistant clinical professor in the School of Rehabilitation Science at McMaster University, co-investigator with the CanChild Centre for Childhood Disability Research at McMaster University, and owner of a research consulting firm located in Hamilton, Ontario. She has worked, taught occupational therapy, and conducted research in the United States and Canada. Her research and publications have contributed to several areas of practice, including homelessness, childhood disability and poverty, out-of-school time activity participation, and trauma-informed care.

Throughout her career, Petrenchik has been actively involved in the development and evaluation of strategic alliances concerned with promoting health, social participation, and quality of life in vulnerable populations, including at-risk youth and children and families experiencing chronic poverty and homelessness. She has worked in a variety of settings, including homeless shelters and youth development centers, and with community collaborations serving low-income children, families, and single adults. Immediately following Hurricane Katrina, Petrenchik worked with displaced families and adults as a member of an American Red Cross Disaster Mental Health Team stationed in Louisiana.

Andrea B. Sherwin, PhD, OTR/L, served as assistant professor in the Department of Occupational Therapy and Occupational Science at Towson University. She earned a BA in French language and literature from Tufts University; an MS in occupational therapy from Columbia University, College of Physicians and Surgeons; and an EdM in educational administration and a PhD in special education from Teachers College, Columbia University. An occupational therapist for more than 15 years, she practiced in a wide variety of settings, including school-based practice, home health, early intervention, and transitional group homes in New York, Massachusetts, and Maryland. Sherwin focused her research on parent and family advocacy, empowerment, self-determination, and occupational balance, and she presented on those topics at local and national conferences. She also was interested in emerging technologies and Internet-based experimental designs.

Anne A. Poulsen, PhD, is a director of Work Life Balance Solutions–Queensland and is a senior research officer at the University of Queensland, St. Lucia, Brisbane, Australia. Additionally, she works at the Mater Children's Hospital, South Brisbane, on a research team called KOALA (*Kinder:* for children and families; *Overweight:* for overcoming and being OK!; *Activity:* for an active mind and an active body; *Lifestyle:* for a living, life-giving diet; *Actions:* for all together and ahead we look). She is recognized for interdisciplinary collaborative work in the emerging area of childhood obesity, having recently completed a project at Ipswich Healthy Communities Research Centre, South-East Queensland, where she developed the Research Around Practice in Childhood Obesity Model with an experienced group of clinical and research scientists, public health policymakers, and health practitioners. Poulsen has more than 30 years of experience as an occupational therapist working in pediatric public and private practice. Her PhD focused on leisure pursuits of boys with developmental coordination disorders, a lifelong clinical and research interest that has led to publication of scholarly articles and chapters in nationally and internationally acclaimed works. For this body of literature, she was awarded the OT Australia Postgraduate Research Award.

Poulsen has presented keynote speeches, conference presentations, and workshops within Australia and overseas on topics such as motivation, resilience and flourishing, positive organizational scholarship, work–life balance, leisure participation, and well-being. Her Synthesis of Child, Occupational Performance and Environment–In Time (SCOPE–IT) Model has received international recognition and was further developed for inclusion in the third edition of Kramer and Hinojosa's (2010) text devoted to pediatric frames of reference. She has recently completed a randomized controlled trial demonstrating the effectiveness of driving hazard perception training for men with attention deficit hyperactivity disorder.

Kimberly Vogel, EdD, OTR, is associate professor in the Department of Occupational Therapy at the University of Texas Health Science Center, San Antonio. She earned a BFA in painting from Kutztown University, an MS in occupational therapy from Columbia University, and an EdD in allied health teacher education and administration from the University of Houston/Baylor College of Medicine. Her clinical practice has been in adult psychiatric units. Vogel's research includes fieldwork issues, critical thinking skills, occupational therapy services for children with emotional disturbance, and participation of children with burns in out-of-school activities.

Mental Health Promotion, Prevention, and Intervention With Children and Youth: A Guiding Framework for Occupational Therapy

Reviewers

Rebecca E. Argabrite Grove, MS, OTR/L
Special Education Supervisor
Loudoun County Public Schools
Ashburn, VA

Jean E. Polichino, MS, OTR, FAOTA
Senior Director, Therapy Services Division and ECI Keep Pace
Harris County Department of Education
Houston, TX

Sarah Bream, OTD, OTR/L
Division Director
Special Service for Groups/Occupational Therapy Training Program
Torrance, CA

List of Boxes, Figures, Resources, Reflections, and Tables

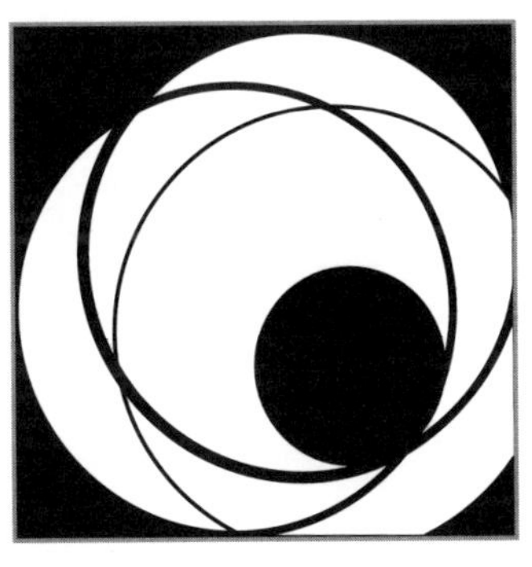

Chapter 1

Chapter 2

Chapter 3

Chapter 4

Chapter 5

Chapter 6

Chapter 7

Chapter 8

Chapter 9

Chapter 10

Chapter 11

Chapter 12

Preface

Susan Bazyk, PhD, OTR/L, FAOTA

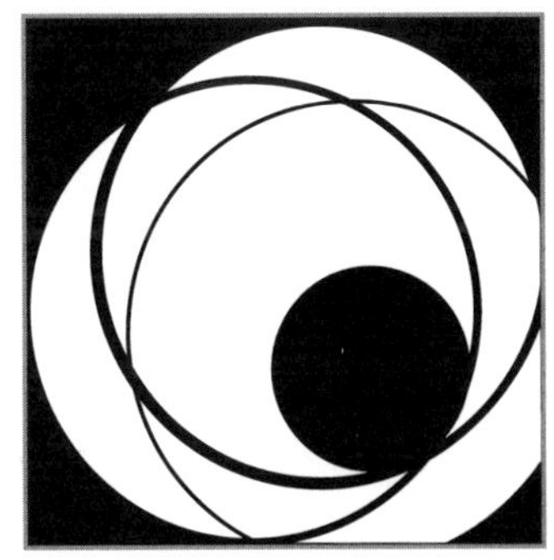

Do not go where the path may lead; go instead where there is no path and leave a trail.

—Attributed to Ralph Waldo Emerson (1803–1882)

My commitment to children's mental health was prompted by an invitation to participate in an American Occupational Therapy Association (AOTA)–sponsored workgroup organized by Leslie Jackson and facilitated by Barbara Hanft in 2000. For 2 days, approximately 20 occupational therapy practitioners and academicians from across the United States discussed occupational therapy's role in addressing the psychosocial and mental health needs of children, the barriers to providing such services, and how to better prepare therapists to work in this area. Participation in this group fueled my commitment to better prepare entry-level and practicing therapists to effectively address children's mental health in all settings and to educate other professionals about occupational therapy's role.

During the past 10 years, with the support of AOTA, a growing coalition of occupational therapists has worked diligently to provide a range of educational materials to help occupational therapists and occupational therapy assistants develop the knowledge and skills needed to promote mental health in all children and youth. In 2005, for example, Jackson and Arbesman wrote the *Occupational Therapy Practice Guidelines for Children With Behavioral and Psychosocial Needs.* A chapter on occupational therapy's role in school mental health (Bazyk, 2007) was added to the 3rd edition of *Occupational Therapy Services for Children and Youth Under IDEA,* edited by Leslie Jackson (2007). More recently, under the leadership of Sandy Schefkind, MS, OTR (pediatric coordinator at AOTA), the School Mental Health workgroup developed several educational resources, including a fact sheet, FAQ, and Webinar (AOTA, 2008, 2009b, 2009c). This book extends these efforts by providing a framework that occupational therapists can apply in all practice settings to promote positive mental health in all children and youth.

Purpose

The aim of *Mental Health Promotion, Prevention, and Intervention in Children and Youth: A Guiding Framework for Occupational Therapy* is to provide a foundation for conceptualizing occupational therapy's role in promoting mental health when working with all children and youth in schools and community settings. The content reflects a public health approach to occupational therapy services at the universal, targeted, and individualized levels. As such, this book emphasizes helping all children develop and maintain positive mental health, which is reflected in the presence of positive affect, positive psychological and social functioning, productive activities, and resilience in the face of adversity. Occupational therapists may need assistance in expanding services to include promotion and prevention activities in addition to intervention with mental health disorders; the information included in this book is intended to assist occupational therapists in doing just that. To that end, the book sets forth the following objectives for readers:

- Delineate how occupational therapists working with children and youth can contribute to mental health promotion, prevention, and intervention in school and community settings;
- Delineate occupational therapy services related to mental health within a public health framework at the universal (Tier 1), targeted (Tier 2), and individualized (Tier 3) levels;
- Recognize current approaches both within and outside the profession relevant to mental health promotion, prevention, and intervention for meeting the diverse needs of children and youth with and without disabilities or mental illness; and
- Identify practical information regarding mental health promotion, prevention, and intervention in everyday occupational therapy practice with children and youth.

Overview of the Book

This publication has been designed as both an AOTA Self-Paced Clinical Course (SPCC) and an AOTA Press textbook. SPCCs are a means for occupational therapists to develop perspective, knowledge, and skills to improve their ability to have a positive impact on the lives of the recipients of their services, including children and their families, teachers, and child care providers. Readers who successfully complete the SPCC exam can obtain continuing education credit for their efforts (continuing education materials and exam are in a separate packet). As a textbook, the content can be used in the classroom or on its own to provide information and serve as a resource.

Note that the text refers specifically to *occupational therapists* rather than to *occupational therapy practitioners* or *occupational therapy assistants*. This choice is for ease of reading, because the occupational therapist has the primary responsibility for evaluation in the occupational therapy process; it in no way negates or diminishes the contribution of occupational therapy assistants in the evaluation and service delivery process, as outlined in the *Guidelines for Supervision, Roles, and Responsibilities During the Delivery of Occupational Therapy Services* (AOTA, 2009a).

The occupational therapy assistant delivers occupational therapy services under the supervision of and in partnership with the occupational therapist in accordance with state regulations, the *Standards of Practice for Occupational Therapy* (AOTA, 2010d), the *Occupational Therapy Code of Ethics and Ethics Standards (2010)* (AOTA, 2010a), the *Standards for Continuing Competence* (AOTA, 2010c), and the *Scope of Practice* (AOTA, 2010b). The course is directed toward occupational therapy assistants as well as occupational therapists.

The sections that follow summarize the purpose of each chapter.

Part 1. Laying the Foundation—Reframing Occupational Therapy

The first five chapters provide foundational information on mental health promotion, prevention, and intervention with children and youth and introduce a public health approach to mental health for occupational therapy. Chapter 1, "Promotion of Positive Mental Health in Children and Youth: A Guiding Framework for Occupational Therapy" (Bazyk), synthesizes current information related to mental health (e.g., positive psychology, mental health continuum, positive youth development) to lay a foundation for the thinking reflected in subsequent chapters about mental health promotion—what it means, who it involves, where and how it is provided, and occupational therapy's unique contributions to it. Chapter 2, "Occupational Therapy Process: A Public Health Approach to Promoting Mental Health in Children and Youth" (Bazyk), presents a discussion of how to apply a public health approach to mental health promotion to the occupational therapy process, and Chapter 3, "Major Approaches Useful in Addressing the Mental Health Needs of Children and Youth: Minimizing Risks, Reducing Symptoms, and Building Competencies" (Bazyk and Brandenburger Shasby), synthesizes major approaches that may be useful in promoting positive mental health, preventing mental ill health, and intervening with the presence of mental health challenges. Some content reflects approaches already used by occupational therapists (e.g., sensory processing) but specifically applied to mental health promotion, whereas other content introduces approaches developed and used outside the field and, as such, is meant to envision new ways of thinking about and providing services within occupational therapy's scope of practice.

Chapter 4, "Pathways to Positive Development: Childhood Participation in Everyday Places and Activities" (Petrenchik and King), presents an integrated view of the concepts of participation, environments, and positive development, emphasizing the importance of children's participation in everyday places and patterns of participation. The final chapter in Part 1, Chapter 5, "Development and Implementation of Groups to Foster Social Participation and Mental Health" (Olson), provides an overview of the development and implementation of occupational therapy groups to promote social participation and mental health.

Part 2. Addressing the Mental Health Needs of Diverse Groups of Children and Youth

The seven chapters in Part 2 present information specific to children and youth with diverse mental health needs—those faced with situational stressors such as poverty, bullying, obesity, loss, and participation in risky behaviors (Chapter 6, "Enduring Challenges and Situational Stressors During the School Years: Risk Reduction and

Competence Enhancement," Bazyk); youth at risk of psychosis and those identified with mental illness (Chapter 7, "Occupational Therapy for Youth at Risk of Psychosis and Those With Identified Mental Illness," Downing); autism (Chapter 8, "Autism: Promoting Social Participation and Mental Health," Crabtree and DeLany); physical and developmental disabilities (Chapter 9, "Children and Youth With Disabilities: Enhancing Mental Health Through Positive Experiences of Doing and Belonging," Petrenchik, King, and Batorowicz); severe emotional disturbance (Chapter 10, "Occupational Therapy for Children With Severe Emotional Disturbance in Alternative Educational Settings," Barnes, Vogel, and Beck); and attention deficit hyperactivity disorder, learning disability, and development coordination disorder (Chapter 11, "Children With Attention Deficit Hyperactivity Disorder, Developmental Coordination Disorder, and Learning Disabilities," Poulsen). Chapter 12, "Begin With the End in Mind: Promoting Mental Health, Social Participation, and Self-Determination in the Transition From School to Adult Life" (Crabtree and Sherwin), the final chapter of the book, addresses transition for youth with disabilities and mental health challenges.

I am fortunate that these 13 contributors, representing the United States, Canada, and Australia, have joined me in the creation of this book. Their combined knowledge and expertise allowed us to develop a comprehensive and practical collection of information and resources to assist occupational therapists and occupational therapy assistants in promoting positive mental health in all children and youth.

References

American Occupational Therapy Association. (2008). *FAQ on school mental health.* Retrieved July 29, 2009, from www.aota.org/Practitioners/PracticeAreas/Pediatrics/Browse/MH/FAQSchoolMH.aspx

American Occupational Therapy Association. (2009a). Guidelines for supervision, roles, and responsibilities during the delivery of occupational therapy services. *American Journal of Occupational Therapy, 63,* 797–803.

American Occupational Therapy Association. (2009b). *Occupational therapy and school mental health* (AOTA Fact Sheet). Retrieved April 2, 2010, from www.aota.org/Practitioners/PracticeAreas/MentalHealth/Fact-Sheets/School-MH.aspx

American Occupational Therapy Association. (2009c). *Raising the bar: Elevating knowledge in school mental health.* Retrieved August 3, 2009, from www.aota.org/Practitioners/ProfDev/CE/AOTA/Webcasts/School-MH.aspx

American Occupational Therapy Association. (2010a). Occupational therapy code of ethics and ethics standards (2010). *American Journal of Occupational Therapy, 64*(Suppl.), S17–S26. doi: 10.5014/ajot.2010.64S17-64S26

American Occupational Therapy Association. (2010b). Scope of practice. *American Journal of Occupational Therapy, 64*(Suppl.), S70–S77. doi: 10.5014/ajot.2010.64S70-64S77

American Occupational Therapy Association. (2010c). Standards for continuing competence. *American Journal of Occupational Therapy, 64*(Suppl.), S103–S105. doi: 10.5014/ajot.2010.64S103-64S105

American Occupational Therapy Association. (2010d). Standards of practice for occupational therapy. *American Journal of Occupational Therapy, 64*(Suppl.), S106–S111. doi: 10.5014/ajot.2010.64S106-64S111

Bazyk, S. (2007). Addressing the mental health needs of children in schools. In L. Jackson (Ed.), *Occupational therapy services for children and youth under IDEA* (3rd ed., pp. 99–121). Bethesda, MD: AOTA Press.

Jackson, L. L. (Ed.). (2007). *Occupational therapy services for children and youth under IDEA* (3rd ed.). Bethesda, MD: AOTA Press.

Jackson, L. L., & Arbesman, M. (2005). *Occupational therapy practice guidelines for children with behavioral and psychosocial needs.* Bethesda, MD: AOTA Press.

PART 1

Laying the Foundation—Reframing Occupational Therapy

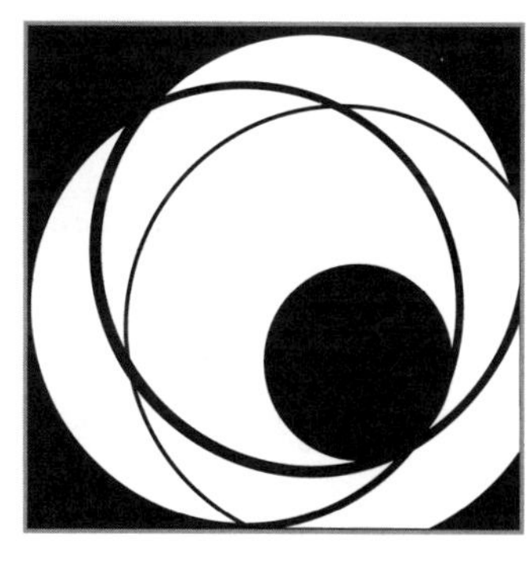

CHAPTER 1

Promotion of Positive Mental Health in Children and Youth: A Guiding Framework for Occupational Therapy

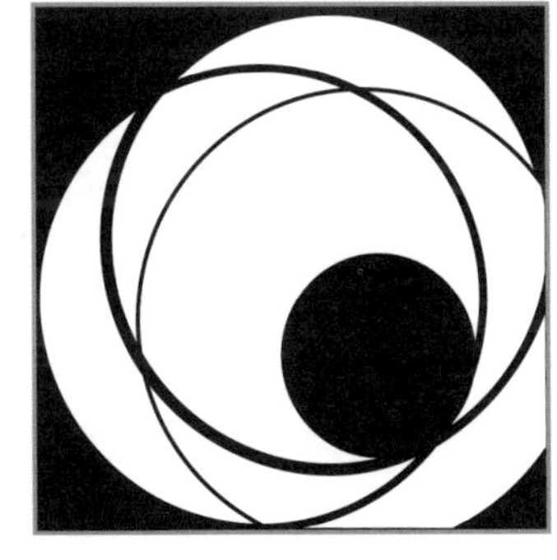

Susan Bazyk, PhD, OTR/L, FAOTA

Learning Objectives

After reading this material and completing the examination, readers will be able to

- Differentiate the meaning of the terms *mental health* and *mental illness;*
- Identify what is meant by *positive psychology, mental health continuum,* and *positive youth development;*
- Recognize leaders in the field of positive psychology and positive youth development;
- Identify the three pillars of positive psychology as defined by Seligman (2002);
- Differentiate mental health promotion and prevention efforts;
- Recognize factors associated with a socioecological framework for mental health promotion; and
- Delineate what a public health model of occupational therapy services to promote children's mental health would encompass in schools and community settings.

When ordinary people are asked to ponder what it means to be healthy, concerns about avoiding illness, disability and suffering are not necessarily the first thoughts that come to mind. As or more likely to be mentioned are the ability to participate in one's chosen form of life, to extract joy and meaning from doing so, and to experience satisfaction and zest with life despite its normal adversities.

—Mittlemark (2007, p. ix)

Occupational therapy has a rich history of promoting mental health in all areas of practice. "The psychosocial perspective in occupational therapy is not an add-on or special technique but is rather an integrated, everyday way of thinking about what the client needs and wants to do" (Jackson & Arbesman, 2005, p. 5). Despite this long-standing perspective, reference to *mental health* is often interpreted to mean intervention to prevent and to treat mental health problems (Barry & Jenkins, 2007). Much of the literature on occupational therapy's role in children's mental health has focused on intervention to address mental ill health (Davidson, 2005; Fette, 2009; Lougher, 2001). Similarly, mental health research in other fields has also focused heavily on healing pathology (Keyes, 2007; Seligman & Csikszentmihalyi, 2000). Recently, for example, the National Institute of Mental Health declared cure therapeutics as a goal of its research to reduce the number of cases of mental illness (Insel & Scolnick, 2006). This focus rests on the assumption that the "absence of mental illness is the presence of mental health" (Keyes, 2007, p. 95).

Within the past 10 years, however, there has been growing attention to the promotion of positive mental health among leaders in psychology and sociology, leading to a paradigm shift reflected in new areas of study and terminology: *mental health continuum, public health approach to mental health, positive psychology,* and *positive youth development* (Barry & Jenkins, 2007; Keyes, 2007; Larson, 2000; Seligman & Csikszentmihalyi, 2000). The purpose of this chapter is to lay a foundation for the thinking reflected in subsequent chapters about mental health promotion—what it means, who it involves, where and how it is provided, and occupational therapy's unique contributions to it.

Framing Mental Health

"The social science literature of the past two decades has confirmed that the perspective from which stories are told, or how they are framed, is a powerful influence in assigning responsibility for an issue or problem" (Lochner & Bales, 2006, p. 15). Frames are organizing principles that are socially shared, persist over time, and provide a way to meaningfully structure the social world (Reese, Grandy, & Grant, 2001). Such "habits of thought" are mental shortcuts used to make sense of the world. How occupational therapists think about mental health has a powerful influence in how their services are perceived, articulated to others, and implemented. If, for example, *working in children's mental health* refers to intervention provided to children with diagnosed psychiatric conditions in a psychiatric setting, then occupational therapy services will be limited to this population and setting. In contrast, if *working in children's mental health* means helping children develop and maintain mental health, then such services might extend to all children with and without identified mental illness and occur in a variety of medical and community-based settings.

Additionally, another habit of thought one may have observed in occupational therapy is the tendency to differentiate areas of practice with labels such as *pediatric, school-based, mental health, rehabilitation, acute care,* and the like. This framing of specialty areas within occupational therapy may also contribute to the habit of narrowly defining *mental health* to mean that which takes place in traditional mental health settings. A case for framing mental health more broadly is proposed in the following sections.

Mental Health Continuum

Keyes (2007) has advocated for the adoption of a two-continua model with mental health belonging to a continuum separate from mental illness. *Mental health* remained undefined and therefore unmeasured until recently. In 1999, *mental health* was defined by David Satcher, the U.S. Surgeon General at the time, as "a state of successful performance of mental function, resulting in productive activities, fulfilling relationships with people, and the ability to adapt to change and cope with adversity" (U.S. Department of Health and Human Services, 1999, p. 4). This definition asserts that mental health is not merely the absence of mental illness but the presence of something positive. Thus, the "U.S. strategy for mental health must simultaneously (a) continue to seek to prevent and treat cases of mental illness and (b) seek to understand how to promote flourishing in individuals otherwise free of mental illness but not mentally healthy" (Keyes, 2007, p. 95).

Over the past several years, Keyes (2002, 2005, 2006, 2007) has studied the dimensions of mental health and its measurement and has proposed a cluster of symptoms and diagnostic criteria for mental health. In the same way that a diagnosis of major depressive disorder is based on symptoms of *anhedonia* (negative emotions) and malfunctioning, a diagnosis of mental health is proposed to consist of symptoms of *hedonia* (positive emotions) and positive psychological and social functioning. Examples of positive emotions include *positive affect* (regularly cheerful, interested in life, happy). *Positive functioning* includes psychological (e.g., self-acceptance, purpose in life, autonomy) and social (e.g., sense of belonging, meaningful social life, positive attitude toward people) components. The continuum of mental health as described by Keyes (2007) can be viewed as ranging from mental illness, "languishing in life," or both at one end to "moderately mentally healthy" and "complete mental health and flourishing" at the other end (Figure 1.1).

Mental ill health is an umbrella term that includes a continuum from the most severe disorders to mild symptoms of differing duration and intensity (Barry & Jenkins, 2007). The terms *mental illness* and *mental disorders* are commonly used to refer

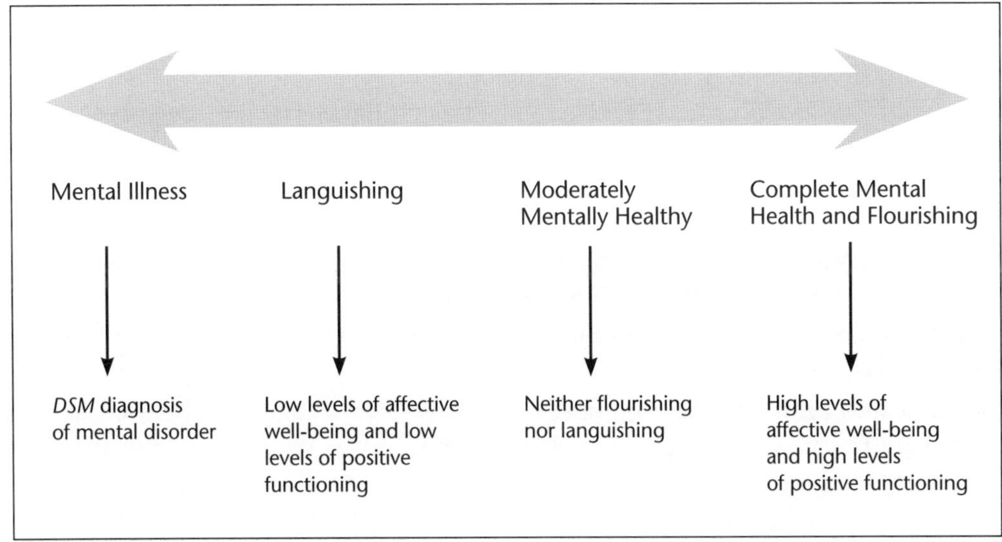

Figure 1.1. Mental health continuum.

Note. DSM = *Diagnostic and Statistical Manual of Mental Disorders* (American Psychiatric Association, 2000).

Source. Based on concepts developed by Keyes (2007).

to diagnosable psychiatric conditions that significantly interfere with a person's functioning, such as bipolar disorder, schizophrenia, and dementia. *Mental health problems* often refers to more common issues, such as anxiety and depression, which may be less severe and of shorter duration, but if left unattended may develop into more serious conditions (Barry & Jenkins, 2007).

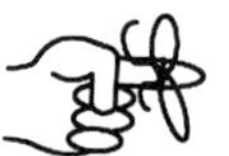

Remember this. . . .
"Evidence indicates that the absence of mental illness does not imply the presence of mental health, and the absence of mental health does not imply the presence of mental illness" (Keyes, 2007, p. 100).

The findings of a large survey study of U.S. adults between the ages of 25 and 74 living in the 48 contiguous states support a two-continua model of mental health and mental illness (Keyes, 2002, 2005). "That is, the evidence indicates that the absence of mental illness does not imply the presence of mental health, and the absence of mental health does not imply the presence of mental illness" (Keyes, 2007, p. 100). Increased impairment and disability was found in adults without complete mental health who were flourishing—even those without a mental illness. Completely mentally healthy adults functioned superior to all the other categories in terms of fewest workdays missed, fewest chronic physical conditions, lowest health care use, and highest levels of psychosocial functioning. In addition, completely mentally healthy adults functioned better than adults with moderate mental health, who functioned better than those who were languishing. Curiously, languishing adults without mental illness reported the same health limitations and worse levels of psychosocial functioning than adults with mental illness who also had moderate mental health or were flourishing. Approximately 20% of the adults were identified as flourishing. In a similar study of mental health in adolescence, Keyes (2006) found that flourishing was most prevalent in youth ages 12 to 14 (approximately 50%), with moderate mental health most prevalent in youth ages 15 to 18 (approximately 55%). These research findings indicate a need for national programs to emphasize mental health promotion in addition to ongoing efforts to prevent and treat mental illness. Positive mental health is associated with greater physical health and everyday functioning.

Positive Psychology

Related to but separate from the literature on the mental health continuum is work derived from the field of positive psychology. In 2000, Seligman and Csikszentmihalyi edited a special issue of *American Psychologist* devoted to positive psychology. "The aim of positive psychology is to begin to catalyze a change in the focus of psychology from preoccupation only with repairing the worst things in life to also building positive qualities" (p. 5). Thus, *positive psychology* is the study of processes and conditions that promote optimal functioning in people (Gable & Haidt, 2005). Since its inception in 2000, the positive psychology movement has grown, resulting in numerous conferences, publications, grants, and university courses (Gable & Haidt, 2005).

Research findings from the field of positive psychology may be used to specifically inform practice regarding how to promote positive mental health. For example, Seligman (2002) proposed three pillars of positive psychology as a framework for mental health and authentic happiness: (1) positive emotion, (2) positive traits, and (3) positive institutions (Figure 1.2). The first pillar emphasizes subjective experiences and positive emotions (joy, happiness, pleasure, contentment).

Positive Emotion and Subjective Experience	Positive Traits and Character Strengths	Positive Institutions
• Joy, contentment, pleasure, optimism • Positive emotions experienced during an activity promote further participation, exploration, and mastery. • *Reflection:* What types of engagement produce positive emotions in the children and youth you work with? • *Suggestion:* Help children explore a range of occupations and identify those that add meaning and joy to their lives.	• Humor, love, kindness, artistic talent, curiosity, persistence • Building and using one's signature strengths foster deep emotional satisfaction. • *Reflection:* What positive qualities are unique to each child you work with? • *Suggestion:* Help all children identify their unique signature strengths and engage in occupations that support and cultivate their expression (e.g., artistic talent, volunteer work)	• Environmental factors such as families, caring adults, and programs that foster character strengths and positive emotions • *Reflection:* Do the settings in which children learn, socialize, and play foster positive emotion and personal strengths? • *Suggestion:* Consult with teachers, administrators, and youth workers to create or adapt activities and the environment to promote positive experiences.

Figure 1.2. Three pillars of positive psychology.
Source. Seligman (2002).

"Experiences that induce positive emotion cause negative emotion to dissipate rapidly" (Seligman, 2002, p. xii). Positive emotion experienced during participation in an activity is thought to be a central factor in promoting further exploration and eventual mastery.

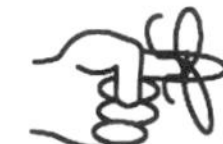

Remember this. . . .
"Experiences that induce positive emotion cause negative emotion to dissipate rapidly" (Seligman, 2002, p. xii).

The second pillar of positive psychology emphasizes the importance of developing individual traits—personal strengths and virtues such as persistence, optimism, self-control, and social skills, to name a few. Six core virtues have been identified: wisdom and knowledge, courage, love and humanity, justice, temperance, and spirituality and transcendence (Seligman, 2002). Each core virtue can be broken down into a number of strengths. For example, wisdom can be broken down into love of learning, curiosity, social intelligence, and perspective. Strengths and virtues serve people during good times and during life's challenges. A person's signature strengths are those that are deeply characteristic of the person. According to Seligman (2002), a person's highest success in living and deepest emotional satisfaction is derived from building and using one's signature strengths.

The third pillar of positive psychology focuses on positive institutions—environmental factors such as families, caring adults, and programs that foster character strengths and positive emotions (Seligman, 2002). Occupational therapists have ample opportunities to promote the three pillars of positive psychology given that their services, through the use of meaningful occupations, foster the development of needed and desired occupations (see Figure 1.2).

Positive Youth Development

Positive psychology has also been applied specifically to children and youth. Interest in helping children develop individual strengths has led to a related area of study described as *positive youth development,* which emphasizes building and improving assets that enable youth to grow and flourish throughout life (Park, 2004). Seligman (2002) proposed that positive youth development can be fostered when traits (e.g., character strengths), subjective experiences (e.g., happiness), and institutions are in alignment. Larson (2000) emphasized the development of initiative as a core quality of positive youth development and made a case for participation in structured leisure activities (e.g., sports, arts, organized clubs) as an important context for such development. Although school-age children in the United States spend approximately half of their waking hours in leisure activities, most research has tended to ignore this out-of-school time (Mahoney, Larson, Eccles, & Lord, 2005). The importance of children's participation in out-of-school leisure activities is discussed in further detail in the "Mental Health Promotion in the Community" section.

Mental Health Promotion

"*Mental health promotion* [italics added] focuses on promoting positive mental health among the general population and addresses the needs of those at risk from, or experiencing, mental health problems" (Barry & Jenkins, 2007, p. 2). Information on the mental health continuum, positive psychology, and positive youth development shares a common view of mental health as a separate state representing the presence of something positive and, thus, provides a foundation for mental health promotion. Although *mental health* has multiple definitions, most reflect the presence of four characteristics: (1) positive affective or emotional state (e.g., subjective sense of well-being, feeling happy), (2) positive psychological and social function (e.g., self-acceptance, fulfilling relationships, self-control), (3) productive activities, and (4) resilience in the face of adversity and the ability to cope with life stressors (U.S. Department of Health and Human Services, 1999; World Health Organization [WHO], 2001).

Mental health is determined by multiple factors that reside in the person (biological, psychological) and in the environment (social, cultural, economic; Barry & Jenkins, 2007). Risk factors increase the likelihood that mental health problems will develop and may also increase the disorder's duration and severity. Protective factors enhance positive mental health and reduce the likelihood that a disorder will develop. Risk and protective factors are present at multiple levels, including the individual, family, community, and society levels (Table 1.1). When considering the range of factors influencing mental health, it is not surprising that a call for comprehensive mental health promotion and prevention programs extends beyond an individual focus to address wider social factors (Barry & Jenkins, 2007; WHO, 2001).

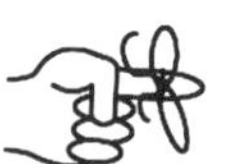

Remember this. . . .
Positive mental health contains the following characteristics:
- **Positive affect**
- **Positive psychological and social function**
- **Productive activities**
- **Resilience in the face of adversity and coping with life stressors.**

Given what is known about mental health, WHO (2001) has advocated a public health approach to mental health that emphasizes the promotion of mental health and the prevention of and intervention with mental illness. Positive mental health is considered fundamental to overall health and quality of life and contributes to the functioning of individuals, families, communities, and societies (Barry & Jenkins, 2007). As such, mental health can be located within a health promotion framework that is based on an empowering, participative, and collaborative process to help people take control of and improve their health (WHO, 2001). Barry and Jenkins (2007) have applied this framework to the promotion of mental health in the following five areas: (1) building healthy public policy, (2) creating supportive

Table 1.1. Risk and Protective Factors Associated With Positive Mental Health

Level	Protective Factors	Risk Factors
Individual	Positive sense of self Good physical health Effective social skills Close relationship to family Good coping skills	Low self-esteem Chronic illness or physical disability Poor social skills Insecure attachment to family Poor coping skills
Social	Caring and supportive parents Positive early attachment Sense of social belonging Supportive relationships Participation in the community	Social isolation Abuse, neglect, violence, or all of these Peer rejection Separation and loss
Structural	Safe living environment Economic security Positive educational experience Access to health and other supports	Neighborhood violence and crime Poverty Unemployment Homelessness School failure Lack of health and other support services

Source. From *Implementing Mental Health Promotion* (p. 6), by M. M. Barry & R. Jenkins, 2007, Edinburgh, Scotland: Churchill Livingstone/Elsevier. Copyright © 2007 by Elsevier. Adapted with permission.

environments, (3) strengthening community action, (4) developing personal skills, and (5) reorienting health services (Box 1.1).

Because a public health approach to mental health involves promotion, prevention, and intervention, it is important to make distinctions among these practices. Prevention frameworks developed over the past 2 decades have traditionally focused on reducing the incidence and seriousness of problem behaviors and mental health disorders (Barry & Jenkins, 2007; Catalano, Hawkins, Berglund, Pollard, & Arthur, 2002). Early prevention programs tended to focus primarily on reducing risk factors (e.g., family history of substance abuse, poverty); however, current approaches recognize the importance of enhancing protective factors as well (e.g., social and emotional competencies, clear standards for behavior). Although a number of prevention frameworks have been proposed, one that has been widely applied in the area of behavior management is positive behavioral interventions and supports (PBIS; U.S. Department of Education, 2010). This three-tiered prevention framework has been depicted as a pyramid, including primary prevention (to reduce incidence of problems targeting the whole school population and teach positive behaviors), secondary prevention (to reduce prevalence and duration of problems targeting high-risk groups), and tertiary prevention (to reduce impaired function by targeting groups with symptoms of behavior problems; see www.PBIS.org).

Although prevention frameworks focus on reducing problems, promotion frameworks emphasize competence enhancement: building strengths and resources (Barry & Jenkins, 2007). Mental health promotion is viewed as a multidisciplinary area of practice emphasizing mental health promotion in the whole population—those with and without mental health problems. As such, this framework emphasizes improving the social, physical, and economic environments that determine the mental health of people and populations.

Box 1.1. Socioecological Framework for Mental Health Promotion

The Ottawa Charter for Health Promotion [World Health Organization, 1986] outlines the following five areas as important for mental health promotion:

1. *Building healthy public policy:* Calls all policymakers to put mental health promotion on the agenda to foster coordinated action across health, economic, and social policies to improve mental health. Policies related to employment, housing, education, and child care, for example, are viewed as affecting the mental health of the whole population.
2. *Creating supportive environments:* Focuses on the interaction between people and their environments, including the social, physical, cultural, and economic aspects of the environment. Key contexts for creating and promoting positive mental health include homes, schools, workplaces, and community settings. *Examples:* Promote mental health in schools; reduce disadvantage and prevent stigma.
3. *Strengthening community action:* Emphasizes the empowerment of communities through active efforts to identify their own needs, set priorities, and plan and implement action to promote optimal health. Community development approaches promote public participation and increased capacity to improve mental health at the community level.
4. *Developing personal skills:* Involves promoting personal and social development by providing information, education, and skill training. Information and education to foster mental health literacy can target schools and families so that children and youth understand positive mental health as an integral part of overall health. *Examples:* Teach children about positive mental health in schools; educate parents on how to foster mental health in their children.
5. *Reorienting health services:* Calls for mental health services that emphasize promotion and prevention activities and the treatment of mental illness across a variety of groups, for example, children, young mothers, and people with chronic health problems, disabilities, or both. Reorienting health services to promote mental health requires greater attention to education of health care providers and reorganization of health services.

Source. From *Implementing Mental Health Promotion* (p. 16), by M. M. Barry and R. Jenkins, 2007, Edinburgh, Scotland: Churchill Livingstone/Elsevier. Copyright © 2007 by Elsevier. Adapted with permission.

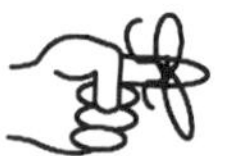

Remember this. . . .
Mental health prevention focuses on efforts to reduce the incidence and seriousness of mental health problems. Mental health promotion focuses on building strengths and resources to foster mental health and well-being.

> Thus, mental health promotion is mostly undertaken by people who do not claim to be mental health promoters, and most professionals who engage in purposive mental health promotion do so not under the title "mental health promoter," but rather as teacher, social worker, physician, occupational therapist, politician, among other vocations. (Mittlemark, 2007, p. x)

Mental health promotion, although addressing the needs of the whole population, also addresses the needs of those experiencing mental ill health, which includes creating supportive environments, reducing stigma and discrimination, and supporting the social and emotional health of clients and their families (Barry & Jenkins, 2007). Mental health promotion is enhanced by having a skilled and informed workforce drawn from different sectors, including health, education, and community organizations. Workforce training and education should promote collaboration among multiple disciplines and include awareness raising about the promotion of mental health and the development of specific strategies (Barry & Jenkins, 2007). Health care providers may, for example, need assistance in expanding services to include promotion and prevention activities in addition to the treatment of mental health disorders. Information included in this book is intended to assist occupational therapists with expanding existing services to include promotion and prevention strategies.

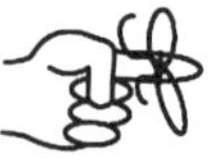

Remember this. . . .
Mental health promotion is enhanced by having a skilled and informed workforce drawn from different sectors, including health, education, and community organizations.

In terms of evidence, programs promoting mental health have reported long-lasting positive effects on multiple areas of function and have also reported the dual effect of reducing risks of mental illness (Hosman & Jané-Llopis, 1999). A recent evidence-based review of mental health promotion programs indicated that sufficient knowledge exists to move evidence into practice (Jané-Lopis, Barry, Hosman, & Patel, 2005). Suggestions for action to improve the quality of program implementation, integrate mental health into health promotion, and move mental health into the government agenda were also proposed.

Occupational Therapy's Role in the Promotion of Children's Mental Health

The frameworks described in the preceding section share a common focus on the promotion of mental health for all people—on building positive qualities and personal strengths in addition to remediating problems. Given this paradigm shift, it is timely for occupational therapists to consider reframing mental health services for children to include promotion and prevention in addition to occupational therapy's traditional focus on intervention. Such a shift in thinking requires careful reflection on several questions related to who therapists should serve and where, followed by a strategic conceptualization of what services might entail. In terms of who, when adopting a public health approach to mental health, occupational therapists can serve all children—those with and without disabilities and mental health disorders. In addition, although services can be offered in a variety of settings, school and community settings are prominent contexts for the provision of occupational therapy services for children and youth and, as such, are emphasized in the following sections. Factors associated with context can significantly affect occupational therapy services, especially when it comes to school practice. For this reason, I discuss envisioning and articulating occupational therapy's role in promoting children's mental health in school and community settings in separate sections.

In terms of what occupational therapy services entail, although occupational therapy's emphasis will vary depending on context, all efforts share a common belief in the positive relationship between participation in a balance of meaningful occupations and health. Although the *Occupational Therapy Practice Framework: Domain and Process* (2nd ed.; American Occupational Therapy Association [AOTA], 2008) is not considered a theory or model, it provides a useful tool for framing occupational therapy practice and is applied throughout this chapter and others to envision and articulate occupational therapy services. This framework broadly describes occupational therapy's contribution to promoting the health and participation of people, organizations, and populations through engagement in occupation and, as such, is compatible with a public health approach to mental health. Letts, Fraser, Finlayson, and Walls (1993) specifically proposed that occupational therapists frame "doing" occupational therapy within a health promotion framework, enabling people to increase control over and improve their health. In addition, the *Framework* embraces *occupational justice*—that all people need to be given opportunities to engage in needed or chosen occupations, to grow through participation, and to experience independence or interdependence, health, security, and well-being (Wilcock & Townsend, 2008).

The *domain of occupational therapy,* supporting health and participation in life through engagement in occupation, focuses on the major areas of education, play, leisure, social participation, activities of daily living (ADLs), instrumental activities of daily living (IADLs), rest and sleep, and work (AOTA, 2008). The *Framework* also describes the client-centered process of occupational therapy service delivery, which includes evaluation, intervention, and outcome monitoring. This process as it relates to children's mental health is discussed in detail in Chapter 2.

In combination, the domain and process of occupational therapy guide practitioners in promoting occupational performance, which results from the dynamic intersection of the client, context, and occupation (AOTA, 2008). This ecological model, reflecting a long-standing and prominent understanding of the relationship among person, occupation, and environment, has been described from numerous perspectives both within and outside of occupational therapy (Dunn, Brown, & Youngstrom, 2003; Law et al., 1996; Rogers & Holm, 2009). Just as factors within the person may support or impede occupational performance, so too can the environment have a positive or negative influence. A core skill for all occupational therapists is *task analysis*—the ability to analyze the relationship among the person, environment, and activity and determine factors needed for successful participation. When the task–environment demands are greater than the person's abilities, then adaptation of the environment or the task may be provided to foster successful participation (Rogers & Holm, 2009). In addition to considering the relationship among the person, occupation, and environment, occupational therapists view occupation as means and end in the therapy process. In other words, the therapeutic use of occupation is a means to bring about occupational performance.

Public Health Model of Occupational Therapy Services to Promote Mental Health in Children and Youth

A three-tiered model focusing on a public health and primary prevention framework is proposed to envision and guide occupational therapy in the promotion of mental health and prevention and intervention for mental ill health for both school and community settings (Figure 1.3). This framework supports a change in thinking from the traditional, individually focused deficit-driven model of mental health intervention to a whole-population strength-based approach. The three major tiers of service include (1) universal, or whole population; (2) targeted, or selective; and (3) intensive, individualized. The left side of the pyramid represents occupational therapy services in school settings, and the right side represents community settings. Although the domain and process of occupational therapy services will be similar in each setting, the focus will differ. For example, in schools the role of occupational therapy is to help children benefit from their education and function successfully in the school environment. In contrast, services provided in the community will likely occur during out-of-school time, warranting attention to the development of meaningful structured leisure interests, friendships, independent living skills, and beginning work skills. A full discussion of the focus of occupational therapy and process of service provision for children and youth at each tier is presented in Chapter 2.

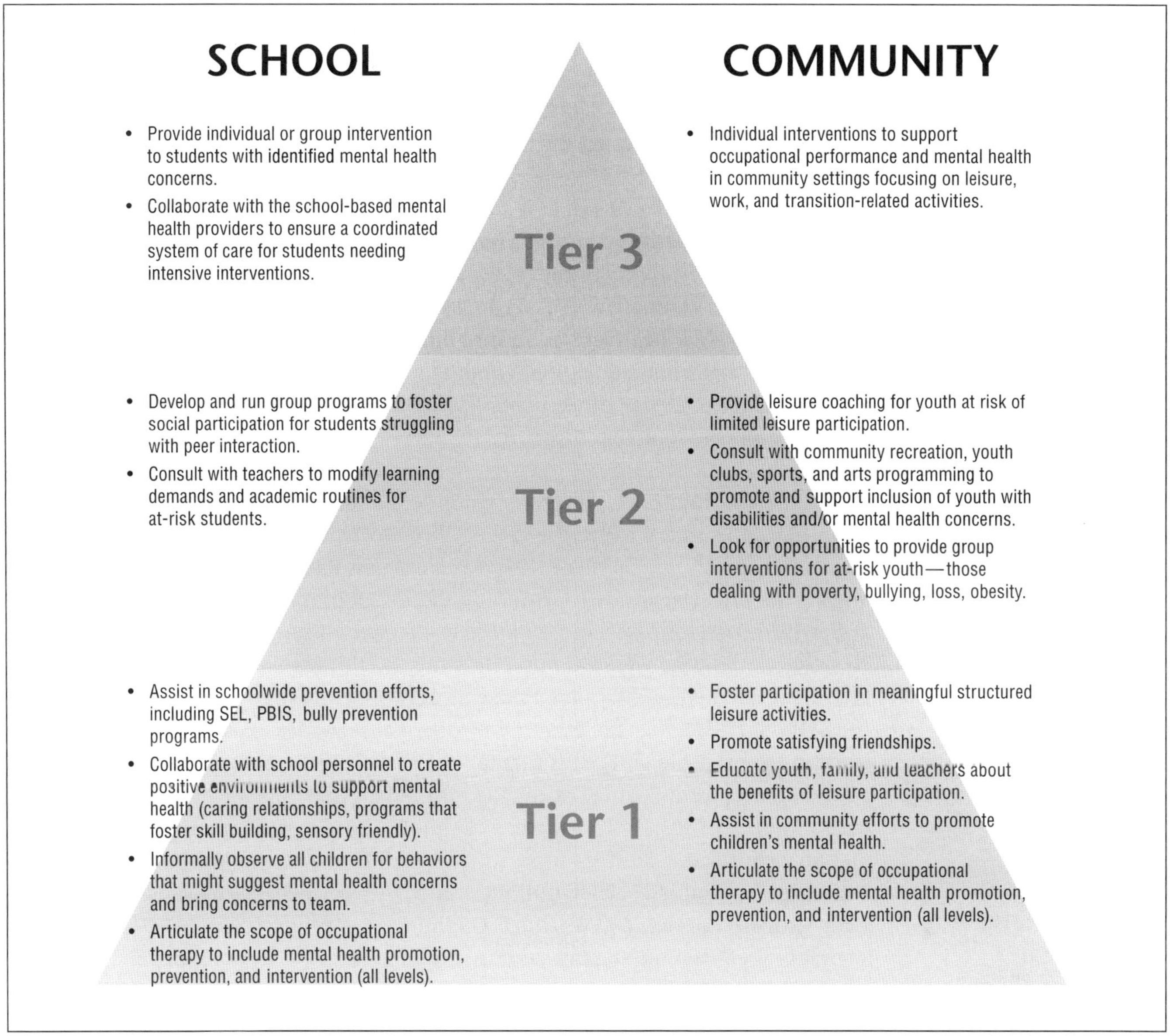

Figure 1.3. Public health model of occupational therapy services to promote mental health in children and youth.

Note. PBIS = positive behavioral interventions and supports; SEL = social and emotional learning.

A discussion of occupational therapy's role in mental health promotion in school and community settings follows.

Mental Health Promotion in Schools

Although mental health services for children have historically been provided in hospitals and community mental health centers, the Education for All Handicapped Children Act of 1975 was the first federal initiative that required schools to meet the mental health needs of students with emotional disturbance, playing a key role in blurring the lines of responsibility for where such services should be provided

(Bazyk, 2007; Kutash, Duchnowski, & Lynn, 2006). However, because the Individuals With Disabilities Education Improvement Act of 2004 (IDEA) focuses solely on students with identifiable disabilities that interfere with academic achievement, only a small percentage of children needing mental health services actually receive such care in school. Nonetheless, most children receiving mental health services obtain care in schools, making schools the "de facto mental health system for children in this country" (Kutash et al., 2006, p. 62).

A national movement to develop and expand school mental health (SMH) services has grown during the past 2 decades as a result of the high prevalence of mental health needs among youth and the awareness that more youth can be reached in schools (Masia-Warner, Nangle, & Hansen, 2006; Weist & Paternite, 2006). Prominent federal initiatives, such as *Mental Health: A Report of the Surgeon General* (U.S. Department of Health and Human Services, 1999) and the President's New Freedom Commission on Mental Health (2003), have identified gaps in services, forcing federal, state, and local child-serving agencies to address the mental health needs of children attending school (Weist & Paternite, 2006). As a result of federal support, two national technical assistance centers were developed in 1995 to promote mental health in schools—the Center for Mental Health in Schools at the University of California, Los Angeles, and the Center for School Mental Health Analysis and Action at the University of Maryland. Despite the recent emphasis on SMH, the field can be viewed as underdeveloped and emerging; far too many children continue to be underidentified and underserved in schools (Koppelman, 2004).

SMH can be thought of as a framework of approaches expanding on traditional methods to promote children's mental health by emphasizing prevention, positive youth development, and schoolwide approaches (see www.schoolmentalhealth.org/Resources/ESMH/DefESMH.html). Schools must be active partners in children's mental health because it is currently accepted that a major barrier to learning is immature or limited social–emotional skills and not necessarily cognitive impairment (Koller & Bertel, 2006). This SMH framework promotes interdisciplinary collaboration between mental health providers, related service providers, teachers, and school administrators to meet the mental health needs of all students.

Multitiered Public Health Model

Legislative changes have prompted schools to shift to a multitiered model of services, committing to the success of all students by providing early identification and intervening services. The 1997 reauthorization of IDEA ended a long period during which special education and general education were viewed as separate programs serving separate populations (Spencer, Turkett, Vaughan, & Koenig, 2006). IDEA 1997 placed greater emphasis on the inclusion of students with disabilities in general education by embedding special education and related services in the classroom and extracurricular activities when possible. General and special education practices have further aligned as a result of IDEA 2004 and the No Child Left Behind Act of 2001, providing school personnel, including occupational therapists, with increasing opportunities to expand their role in schools, particularly in the area of prevention (Cahill, 2007).

Adoption of three-tiered models of supports and services has been evident with the application of both response to intervention (RtI) and PBIS. In an effort to prevent school failure, IDEA 2004 included RtI as a framework for early identification of and intervention for academic and behavior problems. Similarly, schoolwide PBIS supports all students along a continuum of need on the basis of the three-tiered prevention model (see www.pbis.org/). Although PBIS has been widely applied in schools, the focus is primarily on promotion of positive behavior and prevention–intervention of behavior problems (Safran & Oswald, 2003). What is needed in schools is a greater focus on the early detection of and intervention for social–emotional issues that might be experienced by any students, including grieving issues, abuse or neglect, and prodromal signs of a possible psychiatric disorder.

Role of Occupational Therapy

Although the mental health field has traditionally been viewed as the domain of mental health specialists, addressing mental health issues is now recognized as too complex to relegate to a few professionals. Experts are calling for a paradigm shift to better prepare all school personnel (teachers, administrators, psychologists, social workers, related service providers) to proactively address the mental health needs of all students (Koller & Bertel, 2006). Teachers and other frontline personnel, including occupational therapists, play a crucial role in the development of children from both academic and personal, social, and emotional perspectives. Currently, however, no universal mandate exists for preservice teacher education in the area of children's mental health. Providing teachers with a fundamental knowledge of factors that influence the development of mental illness in children and proactive strength based prevention efforts that promote mental health is essential (Koller & Bertel, 2006; Weist & Paternite, 2006). For example, teachers and other school personnel need competencies in the importance of social–emotional health, creating an emotionally healthy classroom, crisis intervention, and mental health interventions in schools. True interdisciplinary training in which school personnel are trained with staff from traditional mental health disciplines is critically needed (Weist & Paternite, 2006).

Occupational therapists have specialized knowledge and skills in addressing people's social participation and mental health needs and, thus, are well positioned to contribute to all three levels of prevention and intervention. For example, services may focus on enhancing social participation in a variety of settings, including the classroom, cafeteria, playground, and school bus (Davidson, 2005). A continuum of occupational therapy early intervening services aimed at social–emotional and mental health promotion, prevention of problem behaviors, early detection through screening, and intensive intervention is recommended. Depending on state guidelines, these services could involve occupational therapists working directly with students, consulting with teachers and parents, providing professional development for school personnel, or all of these.

Occupational therapists can use a number of traditional approaches to guide service provision within a public health model, including the use of meaningful occupations. Findings of a recent evidence-based literature review, for example, have indicated that activity-based interventions help improve children's peer interactions, task-focused behaviors, and social behaviors (Jackson & Arbesman, 2005). Using task analysis, an activity-based approach might involve analyzing and modifying homework requirements for a child experiencing anxiety to foster successful completion and minimize symptoms associated with anxiety. Other traditional occupational therapy approaches used to evaluate and address children's psychosocial needs include sensory-based interventions and social learning theory. In addition to traditional occupational therapy intervention approaches, other approaches developed in the fields of psychology and education ought to be applied by occupational therapists: social and emotional learning and PBIS. The application of these approaches is discussed in detail in Chapter 3.

Mental Health Promotion in the Community

Larson (2000) wrote, "A central question of youth development is how to get adolescents' fires lit, how to have them develop the complex set of dispositions and skills needed to take charge of their lives" (p. 170). Although occupational therapy's role with children and youth in community settings is limited compared with school settings, the need for community-based occupational therapy services and potential for growth is significant. Occupational therapy's role in fostering participation in structured leisure, work, and independent living activities can play a pivotal role in mental health promotion. Although the gradual development of work behaviors and independent living skills in youth are important contributors to positive mental health and the transition to adult life, occupational therapy services and publications in these areas are sparse. Literature outside the field of occupational therapy on the development of work has been synthesized along with implications for practice (Bazyk, 2005; Larson, 2000); however, the few examples of youth services actually geared toward work promotion and independent living appear in publications spanning 2 decades (Evans, McDougall, & Baldwin, 2006; Jackson, Rankin, Siefken, & Clark, 1989). Today, youth face greater challenges in finding meaningful work because the transition to adult work is more complex, offering additional options without structured pathways. Thus, youth must invest more energy into developing the skills and self-knowledge needed to make meaningful decisions about future work (Bazyk, 2005). Occupational therapists' attention to the development of meaningful work is important.

Although work has received little attention, growing interest in children's leisure participation is evident in the profession's publications during the past decade. Researchers have explored leisure participation for youth with disabilities (Hackett, 2003; Howard, 1996; King et al., 2003; Law, Petrenchik, King, & Hurley, 2007; Poulsen, Ziviani, & Cuskelly, 2008; Rosenberg, 2000; Shikako-Thomas, Majnemer, Law, & Lach, 2008) and those living in homeless shelters (Petrenchik, 2006). Others have written about occupational therapy's role in after-school care (Bazyk, 2005; Carter et al., 2004), summer camps (Banet, Gilbert, Gmytrasiewicz, Pereyra, & Reynolds, 2008; Candler, 2003; Loukas & Cote, 2005; Schmelzer, 2006), and urban contexts (Cahill & Suarez-Balcazar, 2009). This work underscores the importance of leisure participation for all children and informs practitioners about programs that foster such participation. Given the relevance of participation in structured leisure to positive youth development and mental health (Larson, 2000), a detailed discussion of supporting literature and implications for occupational therapy in community settings is provided in Chapter 3.

Examples of occupational therapy's role in fostering participation in community-based structured leisure, work, and independent living activities and the contributions to positive mental health are embedded throughout this book. A detailed discussion of the occupational therapy process specific to mental health promotion in schools and community is presented in Chapter 2.

Summary

> Raising children . . . is vastly more than fixing what is wrong with them. It is about identifying and nurturing their strongest qualities, what they own and are best at, and helping them find niches in which they can best live out these strengths. (Seligman & Csikszentmihalyi, 2000, p. 6)

This chapter has provided a foundation for reframing occupational therapy's role in children's mental health on the basis of recent contributions in the areas of positive psychology, positive youth development, and mental health promotion. In addition to addressing the needs of youth with identified psychiatric conditions, promoting positive mental health in all children and in multiple settings is critically needed—building positive qualities and personal strengths in addition to remediating problems. A three-tiered model focusing on a public health and primary prevention framework for occupational therapy services specific to school and community settings was introduced. This framework was used to envision a shift in occupational therapy service provision—serving all children, in school and community settings, and focusing on health-promoting occupations. Although some examples of service provision reflecting promotion, prevention, and intervention were provided, the remaining chapters will further delineate occupational therapy's role relative to specific service delivery models (e.g., consultation, therapeutic groups) and populations (e.g., children at risk of psychosis, those with disabilities).

References

American Occupational Therapy Association. (2008). Occupational therapy practice framework: Domain and process (2nd ed.). *American Journal of Occupational Therapy, 62,* 625–683.

American Psychiatric Association. (2000). *Diagnostic and statistical manual of mental disorders* (4th ed., text rev.). Washington, DC: Author.

Banet, J., Gilbert, J., Gmytrasiewicz, M., Pereyra, M., Reynolds, K., & Taylor, K. (2008). Creating participation at a camp for children with autism and Asperger syndrome. *Developmental Disabilities Special Interest Section Quarterly, 31*(4), 1–3.

Barry, M. M., & Jenkins, R. (2007). *Implementing mental health promotion.* Edinburgh, Scotland: Churchill Livingstone/Elsevier.

Bazyk, S. (2005). Creating occupation-based social skills groups in after-school care. *OT Practice, 11*(17), 13–18.

Bazyk, S. (2007). Addressing the mental health needs of children in schools. In L. Jackson (Ed.), *Occupational therapy services for children and youth under IDEA* (3rd ed., pp. 99–121). Bethesda, MD: AOTA Press.

Cahill, S. M. (2007). A perspective on response to intervention. *Special Interest Section Quarterly School System, 14*(3), 1–4.

Cahill, S. M., & Suarez-Balcazar, Y. (2009). Promoting children's nutrition and fitness in the urban context. *American Journal of Occupational Therapy, 63,* 113–116.

Candler, C. (2003). Sensory integration and therapeutic riding at summer camp: Occupational performance outcomes. *Physical and Occupational Therapy in Pediatrics, 23,* 51–64.

Carter, C., Meckes, L., Pritchard, L., Swensen, S., Wittman, P. P., & Velde, B. P. (2004, April–June). The Friendship Club: An after-school program for children with Asperger syndrome. *Family and Community Health, 27,* 143–150.

Catalano, R. F., Hawkins, D., Berglund, M. L., Pollard, J. A., & Arthur, M. W. (2002). Prevention science and positive youth development: Competitive or cooperative frameworks? *Journal of Adolescent Health, 31,* 230–239.

Davidson, D. A. (2005). Psychosocial issues affecting social participation. In J. Case-Smith (Ed.), *Occupational therapy for children* (5th ed., pp. 449–480). St. Louis, MO: Elsevier/Mosby.

Dunn, W., Brown, C., & Youngstrom, M. J. (2003). Ecological model of occupation. In P. Kramer, J. Hinojosa, & C. B. Royeen (Eds.), *Perspectives on human occupation: Participation in life* (pp. 222–263). Philadelphia: Lippincott Williams & Wilkins.

Education for All Handicapped Children Act of 1975, Pub. L. 94–142, 20 U.S.C. § 1400 *et seq.*

Evans, J., McDougall, J., & Baldwin, P. (2006). An evaluation of the "Youth en Route" program. *Physical and Occupational Therapy in Pediatrics, 26,* 63–87.

Fette, C. V. (2009). Community participation needs of families with children with behavioral disorders: A systems of care approach. *Occupational Therapy in Mental Health, 25,* 44–61.

Gable, S. L., & Haidt, J. (2005). What (and why) is positive psychology? *Review of General Psychology, 9,* 103–110.

Hackett, J. (2003). Perceptions of play and leisure in junior school aged children with juvenile idiopathic arthritis: What are the implications for occupational therapy? *British Journal of Occupational Therapy, 66,* 303–310.

Hosman, C., & Jané-Llopis, E. (1999). Political challenges 2: Mental health. In *The evidence of health promotion effectiveness: Shaping public health in a new Europe* (Report for the European Commission, pp. 29–41). Paris: International Union for Health Promotion and Education.

Howard, L. (1996). A comparison of leisure-time activities between able-bodied children and children with physical disabilities. *British Journal of Occupational Therapy, 59,* 570–574.

Individuals With Disabilities Education Act of 1997, Pub. L. 105–117.

Individuals With Disabilities Education Improvement Act of 2004, Pub. L. 108–446, 20 U.S.C. § 1400 *et seq.*

Insel, T. R., & Scolnick, E. M. (2006). Cure therapeutics and strategic prevention: Raising the bar for mental health research. *Molecular Psychiatry, 11,* 11–17.

Jackson, J., Rankin, A., Siefken, S., & Clark, F. (1989). Options: An occupational therapy transition program for adolescents with developmental disabilities. *Occupational Therapy in Health Care, 6,* 197–214.

Jackson, L. L., & Arbesman, M. (2005). *Occupational therapy practice guidelines for children with behavioral and psychosocial needs.* Bethesda, MD: AOTA Press.

Jané-Llopis, E., Barry, M., Hosman, C., & Patel, V. (2005). Mental health promotion works: A review. *Promotion and Education, 2*(Suppl.), 9–25.

Keyes, C. L. M. (2002). The mental health continuum: From languishing to flourishing in life. *Journal of Health and Social Behavior, 43,* 207–222.

Keyes, C. L. M. (2005). Mental illness and/or mental health? Investigating axioms of the complete state model of health. *Journal of Consulting and Clinical Psychology, 73,* 539–548.

Keyes, C. L. M. (2006). Mental health in adolescence: Is America's youth flourishing? *American Journal of Orthopsychiatry, 76,* 395–402.

Keyes, C. L. (2007). Promoting and protecting mental health as flourishing: A complementary strategy for improving national mental health. *American Psychologist, 62,* 95–108.

King, G., Law, M., King, S., Rosenbaum, P., Kertoy, M. K., & Young, N. L. (2003). A conceptual model of the factors affecting the recreation and leisure participation of children with disabilities. *Physical and Occupational Therapy in Pediatrics, 23,* 63–90.

Koller, J. R., & Bertel, J. M. (2006). Responding to today's mental health needs of children, families, and schools: Revisiting the preservice training and preparation of school-based personnel. *Education and Treatment of Children, 29,* 197–217.

Koppelman, J. (2004). *Children with mental disorders: Making sense of their needs and systems that help them* (NHPF Issue Brief No. 799). Washington, DC: George Washington University, National Health Policy Forum.

Kutash, K., Duchnowski, A. J., & Lynn, N. (2006). *School-based mental health: An empirical guide for decision-makers.* Tampa: University of South Florida, Louis de la Parte Florida Mental Health Institute, Research and Training Center for Children's Mental Health.

Larson, R. W. (2000). Toward a psychology of positive youth development. *American Psychologist, 55,* 170–183.

Law, M., Cooper, B., Strong, S., Stewart, D., Rigby, P., & Letts, L. (1996). The Person–Environment–Occupation model: A transactive approach to occupational therapy performance. *Canadian Journal of Occupational Therapy, 63,* 9–23.

Law, M., Petrenchik, T., King, G., & Hurley, P. (2007). Perceived environmental barriers to recreational, community, and school participation for children and youth with physical disabilities. *Archives of Physical Medicine and Rehabilitation, 88,* 1636–1642.

Letts, L., Fraser, B., Finlayson, M., & Walls, J. (1993). *For the health of it! Occupational therapy within a health promotion framework.* Ottawa, Ontario: CAOT Publications.

Lochner, A., & Bales, S. N. (2006, Winter). Framing youth issues for public support. *New Directions for Youth Development,* pp. 11–23.

Lougher, L. (2001). *Occupational therapy for children and adolescent mental health.* Edinburgh: Churchill Livingstone.

Loukas, K. M., & Cote, T. L. (2005). Sports as occupation: A sports camp experience for children who are blind or have visual impairment. *OT Practice, 10,* 15–19.

Mahoney, J. L., Larson, R. W., Eccles, J. S., & Lord, H. (2005). Organized activities as development contexts for children and adolescents. In J. Mahoney, R. Larson, & J. Eccles (Eds.), *Organized activities as contexts of development: Extracurricular activities, after-school, and community programs* (pp. 3–23). Mahwah, NJ: Lawrence Erlbaum.

Masia-Warner, C., Nangle, D. W., & Hansen, D. J. (2006). Bringing evidence-based child mental health services to the schools: General issues and specific populations. *Education and Treatment of Children, 29,* 165–172.

Mittlemark, M. B. (2007). Foreword. In M. Barry & R. Jenkins, *Implementing mental health promotion* (pp. ix–xi). Edinburgh: Churchill Livingstone/Elsevier.

No Child Left Behind Act of 2001, Pub. L. 107–110.

Park, N. (2004). Character strengths and positive youth development. *Annals of the American Academy of Political and Social Science, 591,* 40–54.

Petrenchik, T. (2006). Homelessness: Perspectives, misconceptions, and considerations for occupational therapy. *Occupational Therapy in Health Care, 20,* 9–30.

Poulsen, A. A., Ziviani, J. M., & Cuskelly, M. (2008). Leisure time physical activity energy expenditure in boys with developmental coordination disorder: The role of peer relations self-concept perceptions. *OTJR: Occupation, Participation and Health, 28,* 30–39.

President's New Freedom Commission on Mental Health. (2003). *Achieving the promise: Transforming mental health care in America* (Final Report, DHHS Pub. No. SMA–03–3832). Rockville, MD: Author. Retrieved July 27, 2010, from www.mentalhealthcommission.gov

Reese, S. D., Grandy, O. H., & Grant, A. E. (2001). *Framing public life: Perspectives on media and our understanding of the social world.* Mahwah, NJ: Lawrence Erlbaum.

Rogers, J. C., & Holm, M. B. (2009). The occupational therapy process. In E. B. Crepeau, E. S. Cohn, & B. A. B. Schell (Eds.), *Willard and Spackman's occupational therapy* (11th ed., pp. 479–518). Philadelphia: Lippincott Williams & Wilkins.

Rosenberg, A. E. (2000). Conducting an inventory of informal community-based resources for children with physical disabilities: Enhancing access and creating professional linkages. *Physical and Occupational Therapy in Pediatrics, 20,* 59–79.

Safran, S. P., & Oswald, K. (2003). Positive behavior supports: Can schools reshape disciplinary practices? *Exceptional Children, 69,* 361–373.

Schmelzer, L. (2006). An occupation-based camp for healthier children. *OT Practice, 11,* 18–23.

Seligman, M. E. P. (2002). *Authentic happiness.* New York: Free Press.

Seligman, M. E. P., & Csikszentmihalyi, M. (2000). Positive psychology: An introduction. *American Psychologist, 55,* 5–14.

Shikako-Thomas, K., Majnemer, A., Law, M., & Lach, L. (2008). Determinants of participation in leisure activities in children and youth with cerebral palsy: A systematic review. *Physical and Occupational Therapy in Pediatrics, 28,* 155–170.

Spencer, K. C., Turkett, A., Vaughan, R., & Koenig, S. (2006). School-based practice patterns: A survey of occupational therapists in Colorado. *American Journal of Occupational Therapy, 60,* 81–90.

U.S. Department of Education, Office of Special Education Programs Center on Positive Behavioral Interventions and Supports. (2010). Retrieved July 27, 2010, from www.pbis.org/default.aspx

U.S. Department of Health and Human Services. (1999). *Mental health: A report of the Surgeon General* (Executive summary). Rockville, MD: U.S. Department of Health and Human Services, Substance Abuse and Mental Health Services Administration, Center for Mental Health Services, & National Institute of Mental Health.

Weist, M. D., & Paternite, C. E. (2006). Building an interconnected policy-training-practice-research agenda to advance school mental health. *Education and Treatment of Children, 29,* 173–196.

Wilcock, A. A., & Townsend, E. A. (2008). Occupational justice. In E. B. Crepeau, E. S. Cohn, & B. B. Schell (Eds.), *Willard and Spackman's occupational therapy* (11th ed., pp. 192–199). Baltimore: Lippincott Williams & Wilkins.

World Health Organization. (1986, November 21). *Ottawa charter for health promotion.* Retrieved January 11, 2001, from www.who.int/healthpromotion/conferences/previous/ottawa/en/

World Health Organization. (2001). *The World Health Report: Mental health: New understanding, new hope:* Geneva: Author.

CHAPTER 2

Occupational Therapy Process: A Public Health Approach to Promoting Mental Health in Children and Youth

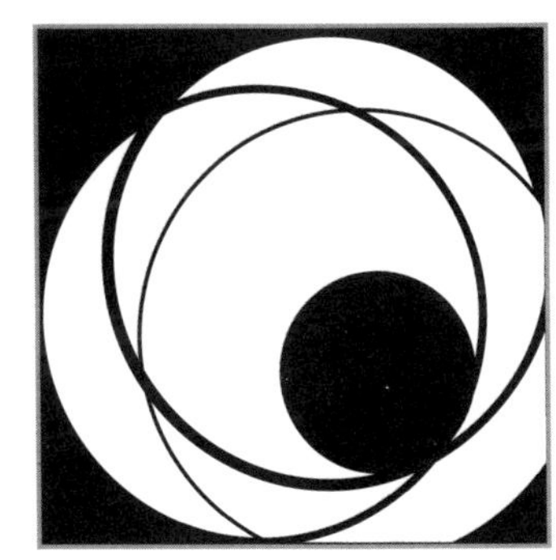

Susan Bazyk, PhD, OTR/L, FAOTA

Learning Objectives

After reading this material and completing the examination, readers will be able to

- Identify the elements of the proposed occupational therapy process (awareness, appraisal, and action) to be applied within a public health framework;
- Identify awareness, appraisal, and action strategies recommended for Tier 1 (universal), Tier 2 (targeted), and Tier 3 (individualized) occupational therapy services;
- Recognize a variety of mental health literacy strategies;
- Recognize strategies for promoting participation in structured leisure occupations for children needing selected or targeted intervention;
- Identify what a systems of care approach is and where it is applied;
- Recognize features of the youth empowerment movement; and
- Recognize strategies for enhancing subjective well-being in people with severe and significant mental illness.

"All people need to be able or enabled to engage in the occupations of their need and choice, to grow through what they do, and to experience independence or interdependence, equality, participation, security, health, and well-being" (Wilcock & Townsend, 2008, p. 198). Applying a public health approach to the promotion of mental health calls for occupational therapists to reframe services for children and youth to include promotion and prevention of problems in addition to remediation. Such a shift in thinking requires a strategic conceptualization of how occupational therapy can serve all children, regardless of disability or mental health status.

This chapter focuses on applying the occupational therapy process within a public health framework (universal, targeted, and individualized services) in schools and community settings. Although occupational therapy's emphasis will vary depending on context, all efforts share a common belief in the positive relationship between participation in a balance of meaningful occupations and health. Occupational therapy promotes the health and participation of people, organizations, and populations through engagement in occupation and emphasizes improving the social, physical, and economic environments that influence the mental health of people and populations (American Occupational Therapy Association [AOTA], 2008).

Occupational Therapy Mental Health Promotion Framework

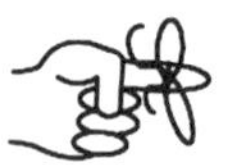

Remember this. . . .
Positive psychology: "[O]ur message is to remind our field that psychology is not just the study of pathology, weakness, and damage; it is also the study of strength and virtue. Treatment is not just fixing problems; it is nurturing what is best . . . work, education, insight, love, growth, and play" (Seligman & Csikszentmihalyi, 2000, p. 7).

An understanding of positive psychology, positive youth development, and mental health promotion is applied to an ecological model of occupational performance to envision occupational therapy services in the promotion of mental health in children and youth (Figure 2.1). Seligman's (2002) three pillars of positive psychology (positive emotions, positive character strengths, and positive institutions), along with Larson's (2000) emphasis on structured leisure participation, are embedded within a person–occupation–environment model of occupational performance.

The proposed occupational therapy process involves (1) awareness (gaining knowledge and skills), (2) appraisal (observation, gathering information, or evaluation), and (3) action (indirect and direct intervention strategies) related to each domain (Table 2.1). For example, in terms of the *person,* occupational therapists need to become *aware* of the mental health continuum, including symptoms associated with various mental illnesses and factors associated with mental health at multiple levels (individual, community). *Appraisal* involves the use of a number of strategies to evaluate the mental health of the person or groups of people and the qualities of physical and social environments. At the most basic level, occupational therapists should pay attention to every child's mental health by specifically observing emotions (Does the child demonstrate periods of happiness, joy, and satisfaction throughout the day?), patterns of occupational participation (Does the child engage in a range of occupations, including play and leisure, work, and rest? Does the child have special interests or hobbies that foster a sense of joy and personal well-being?), and quality of the settings (Do the settings involve caring adults who promote character strengths and positive emotions?). *Actions* are based on the appraisal process and refer to interventions and conditions that promote optimal mental health. Consultation with teachers to understand behaviors associated with sensory defensiveness and to modify interactions to enhance social interaction is an example of an action used to promote a positive setting. Because mental health is perceived as a dynamic state of functioning that can vary throughout a person's life on the basis of many biological (e.g., genetics), environmental (e.g., poverty), or situational (e.g., death of a parent) factors, the occupational therapist must remain vigilant to the impact of such factors on the person's mental health.

As introduced in Chapter 1, a three-tiered public health framework is used to envision and guide occupational therapy in the promotion of mental health and prevention of and intervention with mental ill health for both school and community settings (see Figure 1.3). This framework supports a change in thinking from the traditional, individually focused, deficit-driven model of mental health intervention to a whole-population, strengths-based approach. The aim of occupational therapy

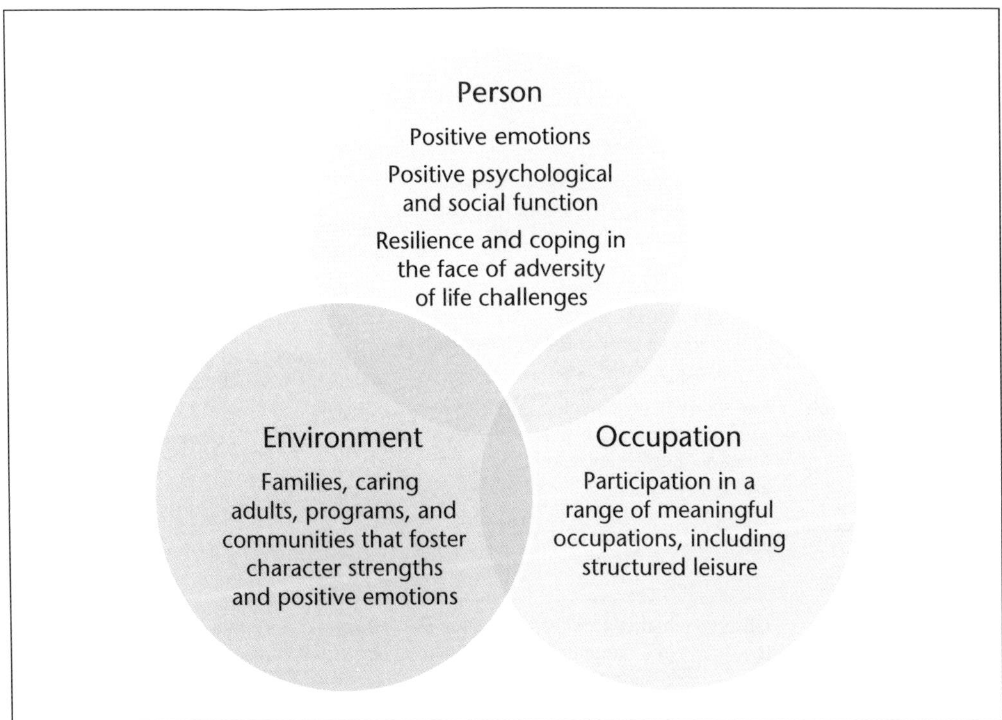

Figure 2.1. Occupational Therapy Mental Health Promotion Framework.

is to promote mental health and flourishing at all tiers, in people with and without mental illness. In addition to reducing problem behaviors, the promotion of mental health and well-being is emphasized when working with people with chronic mental illness. A discussion of the occupational therapy process at each tier in school and community settings follows. Although the domain and process of occupational therapy services is similar in each setting, the focus differs. For example, in schools, occupational therapy services help children benefit from their education and function successfully in the school environment. In contrast, community-based services will likely occur during out-of-school time, warranting attention to the development of meaningful structured leisure interests, friendships, independent living skills, and beginning work skills.

Tier 1 Services: Universal Promotion and Prevention

Services at the universal level are geared toward the entire population, including children and youth with disabilities, illness, or both and the majority who do not demonstrate mental health or behavioral problems. The person–occupation–environment transaction is considered in a broad manner, focusing on the mental health needs of all children and youth. During interactions with children and youth in school and community settings, occupational therapists should make note of children's emotions as they participate in occupations that they need or want to do. Does the physical and social environment support successful participation and enjoyment? If not, what accommodations or adaptations based on analysis of person–occupation–environment might the occupational therapist offer?

Table 2.1. Occupational Therapy Process in the Promotion of Mental Health

	Awareness (Gain Knowledge Base)	Appraisal (Evaluate, Observe)	Action (Intervention)
Person	Gain knowledge of mental health continuum. • Mental illness (psychiatric conditions and associated symptoms in children and youth) • Mental health (emotional, psychological, and social functioning associated with positive mental health). Become familiar with assessment tools used to evaluate behavior, psychological function, social interaction, and participation. Gain knowledge of various approaches used to promote mental health (SEL, PBIS, CBT, and alternative approaches).	Observe emotions. • Does the child demonstrate moments of joy, happiness, and satisfaction throughout the day? • During what activities does the child demonstrate positive emotions? Does he or she have frequent opportunities to engage in these occupations? Use a variety of screening and assessment tools to evaluate psychosocial function, participation in occupation, and quality of life.	Communicate the scope of occupational therapy practice, including mental health promotion to clients (child, parents, teachers, coaches, school administrators). Promote participation in enjoyable occupations. Identify process for referral and intervention to address mental health concerns. Apply a variety of approaches used to promote mental health (SEL, PBIS, CBT, and alternative approaches).
Occupation	Gain knowledge of health benefits of participation in a range of occupations, particularly structured leisure occupations during out-of-school time.	Observe whether child has opportunities to engage in a range of structured leisure occupations during out-of-school time. Identify extracurricular school and community programs.	Educate others about the value of participation in structured leisure interests. Expose and offer supports and scaffolded experiences to foster successful participation. Foster the development of interests through sustained exposure and participation.
Environment	Gain knowledge of school- and community-wide strategies used to promote positive environments (e.g., PBIS, SEL). Become informed about state and federal policies related to children's mental health.	Obtain information about school and community promotion, prevention, and intervention programs. Evaluate the quality of home, school, and community settings for promoting mental health.	Promote successful participation in positive home, school, and community environments. Participate in school committees emphasizing mental health literacy and promotion. Contribute to local, state, and national political action efforts to strengthen mental health programming in schools and the community.

Note. CBT = cognitive–behavioral therapy; PBIS = positive behavioral interventions and supports; SEL = social and emotional learning.

At the universal level, the occupational therapy process focuses less on direct, individualized care and more on indirect services geared to large groups of children and youth. Awareness of schoolwide and community-based promotion and prevention initiatives is critical (e.g., social and emotional learning [SEL], positive behavioral interventions and supports [PBIS]). In addition, it is important to become knowledgeable about key legislation and policies affecting mental health promotion and prevention efforts. For example, the President's New Freedom Commission on Mental Health (2003; Weist & Paternite, 2006) identified fragmentation and gaps in care and specifically recommended that all federal, state, and local child-serving agencies address the mental health needs of youth in the educational system. The commission "emphasized building a mental health system that is evidence-based, recovery-focused and consumer- and family-driven" (Moherek Sopko, 2006, p. 1). Last, it is critical to become familiar with reputable technical assistance centers to develop and maintain information related to mental health promotion (e.g., Center for School Mental Health Services; Box 2.1).

On the basis of a sound awareness of best practice related to mental health promotion and prevention, occupational therapists should appraise school and community settings for the presence and quality of such efforts. Initially, it is important to identify what educational policies and established programs exist so that systematic efforts (action) can be made to ensure that occupational therapy becomes an active and recognized team member within these systems of care. Because at least 80% of the team needs to buy into new approaches to ensure successful implementation, it is critical for occupational therapists to be a part of schoolwide training efforts and actively assist in program implementation (Kutash, Duchnowksi, & Lynn, 2006).

Within schools, occupational therapists can specifically embed services at the universal level in multiple ways. For example, when applying a PBIS framework, occupational therapists should become aware of the school mission statement and descriptions of student expectations to assist educators in creating positive learning environments. When integrating services in the classroom, therapists can encourage students to follow classroom rules and interact with students in ways that help create a positive environment. Because effective classroom instruction is a component of PBIS, therapists can also consult with teachers to ensure that the curriculum and classroom expectations are at an appropriate level for students (Cartledge, 2003). For example, they can be on the lookout for children who have a difficult time regulating arousal to attend during seated classroom work. An in-service on the *Alert Program: How Does Your Engine Run?* (Williams & Shellenberger, 1996) might be one strategy for helping teachers adapt classroom practices on the basis of students' varying sensory needs. Occupational therapists can also assist teachers in embedding SEL activities within classroom learning (Knippenberg & Hanft, 2004).

In addition to schoolwide PBIS and SEL efforts, occupational therapists should become knowledgeable about any other school- and community-based programs developed to foster mental health literacy and promote mental health. This knowledge can be shared with children and families who might potentially benefit from participation.

Tier 1 services reflect a dual commitment to promotion (development of competencies) and prevention (reduction of risks) in the whole population, including the majority of children who do not demonstrate academic or emotional problems (approximately 80%). Research findings have suggested that focusing on both risk reduction and protective factor enhancement is most effective in promoting positive youth development (Catalano, Hawkins, Berglund, Pollard, & Arthur, 2002; Mrazek & Haggerty, 1994). Within both school and community settings, occupational therapists have many opportunities to build competencies and reduce risks in children and youth. A key to moving in this direction is being committed to such efforts and actively seeking opportunities to practice in such a manner.

Box 2.1. Internet Resources on Mental Health

Federal Government

- *Center for Mental Health Services:* Children, adolescents, and family resources.
  www.mentalhealth.samhsa.gov/cmhs
- *National Institute of Mental Health (NIMH):* NIMH's mission is to diminish the burden of mental illness through research.
  www.nimh.nih.gov
- *Office of the U.S. Surgeon General:* In 1999, Surgeon General David Satcher issued a comprehensive report on mental health; Chapter 3 covers children and adolescents.
  www.mentalhealthcommission.gov/reports/reports.htm
- *President's New Freedom Commission on Mental Health:* The commission was created to examine the current gaps in mental illness treatment services and to make recommendations to the President on ways in which the federal government can help states increase access to care and improve quality in their public programs.
  www.mentalhealthcommission.gov

Advocacy Organizations and Technical Assistance Centers

- *Bazelon Center for Mental Health Law:* The Bazelon Center works on a broad array of children's mental health issues.
  www.bazelon.org
- *National Alliance on Mental Illness (NAMI):* NAMI is the nation's largest grassroots mental health organization dedicated to improving the lives of children and adults living with mental illness and their families. Founded in 1979, NAMI has become the nation's voice on mental illness—a national organization that includes NAMI organizations in every state and in more than 1,100 local communities across the country who join together to meet the NAMI mission through advocacy, research, support, and education.
  www.nami.org
- *Centers for School Mental Health—Technical Assistance Centers:* In 1995, two national training and technical assistance centers focused on mental health in schools were established with partial support from the U.S. Department of Health and Human Services and the Center for Mental Health Services. One center is at the University of California, Los Angeles, and the other is at the University of Maryland at Baltimore. Their Web sites include information and resources on school-based mental health programs.
  www.smhp.psych.ucla.edu
  www.csmh.umaryland.edu
- *Minnesota Association for Children's Mental Health:* The association offers practical school mental health resources based on current research and effective programming.
  - Early Childhood Fact Sheets cover a range of conditions (depression, sensory processing disorders) and offer information for parents on such topics as tantrums and toileting.
  - Mental Health Fact Sheets provide information about a variety of conditions (e.g., anxiety disorders, schizophrenia), symptoms, educational implications, instructional strategies, and classroom accommodations.

  www.macmh.org
- *SchoolMentalHealth.org:* This site offers school mental health resources not only for clinicians but also for educators, administrators, parents and caregivers, families, and students. The resources included on the site emphasize practical information and skills based on current research, including prominent evidence-based practices and lessons learned from local, state, and national initiatives.
  www.schoolmentalhealth.org

Approaches Emphasizing Mental Health Promotion

Promotion efforts focus on competence enhancement and positive mental health in the whole population—children with and without disabilities—within the context of their everyday lives. Such an enhancement model assumes that as children become more competent, their psychological well-being improves (Barry & Jenkins, 2007). All children can benefit from home, school, and community resources that help in the development of personal and social skills (e.g., coping, self-awareness, emotional regulation).

Promotion efforts need to involve a comprehensive lifespan approach that considers the age-, situation-, group-, and society-related determinants of and impediments to mental health and wellness. According to Cowen (1991), comprehensive promotion efforts should focus on (1) competence (social–emotional, leisure, and work skills), (2) resilience (ability to cope with life stressors), (3) social system modification (changing social environments to promote mental health), and (4) empowerment (enhancing children's control over their mental health). Occupational therapists, with their commitment to fostering occupational performance, are already offering services emphasizing competence and resilience to the children and youth whom they serve. Such services, however, are generally restricted to a small number of children—those with identified disabilities (typically representing Tier 3), not the whole population. Such restricted services, in part, are influenced by limitations imposed within the setting (e.g., in most schools, children must be eligible for special education and related services) and by insurance companies. Consequently, although occupational therapists are well equipped to provide services to promote mental health in the whole population, social system modifications are needed to support this shift in service provision.

It is essential that occupational therapists look for opportunities to expand services to include mental health promotion and advocate for such shifts in service delivery. Traditionally, an occupational therapist's job expectations have been based on a caseload model of counting the number of children receiving direct intervention as a part of their individualized education program (AOTA, 2006). This model often neglects to account for essential indirect services, including collaborative consultation, team meetings, and in-service trainings. In contrast, the concept of workload encompasses all the direct and indirect services performed to benefit students, making a workload approach helpful for conceptualizing work patterns that optimize effectiveness and impact (AOTA, 2006).

Mental Health Literacy

Although multiple programs and approaches applied in schools and the community focus on the promotion of mental health, this section introduces the concept of mental health literacy. SEL, which emphasizes competency enhancement in recognizing and managing emotions for successful interaction, is presented in Chapter 3.

Mental health literacy focuses on providing all children and youth with a working knowledge of mental health as an integral part of health (Barry & Jenkins, 2007). The term mental health literacy was introduced in Australia by Anthony Jorm and represents a relatively new area of study (Jorm et al., 1997). The concept is derived from the term *health literacy*—the functional capacity to understand and use information for the purpose of personal health promotion. Mental health literacy refers to the knowledge and beliefs about mental health and mental disorders that assist in knowing how to foster mental health and recognize, manage, and seek treatment for mental illness (Griffiths, Christensen, & Jorm, 2009).

Mental health literacy is a relatively new area of investigation, and literature on the topic mostly emanates from Australia, Canada, and Europe. One of the most comprehensive national campaigns to date, "Beyondblue: The National Depression Initiative in Australia," involves multiple targeted strategies. Program evaluations have shown several positive outcomes, including increasing community awareness of depression, increasing the number of early intervention and prevention programs, increasing the capacity of primary caregivers, and reducing stigma (Bourget Management Consulting for the Canadian Alliance on Mental Illness and Mental Health, 2007).

As a Tier 1 service provider, a school-based occupational therapist might collaborate with health educators or school nurses in co-teaching a unit on the mental health continuum, including mental illness, languishing, moderate mental health, and flourishing (Keyes, 2007). Programs that help children learn and talk about mental health, mental illness, and interventions may help reduce the negative stigma associated with mental illness by helping to bring the topic into everyday conversations and framing mental health as a positive state of functioning. Becoming aware of and encouraging use of reliable Internet resources is another strategy for promoting mental health literacy. Santor, Poulin, Leblanc, and Kusumakar (2007) have developed and explored the use and impact of a school-based health information Web site for adolescents. Findings have indicated that the use of such a Web site holds promise for health promotion and early self-identification of emotional problems. Details about *YooMagazine,* an Internet health magazine for youth, are included in Resource 2.1.

Resource 2.1. ***YooMagazine***

YooMagazine, an interactive health magazine for youth, is directed by Darcy Santor at the Centre of Excellence for Child and Youth Mental Health in Ottawa, Ontario, and Alexa Bagnell at the IWK Health Centre in Halifax, Nova Scotia. This Web site is designed to promote health literacy, early detection of difficulties, and help seeking in middle school and high school youth. Specific components of the Web site provide information on developmental, physical health, and mental health topics through static (e.g., information sheets), interactive (e.g., posting questions), and narrative (e.g., viewing answers to previously posted questions) formats. The Web site features monthly information on a key health issue through combinations of these formats. Content for the Web site (i.e., information sheets) was initially developed through a selection of information from a variety of agencies, such as the Centers for Disease Control and Prevention, the U.S. Surgeon's General office, and Statistics Canada; regulatory bodies, such as Health Canada and the U.S. Food and Drug Administration; scientific journals; and professional groups, such as the American Academy of Family Physicians.

YooMagazine can be viewed at www.yoomagazine.net.

Source. Santor et al. (2007).

Prevention

Prevention efforts generally focus on risk reduction—that is, interrupting the processes that lead to a single problem behavior (e.g., drug use, teenage pregnancy, delinquent behavior). Such programs have shown promising results. A recent National Survey on Drug Use and Health (2005) estimated that approximately 78% of 12- to 17-year-old students had heard or seen drug or alcohol prevention messages during the previous year. The survey also found that alcohol, cigarette, and illicit drug use were lower for youth exposed to such messages in school.

Although appropriately designed and implemented school-based prevention programs can prevent or reduce negative behaviors, accumulating evidence has indicated that negative behaviors do not exist in isolation, so programs that address multiple co-occurring negative behaviors are likely to be of greater benefit. The Positive Action program, a comprehensive K–12 social and emotional development program, demonstrated substantial effects on reducing multiple problem behaviors (i.e., substance abuse, violent behavior, sexual activity; Beets et al., 2009). Occupational therapists should become aware of and familiar with the prevention programs offered in their school districts and communities to encourage participation and reinforce the knowledge and skills gained from participation.

Occupational therapists are well equipped to be active participants in the provision of Tier 1 services. Attention to barriers to and opportunities for providing services to promote mental health and prevent risk factors is key to shifting from an emphasis on intervention for children already identified as having mental health or behavior disorders. Although not inclusive, Table 2.2 provides further examples of Tier 1 occupational therapy services emphasizing awareness, appraisal, and action.

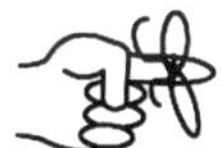

Remember this. . . .
"Prevention researchers have discovered that there are human strengths that act as buffers against mental illness: courage, future mindedness, optimism, interpersonal skill, faith, work ethic, hope, honesty, perseverance and the capacity for flow and insight, to name several" (Seligman & Csikszentmihalyi, 2000, p. 7).

Tier 2 Services: Targeted Mental Health Interventions

Tier 2 services are geared toward students at risk of behavioral and mental health problems, a group that includes children with and without physical or developmental disabilities (about 10% to 15%). Targeted interventions are designed to support children and youth who have learning, emotional, or life experiences that place them at risk of engaging in problematic behavior, developing mental health challenges, or both. For example, children with physical or developmental disabilities might struggle with low self-esteem, issues related to feeling different, or the stress associated with frequent hospitalizations. Children living in poverty are at risk of participating in risky street activities or experiencing chronic anxiety as a result of living in stressful home and neighborhood environments.

Compared with Tier 1 services, the person–occupation–environment transaction focuses more specifically on children and youth at risk of developing mental health problems. At this level, children are generally not identified as having a mental or emotional disorder but often begin to display subtle changes in performance. Services emphasize both prevention of the development of a mental illness and the promotion of competencies to offset early symptoms (e.g., time management, relaxation strategies). Occupational therapists might focus on adapting activities and the environment to foster successful participation and applying strategies to minimize early symptoms and promote positive psychological functioning (e.g., breaking down school assignments and giving one part at a time to minimize anxiety, teaching relaxation strategies). Chapter 3 has more information on developmental psychopathology.

School Settings

Awareness

To address the needs of youth at risk of developing mental illness, occupational therapists must develop an awareness of this population's specific needs. Although strategies to prevent problem behaviors have received significant attention in school settings, the prevention of mental illness through early identification and intervention has not. Forness (2003) suggested that applying the concept of developmental psychopathology supports a public health framework of children's mental health and, as such, can assist families and professionals in being more proactive in the early detection of emotional or behavioral disorders. *Developmental psychopathology*

Table 2.2. Examples of Occupational Therapy Tier 1 Services

<table>
<tr>
<td rowspan="2">

Tier 1 Services
Universal

Target
All children with and without disabilities.

Occupational therapy services
Efforts focus on
• Creating positive environments;
• Promoting mental health literacy;
• Collaborating with caregivers, youth, and teams to promote mental health awareness (e.g., serve on committees related to promoting positive mental health);
• Observing affect and participation patterns in all children; and
• Promoting successful and enjoyable participation in occupational performance areas, including structured leisure pursuits.

</td>
<td>

School Level

Awareness
• *Become knowledgeable* about state-of-the-art mental health promotion and prevention programs using reputable technical assistance centers (e.g., CASEL) and current literature.
• *Learn* about public policy affecting children's mental health at the local, state, and national levels.

Appraisal
• *Identify* school efforts to promote mental health literacy, SEL, and the use of PBIS. Support implementation in a variety of contexts (classroom, hallways, lunchroom, playground, and restrooms).
• *Become aware* of school prevention programs focusing on risk reduction (e.g., teen pregnancy, drug use, suicide, bullying), encourage participation, and reinforce message.
• *Evaluate* lunch and recess for factors that may impede social participation for any student.
• Informally *observe* all children for behaviors that might suggest mental health concerns or limitations in social–emotional development. Bring concerns to the educational team.

Action
• *Promote* mental health literacy efforts offered in the school. Collaborate with health educators and school nurses to promote schoolwide mental health literacy activities.
• *Provide* in-service education to teachers and staff on the following topics:
1. *Sensory processing*—how to adapt classroom practices on the basis of students' varying sensory needs to enhance attending and behavior regulation (e.g., the Alert Program)
2. *SEL*—How to embed SEL activities within classroom routines and activities (e.g., identifying feelings, thinking about how feelings influence behavior, perspective taking).
3. *Positive mental health* and the type of activity participation that helps foster it.
• *Consult* with teachers to help them recognize the student's most effective learning styles. Ensure that students are able to meet classroom demands and create modifications if needed.
• Clearly *articulate* the scope of occupational therapy practice, including social participation, social–emotional function, and mental health (all tiers).

</td>
</tr>
<tr>
<td>

Community Level

Awareness
• *Learn* about mental health literacy initiatives at the national, state, and local levels.

Appraisal
• *Identify* community opportunities for inclusive participation in mental health literacy efforts and foster participation.

Action
• *Promote* opportunities for all children and youth to participate in structured leisure occupations in a variety of community settings. Help children recognize the relationship between participation in meaningful leisure interests and positive mental health.
• *Advocate* for inclusive structured leisure opportunities (arts, music, theater, sports, clubs).

</td>
</tr>
</table>

Note. CASEL = Collaborative for Academic, Social, and Emotional Learning; PBIS = positive behavioral interventions and supports; SEL = social and emotional learning.

presumes that the trajectory of such disorders results from a variety of early genetic or environmental factors that are often overlooked (Forness, Kavale, MacMillan, Asarnow, & Duncan, 1996). Parents, teachers, and service providers who interact with youth on a daily basis may become aware of and concerned about early symptoms, mild functional impairments, or both but may not recognize them as *prodromal*—that is, as early symptoms of a psychiatric disorder. Inherent in the concept of developmental psychopathology is the need for early detection and primary prevention—of "front-loading" efforts at the earliest signs of trouble instead of "back-loading" efforts long after a diagnosis is confirmed (Forness, 2003).

Retrospective studies have indicated that children with prodromal signs of emotional disorders are often misidentified as having a learning disability or related problems in schools (Lopez, Forness, MacMillan, Bocian, & Gresham, 1996). Certain special education designations, such as learning disability or speech–language problems, tend to serve as the gatekeeping categories of first resort for students with mental health problems (Hoagwood & Johnson, 2003). In addition, Duncan, Forness, and Harsough (1995) found that although eligibility for special education occurred at a mean age of 7 years, 8 months, parents reported recognizing that something was wrong at age 3 years, 5 months.

Although the functional analysis of behavior and positive behavioral supports have been widely applied in schools to address behavior, attention to early detection of prodromal signs of a possible psychiatric disorder has been lacking (Forness, 2003). Tier 1 and Tier 2 services ought to include systematic attention to interdisciplinary screening and referral for mental health disorders. Occupational therapists, with their background in psychopathology and behavior, can play an important role in such early detection, screening, and intervention.

Occupational therapy's role working within the Portland Identification and Early Referral (PIER) Program with youth at risk of psychosis and those experiencing mental illness is addressed in Chapter 7. By applying a public health framework, PIER focuses on communitywide education about early detection of and intervention for severe mental illness, evaluation and monitoring of interventions, access to services, and epidemiological data and analyses.

Children with and without physical or emotional disabilities are likely, at some point in their lives, to struggle with situational stressors such as parental divorce, the death of a family member, living in poverty, friendship issues, bullying, or academic challenges. During such times, character strengths, coping strategies, and environmental supports can serve as important buffers in preventing mental ill health (Catalano et al., 2002). While interacting with and observing children, occupational therapists can make a habit of being aware of possible stressors and advocating for and developing services to counteract stressors and build competencies (e.g., bereavement support groups, participation in after-school clubs). Refer to Chapter 6 to learn about reducing risks and promoting competencies in the presence of situational stressors such as bullying, bereavement, poverty, and obesity.

Appraisal

Appraisal efforts at this level need to emphasize efficient but careful screening for subtle changes in behavior and functional skills. Students at this level are typically not identified as needing special education and, as such, will not be officially included in the therapist's caseload. Specifically, some children with mild mental disorders display symptoms that are not immediately apparent and, thus, often go undetected (Koppelman, 2004). For example, a child who is mildly depressed might be quiet and withdrawn and underperform academically, whereas a child with mild attention deficit hyperactivity disorder (ADHD) may have difficulty focusing on and getting homework completed. Anxiety might cause excessive stress for the child required to speak in front of the class.

Occupational therapists can use both informal and formal evaluation strategies to identify risk, changes in behavior or functional skills, or the early presence of mental health problems. A variety of strategies can be used, including observations of performance and social interaction, informal interviews with the student or teacher, or screening assessments. Evaluation is followed by the development of a support plan that might include environmental modification (e.g., reduction of expectations, modified interactions) or small-group intervention. At this level, occupational therapists might collaborate with teachers, social workers, or other mental health providers to develop and cofacilitate such selective interventions. The number of children with subthreshold mental health issues remains unidentified; thus, early intervention and prevention is needed before problems escalate (Koller & Bertel, 2006).

Action

Because teachers are generally not prepared to recognize mental health problems, occupational therapists can play a role in early identification and psychoeducation (Koller & Bertel, 2006). Educating teachers about the early signs of mental illness and proactive, strengths-based prevention strategies may help them become more involved in early identification of problems and the development of appropriate classroom accommodations.

After the screening process, a range of early intervention activities can be implemented. "Experts say that most children with mild mental disorders could benefit from some form of treatment, whether medication, behavioral or behavioral cognitive therapy, family counseling, or some combination thereof" (Koppelman, 2004, p. 7). General education students demonstrating behavioral or learning difficulties because of such mental health conditions may be provided coordinated early intervention services even if special education is not needed, according to the Individuals With Disabilities Education Improvement Act of 2004 (Jackson & Arbesman, 2005). Another way in which services can be offered for students who do not qualify for special education is through Section 504 of the Rehabilitation Act of 1973. For many students with mild mental disorders, accommodations that are provided under Section 504 are sufficient for enhancing school functioning. For the child with anxiety, the occupational therapist might consult with the teacher and child to discuss realistic expectations and strategies for reducing stress (e.g., break down assignments into manageable pieces).

Small-group interventions can be developed jointly by occupational therapists and other team members to serve students with similar needs (Freeman et al., 2006). SEL groups might be cofacilitated by an occupational therapist and speech–language pathologist for students with Asperger syndrome, for example. Occupation-based

SEL groups can also be offered to other at-risk groups, including low-income urban youth (Bazyk, 2005).

Community Settings

In addition to addressing school function, attention to home and community participation is essential. Close collaboration with caregivers regarding early intervention and carryover into the home must be ongoing. In particular, the promotion of successful participation in social and structured leisure activities during out-of-school time is important for building competencies and offering enjoyable experiences that promote a sense of emotional well-being. Approaches for fostering participation in meaningful community-based occupations have been proposed. For example, Engaging and Coaching for Health (EACH)–Child provides strategies for promoting sustained physical activity in children through a process of exploration and engagement, coaching, and scaffolded experiences (Ziviani, Poulsen, & Hansen, 2008). In a related way, Occupational Performance Coaching has been proposed as an approach to assist parents and their children to participate more successfully in self-identified home and community occupations (Graham, Rodger, & Ziviani, 2009).

Awareness

The first step in promoting participation is developing an awareness of the many intrapersonal and interpersonal benefits of structured leisure participation and communicating these to children, families, and community leaders. A detailed discussion of the contributions of structured leisure participation on promoting mental health is provided in Chapter 3. Special efforts to promote participation might be necessary for children at risk of limited participation because of restricted access and availability (e.g., low-income urban youth). Children and youth with developmental disabilities are also at risk of limited participation in structured leisure, which may lead to feelings of isolation, restricted social interaction, and boredom. Those children experiencing early signs of mental illness (e.g., depression) may display little interest or motivation to participate in extracurricular activities and may need support and encouragement to initiate such participation.

Appraisal

To promote participation in structured leisure, it is important to know one's community. Specifically, becoming aware of the range of activity options is essential, including sports, arts, music, outdoor and community recreation, and club-related options. Personally visiting settings and meeting directors is one strategy that would allow the occupational therapist to assess whether the context is open to children and youth with disabilities or mental health problems and whether the setting might support positive functioning (e.g., physical and psychological safety, appropriate structure, supportive relationships, opportunities for belonging, positive social norms, and opportunities for skill building; Eccles & Gootman, 2002). Once the therapist is aware of community options, a discussion of possible interests can take place on the basis of the child's personality, developmental stage, and ability level. Identifying activities that are meaningful, enjoyable, and interesting and that provide the "just-right" challenge is key to motivating engagement (Poulsen, Rodger, & Ziviani, 2006).

Action

"Identifying an interest is the first step in achieving a goal; however, to engage in an activity relies on sustaining that interest through supportive environments and well-targeted instructional strategies" (Ziviani et al., 2008, p. 264). Adapting initial entry into the activity might be necessary depending on the person's specific needs. For example, a child with anxiety might agree to participate in a new activity if given the option to bring a friend or simply observe the first session. Consulting with the instructor or coach to modify the environment, activity, or interaction to support successful participation is another strategy for ensuring sustained involvement. Being available for ongoing consultation and problem solving is also advised.

When feasible, fostering participation in integrated community settings for children with disabilities is suggested. Wehmeyer and Bolding (1999) found that people who lived or worked in community-based settings were more self-determined, had more choices, and were more satisfied than those living in congregate settings. Refer to Table 2.3 for examples of occupational therapy services at Tier 2 emphasizing awareness, appraisal, and action in schools and the community.

Tier 3 Services: Intensive Mental Health Interventions

Tier 3 services are provided for children and youth with identified mental, emotional, or behavioral disorders that limit participation in needed and desired areas of occupational performance. Approximately 1 in 5 children ages 9 to 17 have a diagnosable emotional or behavioral disorder; the most common are anxiety (8%), substance abuse disorder (10.3%), depression (5.2%), conduct disorders (3.5%), and ADHD (4.5%; Koppelman, 2004; National Research Council [NRC] & Institute of Medicine [IOM], 2009). About half have mild impairment and may be served by Tier 2 services, and the other half have significant impairment. *Serious emotional disturbance (SED)* refers to a range of diagnosable behavioral and mental disorders that severely impair daily functioning in the home, school, and community and affect approximately 5% to 9% of children and youth (U.S. Department of Health and Human Services, 1999). A greater number of children and youth in the child welfare (50%) and juvenile justice (67%–70%) systems than not in those systems have mental health problems (NRC & IOM, 2009). In the population of children with disabilities, approximately 11.5% have been reported to experience psychosocial issues, but only about 42% of those actually receive mental health services (Witt, Kasper, & Riley, 2003). In addition to these statistics, many other children who experience social and emotional challenges that do not meet the criteria for mental health diagnosis experience impaired function and distress (Masia-Warner, Nangle, & Hansen, 2006). Unfortunately, about 70% to 80% of children who need mental health services do not receive such care (Kutash et al., 2006).

Awareness

At Tier 3, the person–occupation–environment transaction requires an in-depth knowledge of a range of mental health and behavioral disorders, how the disorders influence the person's functioning in a variety of occupational areas (education,

Table 2.3. Examples of Occupational Therapy Tier 2 Services

Tier 2 Services **Targeted Intervention for At-Risk Children and Youth**	
Target Children and youth • With any disability (cerebral palsy, autism spectrum disorder, learning disability, attention deficit hyperactivity disorder), • Experiencing loss (e.g., through death, divorce, military deployment), • Who are overweight or obese, • Living in poverty, • Demonstrating early signs of a mental health disorder (e.g., anxiety) or sudden changes in behaviors, or • Who struggle with friendships and appear to be loners. **Occupational therapy services** Efforts involve a more direct role in evaluation and service provision and focus on all Tier 1 services as well as • Screening for early identification of problems in a variety of areas, including social participation, sensory processing, and play and leisure; • Early intervening services to promote successful participation in school, home, and community; • Small-group work; • Coaching; and • Consultation and collaboration.	**School Level** **Awareness** • *Learn* about early signs of a variety of mental illnesses (e.g., depression, anxiety, obsessive–compulsive disorder, schizophrenia) and how such symptoms might manifest themselves in school and home settings. • *Become knowledgeable* about strategies for early intervention. **Appraisal** • *Use* both informal and formal evaluation strategies to identify risk, changes in behavior or functional skills, or the early presence of mental health problems. • *Evaluate* social participation with peers during all school activities, including recess and lunch. • *Analyze* the sensory, social, and cognitive demands of school tasks and recommend adaptations to support a student's participation. **Action** • *Provide* early intervening services or Section 504 accommodations for students demonstrating behavioral or learning difficulties as a result of mild mental health disorders or psychosocial issues. • *Consult* with teachers to modify learning demands and academic routines to support a student's development of specific social–emotional skills. • *Provide* parent education on how to adapt family routines or activities to support children's mental health, especially with high-risk children. • *Develop* and run group programs to foster social participation for students struggling with peer interaction. • *Provide* psychoeducation in-services to educate teachers about the early signs of mental illness and appropriate accommodations.
	Community Level Awareness • *Become knowledgeable* about the benefits of participation in structured leisure and communicate this understanding to children and youth and their families. **Appraisal** • *Identify* community recreation centers, dance studios, sports opportunities, clubs, and other settings that offer inclusive opportunities for participation. **Action** • *Visit* community settings, meet the program directors, and explore options for youth with mental or physical needs to participate. • *Develop* a resource guide of positive settings for youth to participate in structured leisure activities.

leisure, activities of daily living [ADLs], social participation), current medical and psychosocial interventions, and school and community services. Accessing information from reliable technical assistance centers, government reports, and current literature is essential for developing a solid knowledge base (Box 2.1).

Appraisal

The occupational therapist will need to use a variety of evaluation strategies to analyze the person–occupation–environment transaction and factors limiting occupational performance. Observations, interviews, and formal assessments are best conducted in natural school, home, and community contexts. Assessments can be broadly categorized as evaluating occupational participation, limitations in component function (e.g., social skills), functional competencies, or quality of life. Examples are included in Table 2.4.

Action

Although services at Tier 3 are individualized to meet the specific needs of children and youth on the basis of the mental health condition and presenting symptoms, adopting a systems perspective is critical, because children and youth often benefit from supports and services that are intensive and provided by multiple systems in the community. The following sections discuss three key perspectives for guiding service provision for children and youth with mental health disorders: systems of care, youth empowerment, and promotion of subjective well-being.

Systems of Care

Systems-of-care approaches provide a framework for youth, families, schools, and community partners to provide individualized services and supports that help children and youth with SED and their families achieve their desired goals (Sebian et al., 2007). The federal entity that administers the Comprehensive Mental Health Services for Children and Their Families Program (Systems-of-Care) is the Substance Abuse and Mental Health Services Administration. Philosophies guiding systems-of-care approaches emphasize a comprehensive, integrated continuum of mental health and related services and supports that are community based, family driven, youth guided, and culturally and linguistically competent. Such approaches are necessary because youth with serious mental health disorders typically receive services from two or more public agencies such as juvenile justice, child welfare, special education, and state and local mental health departments. Systems-of-care approaches aim to "wrap" families in a comprehensive network of community services with interagency collaboration across agencies. Coordinated services ease the burdens families may experience when services are fragmented and conflicting. Services are intended to be family driven and youth guided. To assist in providing comprehensive, integrated services, occupational therapists need to embrace systems-of-care approaches and work collaboratively with youth, families, and multiple service providers.

Table 2.4. Selection of Assessments Focusing on Social Participation, Occupational Performance, and Quality of Life in Children and Youth

Assessment	Purpose
Assessment Scale for Positive Character Traits for Developmental Disabilities (Woodard, 2009)	Designed to measure the presence and strength of selected strength-based traits in people with developmental disabilities considered to be associated with level of happiness, quality of life, or both.
Children's Assessment of Participation and Enjoyment and Preferences for Activities of Children (King et al., 2004)	Focus is on assessment of participation or engagement in activities: recreational, physical, and social.
Child Health Questionnaire (CHQ; Landgraf, Abetz, & Ware, 1996)	Designed to measure functional health status, well-being, and health outcomes of children ages 0–18 years. The CHQ measures 12 domains of health, such as behavior, bodily pain, general health, and mental health.
Devereux Student Strengths Assessment (K–8; LeBuffe, Shapiro, & Naglieri, 2009) Devereux Early Childhood Assessment for Infants and Toddlers Devereux Early Childhood Assessment for Preschoolers	Strength-based assessments grounded in resiliency theory to measure social–emotional competency and school success. This is a useful assessment to measure changes as a result of social and emotional learning programming.
ITSEA/BITSEA Comprehensive Kit: Infant Toddler Social Emotional Assessment (ITSEA) and Brief Infant Toddler Social Emotional Assessment (BITSEA; Carter & Briggs-Gowan, 2005)	*ITSEA:* Screen for social–emotional problems *BITSEA:* In-depth analysis of emerging social–emotional development and intervention guidance; 17 subscales in four domains; parent form and child care provider form.
Occupational Therapy Psychosocial Assessment of Learning (Townsend et al., 1999)	Assesses the psychosocial aspects of a student's performance within the classroom as a part of the evaluation to determine student–environment fit.
Perceived Efficacy and Goal Setting System (Missiuna, Pollock, & Law, 2004)	An innovative and motivating tool that enables young children to reflect on their strengths and abilities and identify areas of daily challenge. The collaborative goal setting involves children and their families in identifying priorities for intervention.
School Function Assessment (Coster, Deeney, Haltiwanger, & Haley, 1998)	Designed to measure students' performance in functional tasks that support participation in academic and social aspects of elementary school. Focus is on nonacademic aspects of school function that support mastery in academics.
Social Skills Improvement System (Gresham & Elliott, 2008)	Provides an evidence-based, multitiered assessment and intervention system aimed at helping students develop, improve, and maintain important social skills.
School Setting Interview; elementary and high school (Hoffman, Hemmingsson, & Kielhofner, 2000)	Client-centered semistructured interview to assess student–environment fit and identify need for accommodations in physical or social contexts.
Youth Quality of Life Instrument–Research Version (Seattle Quality of Life Group, University of Washington; Topolski et al., 2001)	An easy-to-understand self-administered questionnaire assessing quality of life in youth ages 11–18, including those with and without disabilities.

Youth Empowerment

Youth involvement in systems of care begins with education and leads to opportunities for youth as decision-making partners in their own care and as active partners in helping shape policies and procedures that govern youth in community systems of care. The youth empowerment process supports all students in becoming leaders of mental health promotion in their own lives, in their own schools, and in their communities. *Youth involvement* means that youth voices should be heard, valued, and used in all decisions that affect youth's lives and the lives of their peers and families (Walker, Gowen, & Aue, 2009). Occupational therapists need to become aware of and support national, state, and local youth empowerment initiatives as a strategy for promoting young people's mental health.

Subjective Well-Being

Several terms have been used to describe positive thinking and feelings about one's life, including *subjective well-being* (Diener, 2000) and *authentic happiness* (Seligman, 2002). A sense of emotional well-being or happiness can be characterized by feeling and believing that one's life is satisfying and is associated with frequent experiences of positive affect, low levels of negative affect, and the ability to participate in activities that preserve these states. "Experiences that induce positive emotion cause negative emotion to dissipate rapidly" (Seligman, 2002, p. xii). According to Seligman (2002), authentic happiness comes from identifying and developing one's *signature strengths* (i.e., strengths that are deeply characteristic of the person) and using them every day in work, love, and play. For people with severe and persistent mental illness, developmental disabilities, or both, guarding against focusing solely on the reduction of problem behaviors is important. Attention to participation in meaningful occupations that foster positive emotions and signature strengths will enhance a sense of emotional well-being, happiness, and quality of life. Csikszentmihalyi (2004) acknowledged the importance of passion and joy: "We need joy to keep the dark night of the soul at bay, to feel that life is exciting and expanding, and to grow in the process of living" (p. 364). Occupational therapy's responsibility is to make sure that opportunities for joy exist that lead to growth in all children and youth.

The concept of occupational enrichment can be used to foster participation in occupations that promote subjective well-being and authentic happiness. *Occupational enrichment* involves the deliberate manipulation of the environment to support engagement in a meaningful array of occupations and is especially critical in situations involving occupational deprivation (Molineux & Whiteford, 1999). *Occupational deprivation* has been described as the influence of an environment that keeps a person from developing, using, or enjoying something (Wilcock, 2006). For youth experiencing significant mental health issues or developmental disabilities, ensuring access to a range of community-based leisure occupations and supporting successful participation is recommended (e.g., arts, theater, dance, sports). The example of Seth Chwast (Box 2.2) illustrates the transformative power of painting for a young adult with autism.

Various intervention approaches used to reduce symptoms, minimize risks, and build competencies are included in Table 2.5 and further discussed in Chapter 3. In addition, the Web site www.SchoolMentalHealth.org offers practical information on intervention approaches to address a variety of mental health conditions. Moreover, Part 2 of this book focuses specifically on occupational therapy's role with diverse populations.

Summary

"*Positive psychology* [italics added] is the study of the conditions and processes that contribute to the flourishing or optimal functioning of people, groups, and institutions" (Gable & Haidt, 2005, p. 103). This chapter proposed an occupational therapy

Box 2.2. Participation in Creative Occupations and Emotional Well-Being

Seth Chwast is a young adult who was diagnosed with autism as a very young child. A dramatic change occurred at age 20, when he took an oil painting class at the Cleveland Museum of Art. Seth has an innate ability to mix colors and create amazing works of art that reflect his vision of the world. Although he rarely speaks, Seth began describing his world in paint.

Seth's art can be viewed on his Web site, www.sethchwastart.com. For each painting, Seth has included a statement. For "Three Swimming Sea Turtles with Yellow Stones," he wrote,

> Turtles feel happy swimming in The Ocean! The Turtles' Shells have different hues of Oranges, Golds, Greens, & Blues. The Turtles' Eyes are Gold and Dark Blue. The Turtles' Faces are Sage and Gold. The Turtles' Skin have scales on their Bodies. The Turtles' Shells are hard to Protect their Bodies. The Turtles' Shells have shapes and patterns with lines. The Rain Forest Leaves have veins. Some Leaves are Dark Purple with Gold. The Rain Forest Background has Different Hues of Greens. The Sky is above the Rain Forest. The Ocean is below the Rain Forest. The Ocean's Water is Cool. 3 Swimming Sea Turtles are Beautiful! I feel excited about The 3 Swimming Sea Turtles with Yellow Stones Painting! The 3 Turtles feel calm and comfort in The Ocean. I swim in the Ocean with 3 Sea Turtles! We have a lot of fun!

On his Web site, his mother wrote,

> Seth Chwast is autistic. He cannot safely cross the street. Moms of autistic children know he is autistic in 30 seconds. And they also know his art is powerful and moving in 30 seconds. When he crossed the equator, moms speaking Spanish were stroking Seth and crying with joy and hope. Seth is an icon for anyone who has been in a hopeless situation, was invisible and ignored, and then triumphs and bursts into beauty and glory. He is autistic and he lives in a state of bliss. His art conveys his contagious sense of joy, happiness, and beauty, and his story inspires.

process involving awareness, appraisal, and action for describing services within a public health framework (universal, targeted, and individualized) for school and community settings. In addition, it applied principles of positive psychology (positive emotions, character strengths, and institutions) to the person–occupation–environment transaction to envision occupational therapy services that emphasize mental health promotion and the prevention of and intervention for mental ill health in children and youth.

References

American Occupational Therapy Association. (2006). *Transforming caseload to workload in school-based early intervention occupational therapy services.* Bethesda, MD: Author.

American Occupational Therapy Association. (2008). Occupational therapy practice framework: Domain and process (2nd ed.). *American Journal of Occupational Therapy, 62,* 625–683.

Barry, M. M., & Jenkins, R. (2007). *Implementing mental health promotion.* Edinburgh, Scotland: Churchill Livingstone/Elsevier.

Bazyk, S. (2005). Creating occupation-based social skills groups in after-school care. *OT Practice, 11*(17), 13–18.

Beets, M. W., Flay, B. R., Vuchinich, S., Snyder, F. J., Acock, A., Li, K., et al. (2009). Use of a social and character development program to prevent substance use, violent behaviors, and sexual activity among elementary-school students in Hawaii. *American Journal of Public Health, 99,* 1438–1445.

Bourget Management Consulting for the Canadian Alliance on Mental Illness and Mental Health. (2007). *Mental health literacy: A review of the literature.* Retrieved December 28, 2009, from www.camimh.ca/files/literacy/lit_review_may_6_07.pdf

Cartledge, G. (2003). Promoting nurturing and supportive school environments for students with learning and behavior problems. In L. M. Bullock, R. A. Gable, & K. J. Melloy (Eds.), *Prevention/intervention for noncompliant, acting-out, and aggressive behavior: Promoting positive student outcomes* (pp. 10–15). Arlington, VA: Council for Exceptional Children.

Table 2.5. Examples of Occupational Therapy Tier 3 Services

Tier 3 Services Intensive interventions	
Target Children and youth with identified • Mental health problems or diagnoses, • Behavioral challenges, or • Developmental disabilities. **Occupational therapy services** Efforts involve more direct, individualized services within a systems-of-care philosophy and included all of Tier 1 and 2 services as well as • Direct intervention (individual and group work), • Advocacy, • Community integration, • Consultation and collaboration, and • Accommodations.	**School Level** **Awareness** • *Become knowledgeable* about symptoms, medical management, psychological services, and so forth for a range of mental health disorders and how these present themselves in children and youth. • *Become knowledgeable* about mental health disorders common to children with various developmental disorders such as autism, attention deficit hyperactivity disorder, and intellectual disabilities. • *Identify* reputable and useful Internet resources for accessing current information about mental illness and interventions supported with evidence. **Appraisal** • *Evaluate* school function (classroom participation, activities of daily living [ADLs], play and leisure, social participation, and beginning work skills) in a variety of natural contexts (classroom, lunchroom). • *Assist* in the Functional Behavior Assessment process and contribute to the development and implementation of the Behavioral Intervention Plan. **Action** • *Collaborate* with the school-based mental health providers, teachers, and administrators to ensure a coordinated system of care for students needing intensive interventions. • *Provide* ways to modify or enhance school routines to reduce stress and the likelihood of behavioral outbursts. • *Promote* the development of individual interests by exploring extracurricular activities and providing the necessary supports to enhance successful participation. • *Offer* individual or group interventions for students with serious emotional disturbance either through special education or Section 504 to enhance participation in education, social participation, play and leisure, and ADLs. • *Collaborate* with teachers in modifying classroom expectations based on the student's specific behavioral or mental health needs. • *Analyze* students' unique sensory needs and develop intervention strategies to promote sensory processing and successful function in multiple school contexts (e.g., classroom, cafeteria). • Psychoeducation: *Educate* teachers about the early signs of mental illness and proactive strength-based prevention strategies. • *Provide* tips for promoting successful functioning throughout the school day, including transitioning to classes, organizing work spaces such as desk and locker, handling stress, and developing strategies for time management.
	Community Level **Awareness** • *Become knowledgeable* about the health benefits of creative arts and alternative approaches (e.g., yoga) with children and youth with mental health disorders. **Appraisal** • *Identify* national and local community settings that would welcome children and youth with identified mental health disorders (e.g., arts, theater, music, recreation). **Action** • *Use* coaching models to help youth with mental health and physical challenges participate in meaningful leisure occupations.

Carter, A. S., & Briggs-Gowan, M. (2005). *ITSEA BITSEA: The Infant–Toddler and Brief Infant–Toddler Social Emotional Assessment.* San Antonio, TX: PsychCorp.

Catalano, R. F., Hawkins, D., Berglund, M. L., Pollard, J. A., & Arthur, M. W. (2002). Prevention science and positive youth development: Competitive or cooperative frameworks? *Journal of Adolescent Health, 31,* 230–239.

Coster, W., Deeney, T., Haltiwanger, J., & Haley, S. (1998). *School Function Assessment.* San Antonio, TX: Psychological Corporation.

Cowen, E. (1991). In pursuit of wellness. *American Psychologist, 46,* 404–408.

Csikszentmihalyi, M. (2004). What we must accomplish in the coming decades. *Zygon, 39,* 359–366.

Diener, E. (2000). Subjective well-being: The science of happiness and a proposal for a national index. *American Psychologist, 55,* 34–43.

Duncan, B. B., Forness, S. R., & Harsough, C. (1995). Students identified as seriously emotionally disturbed in school-based day treatment: Cognitive, psychiatric, and special educational characteristics. *Behavioral Disorders, 20,* 238–252.

Eccles, J. S., & Gootman, J. A. (Eds.). (2002). *Community programs to promote youth development.* Washington, DC: National Academies Press.

Forness, S. R. (2003). Barriers to evidence-based treatment: Developmental psychopathology and the interdisciplinary disconnect in school mental health practice. *Journal of School Psychology, 41,* 61–67.

Forness, S. R., Kavale, K. A., MacMillan, D. L., Asarnow, J. R., & Duncan, B. B. (1996). Early detection and prevention of emotional or behavioral disorders: Developmental aspects of systems of care. *Behavioral Disorders, 21,* 226–240.

Freeman, R., Eber, L., Anderson, C., Irvin, L., Bounds, M., Dunlap, G., et al. (2006). Building inclusive school cultures using school-wide PBS: Designing effective individual support systems for students with significant disabilities. *Research and Practice for Persons With Severe Disabilities, 31,* 4–17.

Gable, S. L., & Haidt, D. (2005). What (and why) is positive psychology? *Review of General Psychology, 9,* 103–110.

Graham, F., Rodger, S., & Ziviani, J. (2009). Coaching parents to enable children's participation: An approach for working with parents and their children. *Australian Occupational Therapy Journal, 56,* 16–23.

Gresham, M., & Elliott, S. N. (2008). *Rating Scales Manual. SSIS Social Skills Improvement System.* Minneapolis, MN: Pearson.

Griffiths, K. M., Christensen, H., & Jorm, A. F. (2009). Mental health literacy as a function of remoteness of residence: An Australian national study. *BMC Public Health, 9,* 1–20. Retrieved December 28, 2009, from www.biomedcentral.com/1471-2458/9/92

Hoagwood, K., & Johnson, J. (2003). School psychology: A public health framework: I. From evidence-based practices to evidence-based policies. *Journal of School Psychology, 41,* 3–21.

Hoffman, O. R., Hemmingsson, H., & Kielhofner, G. (2000). *The School Setting Interview: A user's manual.* Chicago: University of Illinois, Department of Occupational Therapy.

Individuals With Disabilities Education Improvement Act of 2004, Pub. L. 108–446, 20 U.S.C. § 1400 *et seq.*

Jackson, L. L., & Arbesman, M. (2005). *Occupational therapy practice guidelines for children with behavioral and psychosocial needs.* Bethesda, MD: AOTA Press.

Jorm, A. F., Korten, A. E., Jacomb, P. A., Christensen, H., Rodgers, B., & Pollitt, P. (1997). "Mental health literacy": A survey of the public's ability to recognize mental disorders and their beliefs about the effectiveness of treatment. *Medical Journal of Australia, 166,* 182–186.

Keyes, C. L. (2007). Promoting and protecting mental health as flourishing: A complementary strategy for improving national mental health. *American Psychologist, 62,* 95–108.

King, G., Law, M., King, S., Hurley, P., Hanna, S., Kertoy, M., et al. (2004). *Children's Assessment of Participation and Enjoyment (CAPE) and Preferences for Activities of Children (PAC).* San Antonio, TX: Harcourt Assessment.

Knippenberg, C., & Hanft, B. (2004). The key to educational relevance: Occupation throughout the school day. *School System Special Interest Section Quarterly, 11*(4), 1–4.

Koller, J. R., & Bertel, J. M. (2006). Responding to today's mental health needs of children, families, and schools: Revisiting the preservice training and preparation of school-based personnel. *Education and Treatment of Children, 29,* 197–217.

Koppelman, J. (2004). *Children with mental disorders: Making sense of their needs and systems that help them* (NHPF Issue Brief No. 799). Washington, DC: George Washington University, National Health Policy Forum.

Kutash, K., Duchnowski, A. J., & Lynn, N. (2006). *School-based mental health: An empirical guide for decision-makers.* Tampa: University of South Florida, Louis de la Parte Florida Mental Health Institute, Research and Training Center for Children's Mental Health.

Landgraf, J. L., Abetz, L., & Ware, J. E. (1996). *The CHQ user's manual.* Boston: New England Medical Center, The Health Institute.

Larson, R. W. (2000). Toward a psychology of positive youth development. *American Psychologist, 55,* 170–183.

LeBuffe, P. A., Shapiro, V. B., & Naglieri, J. A. (2009). *The Devereux Student Strengths Assessment (DESSA).* Lewisville, NC: Kaplan Press.

Lopez, M., Forness, S. R., MacMillan, D. L., Bocian, K., & Gresham, F. M. (1996). Children with attention deficit hyperactivity disorder and emotional or behavioral disorders in the primary grades: Inappropriate placement in the learning disability category. *Educational Treatment of Children, 19,* 286–299.

Masia-Warner, C., Nangle, D. W., & Hansen, D. J. (2006). Bringing evidence-based child mental health services to the schools: General issues and specific populations. *Education and Treatment of Children, 29,* 165–172.

Missiuna, C., Pollock, N., & Law, M. (2004). *Perceived Efficacy and Goal Setting System (PEGS).* San Antonio, TX: Psychological Corporation.

Moherek Sopko, K. (2006, August). School mental health services in the United States. *inForum: Brief Policy Analysis.* Alexandria, VA: National Association of State Directors of Special Education. Retrieved July 27, 2010, from www.projectforum.org/docs/SchoolMentalHealthServicesintheUS.pdf

Molineux, M. L., & Whiteford, G. (1999). Prisons: From occupational deprivation to occupational enrichment. *Journal of Occupational Science, 6*(3), 124–130.

Mrazek, P. J., & Haggerty, R. J. (Eds.). (1994). *Reducing risks for mental disorders.* Washington, DC: National Academies Press.

National Research Council, & Institute of Medicine. (2009). *Preventing mental, emotional, and behavioral disorders among young people: Progress and possibilities.* Washington, DC: National Academies Press.

National Survey on Drug Use and Health. (2005). *Results from the 2004 National Survey on Drug Use and Health: National findings.* Retrieved October 5, 2005, from www.oas.samhsa.gov/NSDUH/2k4NSDUH/2k4results/2k4results.htm#ch6

Poulsen, A., Rodger, S., & Ziviani, J. (2006). Understanding children's motivation from a self-determination theoretical perspective: Implications for practice. *Australian Occupational Therapy Journal, 6,* 78–86.

President's New Freedom Commission on Mental Health. (2003). *Achieving the promise: Transforming mental health care in America.* (Final Report, DHHS Pub. No. SMA–03–3832). Retrieved December 15, 2006, from www.mentalhealthcommission.gov/reports/reports.htm

Rehabilitation Act of 1973, Pub. L. 93–112, 29 U.S.C. § 701 *et seq.*

Santor, D. A., Poulin, C., Leblanc, J., & Kusumakar, V. (2007). Adolescent help-seeking behavior on the Internet: Opportunities for health promotion and early identification of difficulties. *Journal of the American Academy of Child and Adolescent Psychiatry, 46,* 50–59.

Sebian, J., Mettrick, J., Weiss, C., Stephan, S., Lever, N., & Weist, M. (2007). *Education and system-of-care approaches: Solutions for educators and school mental health professionals.* Baltimore: University of Maryland Center for School Mental Health Analysis and Action.

Seligman, M. E. P. (2002). *Authentic happiness.* New York: Free Press.

Seligman, M. E. P., & Csikszentmihalyi, M. (2000). Positive psychology: An introduction. *American Psychologist, 55,* 5–14.

Topolski, T. D., Patrick, D. L., Edwards, T. C., Huebner, C. E., Connell, F. A., & Mount, K. K. (2001). Quality of life and health-risk behaviors among adolescents. *Journal of Adolescent Health, 29*(6), 426–435.

Townsend, S., Carey, P., Hollins, N., Helfrich, C., Blondis, M., & Hoffman, A. (1999). *Occupational therapy psychosocial assessment of learning (OT PAL).* Chicago: Model of Human Occupation Clearinghouse.

U.S. Department of Health and Human Services. (1999). *Mental health: A report of the Surgeon General.* Rockville, MD: U.S. Department of Health and Human Services, Substance Abuse and Mental Health Services Administration, Center for Mental Health Services, & National Institute of Mental Health.

Walker, J. S., Gowen, L. K., & Aue, N. (Eds.). (2009). Research, policy, and practice in children's mental health: Youth empowerment and participation in mental health care. *Focal Point, 23*(2).

Wehmeyer, M. L., & Bolding, N. (1999). Self-determination across living and working environments: A matched samples study of adults with mental retardation. *Mental Retardation, 37,* 353–363.

Weist, M. D., & Paternite, C. E. (2006). Building an interconnected policy–training–practice–research agenda to advance school mental health. *Education and Treatment of Children, 29,* 173–196.

Wilcock, A. A. (2006). *An occupational perspective of health* (2nd ed.). Thorofare, NJ: Slack.

Wilcock, A. A., & Townsend, E. A. (2008). Occupational justice. In E. B. Crepeau, E. S. Cohn, & B. B. Schell (Eds.), *Willard and Spackman's occupational therapy* (11th ed., pp. 192–199). Baltimore: Lippincott Williams & Wilkins.

Woodard, W. (2009). Psychometric properties of the ASPeCT–DD: Measuring positive traits in persons with developmental disabilities. *Journal of Applied Research in Intellectual Disabilities, 22,* 433–444.

Williams, M. S., & Shellenberger, S. (1996). *"How does your engine run?" A leader's guide to the Alert Program for self-regulation.* Albuquerque, NM: Therapy Works.

Witt, W. P., Kasper, J. D., & Riley, A. W. (2003). Mental health services use among school-aged children with disabilities: The role of sociodemographics, functional limitations, family burdens, and care coordination. *Health Services Research, 38,* 1441–1466.

Ziviani, J., Poulsen, A., & Hansen, C. (2008). Movement skills proficiency and physical activity: A case for Engaging and Coaching for Health (EACH)–Child. *Australian Occupational Therapy Journal, 56,* 259–265.

CHAPTER 3

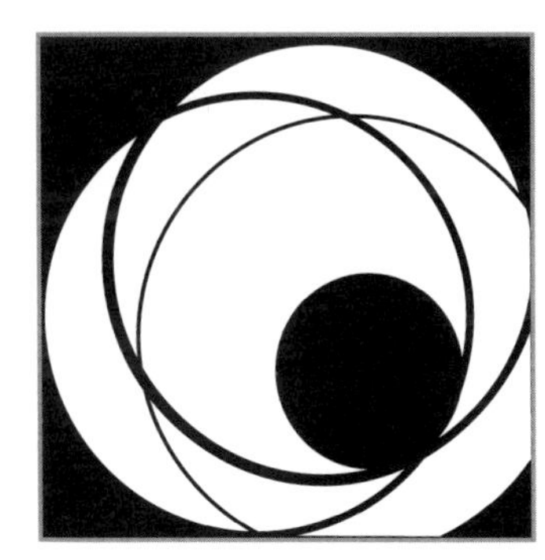

Major Approaches Useful in Addressing the Mental Health Needs of Children and Youth: Minimizing Risks, Reducing Symptoms, and Building Competencies

Susan Bazyk, PhD, OTR/L, FAOTA, and
Sharon Brandenburger Shasby, EdD, OTR/L, FAOTA

Learning Objectives

After reading this material and completing the examination, readers will be able to

- Delineate developmental psychopathology and determine its relevance to occupational therapy practice;
- Recognize features of occupation-based practice and identify the benefits according to an evidence-based review;
- Identify the personal and interpersonal benefits of participation in structured leisure activities;
- Determine the relevance of the Arts in Health movement for occupational therapists working with children and youth;
- Identify how a sensory processing approach can be applied at the universal, targeted, and individualized levels for mental health prevention, promotion, and intervention;
- Differentiate how positive behavioral interventions and supports and social and emotional learning contribute to mental health promotion, prevention, and intervention; and
- Determine how cognitive–behavioral strategies can be applied within an occupational therapy framework of mental health promotion.

As therapists examine the role of occupational therapy in the promotion of children's mental health in the broader context of collaboration with other professionals, areas of study and approaches that guide practice are important to focus on (Cole & Tufano, 2008). Occupational therapists' role in schools and the community is that of therapist, collaborator, advocate, and evidence-based practitioner, each of which requires the ability to communicate intervention strategies and expected outcomes. A variety of intervention approaches from within and outside the field of occupational therapy are available to reduce symptoms, minimize risks, and build competencies specific to children's mental health. Our aim in this chapter is to highlight several approaches, both traditional and recently developed, that are useful in minimizing mental health problems and building competencies within the domain of occupational therapy practice. Our intent is not to provide fully comprehensive and complete information on all possible approaches but to provide foundation information, strategies for implementation, and useful resources for further learning. First, we discuss two broad perspectives related to occupational therapy's role in children's mental health: (1) developmental psychopathology and (2) occupation-based practice. Second, we address several approaches specific to particular areas of functioning: (1) participation in structured leisure activities, (2) Arts in Health, (3) sensory processing, (4) positive behavioral interventions and supports (PBIS), (5) social and emotional learning (SEL), and (6) cognitive–behavioral therapy (CBT).

Developmental Psychopathology

Developmental psychopathology can be viewed as an integrative multidisciplinary perspective and set of continually evolving research strategies focusing on psychological health within a developmental framework (Masten, 2006). More simply, a developmental approach is applied to understanding the pathways toward or away from mental health problems and disorders.

Understanding age-related patterns of competence and disorder is important for developing promotion and prevention interventions (National Research Council & Institute of Medicine, 2009). *Mental health development* is characterized by age-related changes in several areas, including cognitive, emotional, and behavioral abilities. As children mature, successful completion of developmental tasks generally leads to a balanced development of strengths and weaknesses (Catalano, Hawkins, Berglund, Pollard, & Arthur, 2002). Competencies gained at one stage of development provide a foundation for future competencies as the young person faces new challenges and opportunities.

Development is influenced by the complex interaction among biological, psychological, and social factors. Because development occurs in nested contexts of family, school, neighborhood, and the larger society, an ecological perspective of intervention is widely accepted. Understanding the pathways of development enables prevention researchers and practitioners to identify opportunities for modifying pathological developmental trajectories. Individual, family, and school and community characteristics that foster mental health development across different developmental stages are summarized in Table 3.1. Mental health promotion focuses on efforts to enhance the person's ability to gain such developmental competencies.

Understanding the onset of various mental health disorders is also important. For example, longitudinal studies have identified the median age of onset for anxiety and impulse control disorders as 11; substance abuse disorders, 20; and mood disorders, 30 (Kessler et al., 2005). Evidence has indicated that initial symptoms generally appear 2 to 4 years before the onset of a full-blown disorder, suggesting the importance of early screening and intervention. The concept of *developmental cascades* recognizes the interaction between problems and competencies over time

Table 3.1. Factors Associated With Positive Development and Prevention of Mental Health Problems Over Time

Stage	Individual	Family	School and Community
Infancy and early childhood	• Secure attachment • Emotional regulation • Appropriate conduct • Making friends • Understanding self and other's emotions	• Adequate prenatal and postnatal health care • Nurturing relationship with caregiver (reliable, responsive, affectionate) • Support for the development of new skills	• Availability of high-quality child care • Support for early learning • Access to supplemental services, such as screening for vision and hearing • Low ratio of caregivers to children
Middle childhood	• Academic achievement • Appropriate behavior • Positive peer relations • Resilience (ability to adapt to life stressors) • Empathy • Satisfying friendships	• Emotionally responsive interactions with children • Consistent discipline • Language-based rather than physically based discipline • Parental resources, including positive personal efficacy and adaptive coping	• High academic standards and strong leadership • Teacher support • Effective classroom management • Positive family–school relations • School policies and practices to reduce bullying
Adolescence	• Physical health • Intellectual development • Psychological and emotional development • Social development • Connectiveness to peers, family, and community	• Physical and psychological safety • Appropriate structure (limits, rules, predictability) • Supportive relationships • Opportunities to belong • Positive social norms (expectations, values) • Opportunities for skill building • Integration of family, school, and community	• Physical and psychological safety • Appropriate structure (limits, rules, predictability) • Supportive relationships • Opportunities to belong • Positive social norms (expectations, values) • Opportunities for skill building • Integration of family, school, and community
Early adulthood	• Explore identity in love, work, and world view (e.g., values) to obtain a broad range of life experiences and move toward making commitments around which to structure adult life • Subjective sense of adult status in self-sufficiency, making independent decisions, and becoming financially independent • Future orientation and achievement motivation	• Behavioral and emotional autonomy • Balance of autonomy and relatedness to family	• Opportunities for exploration in school and work • Connectiveness to adults outside of family

Source. From "Using a Developmental Framework to Guide Prevention and Promotion," in *Preventing Mental, Emotional, and Behavioral Disorders Among Young People: Progress and Possibilities* (pp. 78–80), by Mary Ellen O'Connell, Thomas Boat, and Kenneth E. Warner (Eds.), 2009, Washington, DC: National Academies Press. Copyright © 2009 by the National Academies Press. Used with permission.

(Masten et al., 2005). For example, externalizing behavioral problems (e.g., conduct disorder) leads to lower academic performance in adolescence, which leads to increased internalizing emotional problems (e.g., anxiety, depression) in young adulthood. Mental health promotion includes efforts to enhance people's ability to achieve developmentally appropriate tasks, whereas prevention programs aim to reduce risks at the biological, psychological, family, and community levels. Interventions might include programming to strengthen family and child protective factors or reduce risk factors.

Developmental psychopathology serves a practical mission of guiding prevention and intervention: "As the developmental patterning and timing of specific problems and disorders is increasingly well-known, particularly in relation to risks, protections, cascades, and progressions, it becomes possible to intervene with increasingly strategic timing and targets" (Masten, 2006, p. 51; Figure 3.1). Because mental health is perceived as a dynamic state of functioning that can vary throughout a person's life on the basis of many biological (e.g., genetics), environmental (e.g., poverty), or situational (e.g., death of a parent) factors, occupational therapists must remain vigilant to the impact of such factors on the person's mental health. With occupational therapy's strong background in lifespan development and an understanding of developmental psychopathology, occupational therapists can be important contributors to both the identification of mental health risks and delays and the promotion of competencies.

Occupation-Based Practice

Although several approaches specific to mental health promotion are important to know about and apply, all occupational therapy services share a common emphasis on the use of meaningful occupation to promote occupational performance (education, play, leisure, work, social participation, activities of daily living [ADLs], instrumental activities of daily living [IADLs], sleep and rest). "As such, occupational therapy practitioners use activities as the means to 'occupation' and for participation within a variety of contexts" (Jackson & Arbesman, 2005, p. 31). In a recent

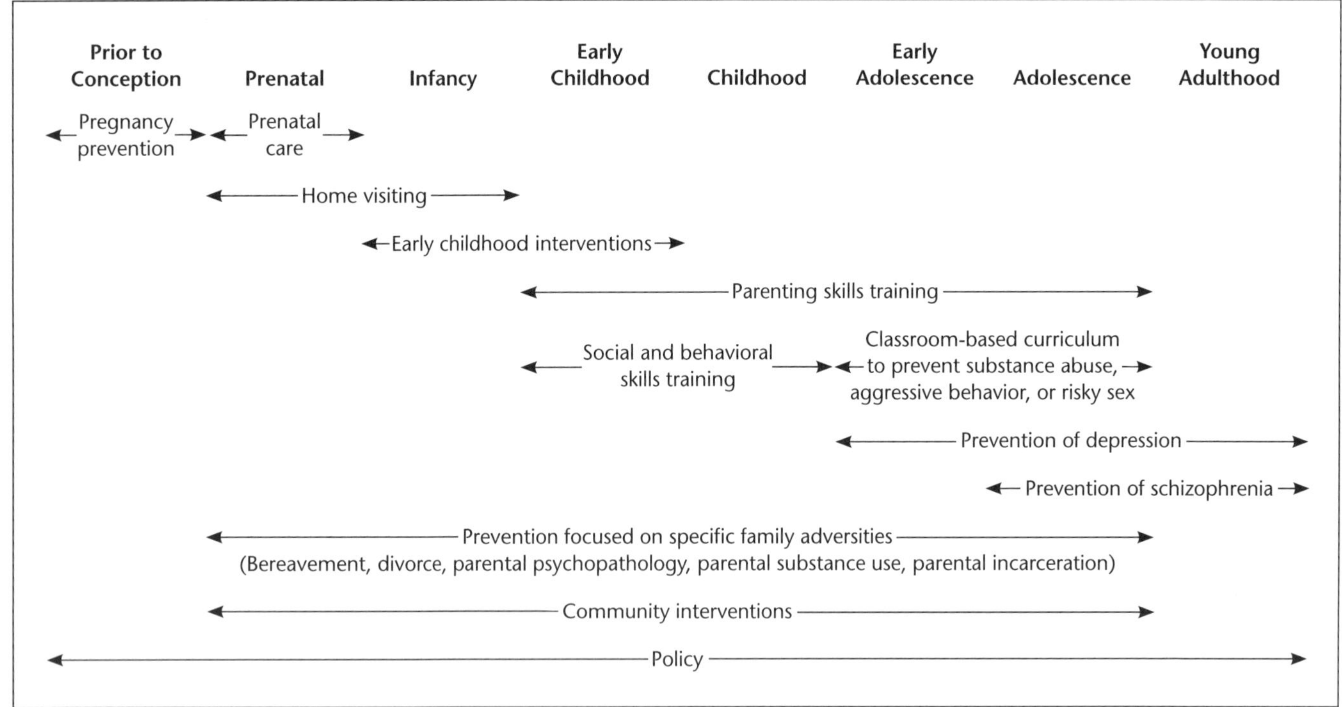

Figure 3.1. Interventions by developmental phase.

Source. From "Using a Developmental Framework to Guide Prevention and Promotion," in *Preventing Mental, Emotional, and Behavioral Disorders Among Young People: Progress and Possibilities* (p. 155), by Mary Ellen O'Connell, Thomas Boat, and Kenneth E. Warner (Eds.), 2009, Washington, DC: National Academies Press. Copyright © 2009 by the National Academies Press. Used with permission.

evidence-based literature review published in the *Occupational Therapy Practice Guidelines for Children With Behavioral and Psychosocial Needs* (Jackson & Arbesman, 2005), the use of activity-based interventions was supported in helping to improve peer and social interaction. Activity-based services were also shown to improve compliance to adult directives, task-focused behaviors, and conformity to social norms (Jackson & Arbesman, 2005). A variety of activities were used in the studies, including play, arts and crafts, board games, role playing, and art–movement programs. Common features among the successful interventions that should be replicated include direct instruction of targeted skills; activities to teach and encourage practice of skills; peer models to foster practice of new skills; supportive adults to provide coaching and reinforcement for appropriate behavior; and a long enough intervention program to allow ample opportunity for practice of emergent skills (Jackson & Arbesman, 2005). Occupational therapists are uniquely equipped to apply this information in practice because of their expertise in activity design, task analysis, child development, and group process. Findings from this evidence-based review support occupational therapy's focus on participation in activities to enhance social interaction and psychosocial function (Jackson & Arbesman, 2005).

On the basis of current evidence, then, the following recommendations have been offered for occupational therapists working with children and youth:

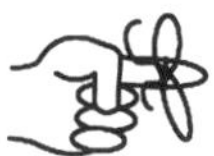

Remember this. . . . **Occupation-based practice is the strategic use of meaningful occupations to promote occupational performance.**

> When planning therapeutic interventions for children who have social, emotional, and behavioral needs, occupational therapists should focus on activities that fit the children's interests and developmental level and that facilitate the social and behavioral skills that have been targeted for improvement. Duo or small-group formats often result in the most powerful interventions, as there are opportunities for positive modeling and skills practice. The therapist should assume the roles of positive model, coach, activity designer and facilitator, and source of emotional support. In addition, occupational therapists must be continually willing to reevaluate their role within the school and provide consultation on classroom-, school-, and community-wide levels. (Jackson & Arbesman, 2005, p. 32)

Seemingly endless opportunities exist for using occupation-based strategies in school, home, and community settings to promote mental health because all occupational therapy services emphasize competency enhancement. In schools, occupation-based services can be embedded in a number of natural contexts, including the cafeteria (lunch groups), recess (game clubs), art, and physical education. Increased emphasis is being placed on participation in extracurricular activities, opening doors for occupational therapists to help children and youth develop and participate in structured leisure interests during after-school hours. Participation in a variety of community-based activities, including the arts, recreation, music, sports, or club activities, can be promoted using coaching strategies.

The vignette in Box 3.1 demonstrates the use of an occupation-based group (Brownie Busters) designed to promote the development of skills in various occupational performance areas, including work, social participation, and IADLs (cooking, shopping, community transportation), for children with multiple developmental

Box 3.1. Brownie Busters—An Occupation-Based Work Group for Children With Multiple Disabilities

Program Development

The purpose of the Brownie Busters program is to (1) provide a community-based functional curriculum for students with multiple disabilities attending elementary school; (2) provide tasks that are meaningful to elementary school students while teaching them skills needed for future employment and independence in their homes and neighborhood community; and (3) encourage collaboration among school team members, including the teacher, teacher assistant, occupational therapist, and parents.

The foundation for the development of the 6-week Brownie Busters work group was based on literature regarding the development of work in children with multiple disabilities indicating that (1) preparation for employment needs to begin at an early age (Jacobs, 1994); (2) participation in meaningful activities within an educational or work context reinforces interest (Bazyk, 2005); and (3) programs for students with moderate intellectual disabilities should emphasize skills that are both functional and longitudinally relevant (Morse & Schuster, 2000). An occupational therapist working in a large Midwestern municipal school district developed and facilitated the 1.5-hour weekly groups over a period of 6 weeks. The classroom teacher, teacher assistant, and parent volunteer served as helpers during the groups.

The overall purpose of the Brownie Busters work group was to have the students make and sell brownie-making kits to teachers, students, and staff at their school. The groups were designed to promote the development of several independent living and work skills, including planning a work task, functional reading (reading labels and recipes), safety issues related to walking in the community, grocery shopping, simple cooking (learning about ingredients, measuring ingredients, pouring ingredients, mixing ingredients), using an oven, sanitary food handling, and selling a product.

Participants

The work group consisted of 8 elementary students, ages 9 to 12, with multiple disabilities, including mild to moderate intellectual impairment and language delays. The diagnoses of the students include cerebral palsy, Down syndrome, and autism.

Group Sessions

The group sessions involved weekly discussions of basic work skills, a trip to the grocery store, making the brownie mixes, putting them in jars, decorating the jars, and selling the brownie mixes. Each session also involved cleanup.

Qualitative Research Findings

Qualitative research methods were used to explore the meaning of group participation from the children's perspective. Each of the 8 group members were interviewed during Weeks 2 and 6 of the program by the occupational therapist to explore the personal meaning ascribed to the group experience. Participant observations served as the second form of data and consisted of weekly observations of the group. On the basis of a qualitative analysis of the interviews and participant observations, three essential themes unfolded—shopping, special ingredients, and doing everything. When asked what comes to mind or what they liked the most when they think of the occupational therapy groups, all of the participants talked about walking to and shopping at the neighborhood grocery store, about ingredients needed for the project, and about doing the tasks necessary for making the brownie jars. By being actively involved in the shopping process, students learned firsthand about how to locate the baking ingredients needed for the brownies. The students began to take on the role of a "shopper" by looking for items needed for baking and using a shopping list. Student also learned about each special ingredient's unique properties by handling, measuring, and tasting them. Last, students expressed joy in "doing everything" and began to function like workers—doing the task, sharing, demonstrating care with the ingredients, using sanitary strategies for handling of food, and preparing the jars to sell. Findings support the importance of occupation-based practice in fostering the link between doing and becoming.

Source. Dixon (2006).

disabilities (Dixon, 2006). Findings from a qualitative study have illustrated that for this group of children, participation resulted in positive emotions—enjoyment from doing everything (Dixon, 2006).

Participation in Structured Leisure Activities

An important aspect of occupation-based practice when working with children and youth is attention to the development of structured leisure participation during out-of-school time. Youth participation in structured leisure (e.g., sports teams, clubs, lessons) is relatively common; approximately 6 in 10 youth participate in organized out-of-school activities at any given time (Mahoney, Harris, & Eccles, 2008; Mahoney, Larson, Eccles, & Lord, 2005). Several terms are used in literature outside of occupational therapy to describe such participation for youth, including *structured leisure activities, voluntary organized activities,* and *extracurricular activities,* to name a few; this discussion uses *structured leisure activities.*

Highly structured leisure activities are associated with the following features: regular participation schedules, rule-guided interaction, direction by one or more adult leaders, an emphasis on skill development that increases in complexity and challenge, and performance that requires sustained active attention and the provision of feedback (Mahoney et al., 2005). A committee of scholars appointed by the National Research Council and Institute of Medicine identified eight key features of contexts as promoting positive youth development: (1) physical and psychological safety; (2) appropriate structure; (3) supportive relationships; (4) opportunities for belonging; (5) positive social norms; (6) support for efficacy and mattering; (7) opportunities for skill building; and (8) integration of family, school, and community efforts (Eccles & Gootman, 2002). Although many organized leisure activities incorporate several, if not all, of those features, occupational therapists can screen and advocate for such features in youth programming.

Benefits of Participation in Structured Leisure Activities

Correlational research has demonstrated a positive relationship between participation in structured leisure activities and positive outcomes such as diminished delinquency, greater achievement, and increased self-efficacy and self-control (Larson, 2000). Research using youth inventories of participation and a qualitative study using focus groups yielded similar findings—that participation in structured leisure activities is associated with both personal and interpersonal development (Dworkin, Larson, & Hansen, 2003; Hansen, Larson, & Dworkin, 2003).

Personal Development

Three domains of personal development have been proposed as benefitting from participation in structured leisure (Hansen et al., 2003). First, participation provides opportunities to facilitate identity work. Exposure to and participation in a variety of leisure activities allows a young person to explore, express, and refine his or her identity and passion (Kleiber, 1999). During such participation, youth assess their talents, interests, values, and place in the social structure. Choices communicate to self and others, "This is who I am" or "This is what I am meant to do" and are based on the person's expectations for successful performance and value of the activity (Barber, Stone, Hunt, & Eccles, 2005, p. 188).

Second, organized activities have been viewed as providing a context for the development of *initiative,* which according to Larson (2000) reflects the self-motivation needed to devote effort over time to achieve a challenging goal—a core quality people need to deal with the complexities of adult life and future work. Three elements of initiative are (1) intrinsic motivation (wanting to do the activity), (2) concerted engagement, and (3) commitment over time.

The third domain of personal development includes cognitive, physical, and emotional skills (Hansen et al., 2003). Participation in organized activities is associated with higher academic achievement (Passmore, 1998); the development of positive habits contributing to physical health, especially with sports (Mahoney et al., 2005); and skill development (e.g., athletic, artistic, homemaking) and beginning work skills (Dworkin, 2003; Mahoney & Stattin, 2000). Several emotional competencies have been associated with participation in structured leisure, including managing feelings, controlling impulses, and increasing self-esteem (Mahoney et al., 2005). In terms of emotional well-being, Csikszentmihalyi (1993) found that when people learn to enjoy complex occupations that provide challenges corresponding to their skills, they are more likely to develop innate abilities, experience a positive self-esteem, and be happier.

Interpersonal Development

The second category, interpersonal development, focuses on the development of social connections. Structured leisure activities involve higher social complexity and thus require peer cooperation and the guidance of adult role models.

Structured leisure activities foster interpersonal development in three ways. First, participation in organized activities provides an important context for the development of new peer friendships, often with youth attending different schools and from different ethnic groups and social classes (Dworkin et al., 2003). Second, youth activities provide opportunities to develop social skills, including working effectively with others, giving and receiving feedback, and acquiring appropriate values about rules and conduct across settings (Hansen et al., 2003; Mahoney et al., 2005). The third attribute of interpersonal development is the growth of close connections to adults with social capital, such as coaches, artists, dancers, musicians, and other valued community members. These relationships can become long-term sources of emotional and social capital (e.g., access to information about future jobs or colleges; McLaughlin, 2000). The benefits of structured leisure activities are summarized in Figure 3.2.

Factors Influencing Participation

Although program features associated with youth development have been identified, to "derive the greatest benefits from organized activities, a youth must participate" (Mahoney et al., 2005, p. 13). Additionally, greater benefits of participation in structured leisure activities are associated with consistent participation over time. Developing new skills, forming new behaviors, and building relationships take time.

Personal development

- Identity work (identify talents and interests)
- Initiative (intrinsic motivation, concerted engagement, and commitment over time)
- Cognitive, physical, and emotional skill
- Emotional well-being (enjoyment)

Interpersonal development

- New peer friendships
- Social skills

Figure 3.2. Benefits of structured leisure participation.

Both exposure to a range of potential leisure occupations and the availability of resources to support engagement are critical factors influencing the likelihood that children and adolescents will develop and maintain healthy leisure interests.

According to Mahoney et al. (2005), "availability and affordability of activities are the most basic factors affecting participation" (p. 14). Resources such as parks, organized sports, and other community programs and competent adults to oversee the activities are essential. In addition, the provision of transportation and financial support are crucial factors influencing participation. Low-income urban and rural youth generally have fewer opportunities to engage in structured leisure activities because of these limitations. A young person's age, developmental status, motivation, and competence may also constrain participation in structured leisure.

Children With Disabilities

Children with disabilities also need opportunities to participate in out-of-school structured leisure occupations to experience the same benefits as their peers. However, environmental barriers and lack of social supports have been linked to decreased participation in leisure activities in this population (Law et al., 2004). Key strategies that communities need to address to enhance the leisure participation of people with disabilities include developing activities of interest in accessible recreational facilities, training staff to safely and effectively foster participation for people with disabilities, and providing activities in integrated community settings (i.e., for people with and without disabilities; French & Hainsworth, 2001).

Implications for Occupational Therapy

Given the developmental and mental health benefits of participation in structured leisure, occupational therapy services can be provided in many ways within a three-tiered system to promote meaningful leisure participation for all children. First, occupational therapists can advocate for participation in structured leisure activities for all children by educating young people, families, teachers, and community leaders about the benefits of leisure participation. Special efforts to promote participation might be necessary for children at risk of limited participation because of restricted access and availability (e.g., low-income urban youth, children with disabilities). Occupational therapists might assume the role of leisure coach with youth deprived of leisure participation opportunities, as described in Chapter 2.

Occupational therapists can systematically evaluate participation in structured leisure activities for qualities reflecting the three pillars of positive psychology—positive emotions, positive character strengths, and positive institutions (see Chapter 2; Seligman, 2002). First, does the young person have some activities outside of school in which he or she is interested, participates routinely, and enjoys? "Experiences that induce positive emotion cause negative emotion to dissipate rapidly" (Seligman, 2002, p. xii). Positive emotion experienced during participation in an activity is thought to be a central factor in promoting further exploration and eventual mastery.

Second, does participation in the activity promote the development of individual traits—personal strengths and virtues such as persistence, optimism, self-control, and social skills? Strengths and virtues help people during good times and during life's challenges. According to Seligman (2002), a person's highest success in living and deepest emotional satisfaction are derived from building and using his or her signature strengths.

Third, does the environment promote the development of character strengths and positive emotions? This analysis can augment the focus on the person–occupation–environment transaction. Occupational therapists have ample opportunities to promote the three pillars of positive psychology, given that their services, through the use of meaningful occupations, foster the development of needed and desired occupations. An exploration of the meaning of long-term participation in dance for teenage girls with and without disabilities is summarized in Box 3.2.

Arts in Health: Participation in Creative Arts Programming

Occupational therapy enjoys a long history of using creative occupations in practice, particularly with people with mental illness. Involvement in art creation has been identified as having a sustained and positive impact on participants' mental and social well-being (Argyle & Bolton, 2005). *Well-being* can be defined as "a state of acceptance with what is—in mind, body and spirit. One can be ill, yet in a state of well-being" (Argyle & Bolton, 2005, p. 341).

The Arts in Health movement was initiated in 2000 by England's National Network for Arts in Health to support artists working in health care settings. The field rapidly diversified and can now be broadly defined as including all activities that aim to use arts-based approaches to improve individual and community health, health promotion, and health care or that seek to enhance the health care environment through provision of artwork or performances (Macnaughton, White, & Stacy, 2006, p. 333). Some projects focus on the therapeutic benefits of the arts, some on supporting health care staff in delivering their services, and others on the concept of *social capital*—that the experience of creativity enhances social relationships and feelings of well-being. Although the traditional use of art therapy is provided by people with specialized training, process-oriented art for health activities is considered more versatile and can involve a variety of practitioners and community artists.

Many community organizations across the United States and internationally exemplify Arts in Health with vulnerable populations, including people with

Box 3.2. Exploration of the Meaning of Long-Term Participation in Dance for Girls With and Without Disabilities

The purpose of this phenomenological study was to explore the perceptions and experiences of long-term participation in dance for teenage girls with and without disabilities attending an integrated studio. Interviews and participant observation were used to study how the youth made sense of their experience.

Participants

Participants were a purposeful sample of 4 girls ages 14 to 15; 2 were without disabilities, and 2 had Down syndrome. All had participated in dance for 10 or more years at the same studio.

Findings

Qualitative data analysis resulted in seven major themes:

1. *Dancers are in tune with their bodies.* Participants expressed being in tune with their bodies and the space around them to complete dance moves and improve skills. They commented on how good it feels to stretch, to be toned, and to use their bodies in new ways.
2. *Dance involves challenge and hard work.* The participants expressed how dance provides an ongoing challenge that requires hard work and dedication. The challenge associated with dance was a reoccurring theme, with 1 participant stating it "never stops giving you a challenge." All 4 participants talked about the value of working hard over time for the desired outcome.
3. *"Doing" dance leads to becoming a dancer.* The participants discussed how their long-term involvement in dance helped them become dancers and take on the persona of a dancer. Observations confirmed that the girls take on a dancer persona from the moment they step into the studio—chins and tummies are tucked and shoulders come down. Both the girls with and without disabilities were observed looking and acting like dancers.
4. *Dancing transforms mood.* When the girls were asked how dance makes them feel, a common theme of happiness emerged. Having fun in dance class is a significant factor contributing to the level of happiness experienced.
5. *Dancing helps develop close friends.* Participation in dance over several years allows the girls to develop close friendships with peers outside of school. The girls used moments in between routines to socialize.
6. *Dance teaches important life skills.* The girls expressed that through their extensive years in dance class they learned many important life skills such as persistence, patience, and delayed gratification. They also indicated how they learned social skills and manners, primarily from the dance instructors.
7. *Dance instructors serve as a role model and coach.* Dance instructors were observed to be firm and clear in their directives as well as nurturing. A comfort level between the teacher and the students was also observed. The participants speak highly of their teachers and appear to regard them as important role models.

Findings suggest that for girls with and without disabilities, the meaning of long-term participation in dance reflected the alignment of the three pillars of positive psychology associated with positive youth development and mental health (Seligman, 2002):

- The first pillar emphasizes subjective experiences and emotions. The dancers were aware that participation in dance transforms mood. A number of positive emotions were noted, including feeling happy, satisfied, and in tune with their bodies. According to Seligman (2002), positive emotion is a central factor in promoting further exploration and eventual mastery.
- The second pillar emphasizes the importance of developing individual traits—strengths and virtues such as persistence, self-control, and social skills. Study findings indicated first that the participants developed a number of personal and interpersonal character strengths thought to promote well-being and buffer against psychological disorders. Personal development reflected identity work by allowing the participants to explore different forms of dance, determine personal preferences, and become a dancer. Second, the participants described the elements of initiative: intrinsic motivation, concerted engagement, and commitment over time (Larson, 2000). Each participant was motivated to continue her pursuit of dance year after year despite the hard work associated

(Continued)

Box 3.2 (*cont.*)

with this leisure pursuit. Last, participation in dance promoted the development of a number of physical and emotional skills. Participants recognized the relationship between hard physical work, improved skill, and health. They also spoke of gaining important emotional competencies such as patience, persistence, and self-confidence. The dancers also noted the development of a number of interpersonal skills. Participants appreciated the development of close friends with peers attending different schools. The dancers also recognized how participation in dance taught important social skills such as listening, respect for authority, and receiving critical feedback.

- The third pillar of positive psychology focuses on positive institutions—environmental factors such as families, caring adults, and programs that foster character strengths and positive emotions (Seligman, 2002). Both the studio setting and dance instructors were viewed by the participants as having a positive influence on their experience of and commitment to dance. The studio provided a safe and inviting place to be a dancer. Instructors were respected role models and coaches.

Conclusion

The experience of dance in this inclusive setting allowed each participant to focus on and nurture the dancer within, which seemed to deemphasize the disability for the girls with Down syndrome. They were young women becoming dancers like all the rest. Occupational therapists can be instrumental in helping all children, including those with disabilities, participate in meaningful structured leisure occupations in inclusive community programs.

Source. Bazyk et al. (2010).

mental illness or developmental disabilities. For example, Pure Vision Arts (www.purevisionart.org), founded in 2002, is New York's first specialized art studio and exhibition space for people with developmental disabilities and mental illness. Beginning, emerging, and established artists attend Pure Vision Arts, contributing to the growing movement of self-taught and visionary art. By creating opportunities for access and inclusion in the arts, Pure Vision Arts is helping to facilitate social change and breaking down stereotypes about people who have disabilities. Many of the artists have experienced remarkable lives as a result of becoming artists. The sheer power and uniqueness of their work helps break down negative public misperceptions and stereotypes about people who have disabilities.

Occupational therapists can inform children, families, and professionals about the health benefits of participation in creative arts and encourage participation. Identifying community programs (dance, arts, music, theater) and making this information available to families is an important step in promoting such participation. Examples of community-based creative arts programs to promote mental health and well-being are described in Boxes 3.3 and 3.4.

Sensory Processing

"There is an accumulating body of literature describing sensory processing as an important factor in human behavior" (Dunn, 2007, p. 84). Many approaches traditional to occupational therapy practice, including sensory processing, may be useful in the promotion of children's mental health. "Occupational therapy practitioners recognize that well-regulated sensory systems can contribute to important outcomes in social–emotional, physical, communication, self-care, cognitive, and adaptive skill development" (American Occupational Therapy Association [AOTA],

Box 3.3. Arts in Health: A Community Example

The Looking Well project in High Bentham, North Yorkshire, England, represents an Arts in Health project working within a social capital model. The project grew out of a community consultation exercise in High Bentham in 1995 that revealed high levels of depression, loneliness, and isolation among people of all ages, particularly women, within the farming community of this small town. Findings also revealed a lack of opportunities for children to participate in physical activity. Social exclusion within this community was identified as a primary factor leading to a cycle of declining health.

In 1997, the Looking Well program was established by Pioneer Projects (Celebratory Arts) Ltd., a charity run by artists living in the local area. The aim of this project is to enhance the health and well-being of people of all ages in the community and to improve their social and physical environment through engagement in creativity and the arts. The project is run on limited funds in a rented shop in town. The shop is furnished mainly with a long table at which participants make their art and by a scattering of easy chairs positioned around a wood-burning stove. Conversations about sensitive issues like depression, stress, and loneliness occur more easily while the participants' eyes are focused on a creative activity and not on each other. Artwork is geared toward the health promotion needs of the community and is displayed and distributed in local health centers and around the town.

Although participation in art provides distraction from the problems of daily living, it also gives participants a sense of individual achievement at having made something that has some value within their community. Since its inception, Looking Well has fostered the regeneration of this deprived community, with more than one-third of the population involved in its activities. One of the young mothers who originally participated while suffering from depression has now become a paid employee. The project has achieved additional funding for five other part-time employees. The local general practitioner has noted several patients who have been transformed by participating in the art activities.

Source. Macnaughton, White, and Stacy (2005).

2008, p. 1). Occupational therapists' specific knowledge and skill in this area can be applied at universal, targeted, and individualized levels to promote successful participation in school and community settings for children with and without disabilities. A guiding belief is that all children and adults are sensory beings responding to everyday sensation in individual ways, resulting in unique sensory preferences that are reflected in what people do and how they interact with others. Although most people demonstrate moderate responses to sensory input, allowing for successful participation throughout the day, those with various disabilities (e.g., autism) or mental illness (e.g., psychosis) may respond to sensory input in more intense ways, resulting in performance challenges (Dunn, 2007). Intense responses to sensory input, for example, can negatively influence a person's emotions (e.g., causing irritability or tantrums) and social interaction (e.g., causing withdrawal or aggression). Occupational therapists can play an important role in helping children, families, and professionals develop a working knowledge of sensory processing in order to understand children's behaviors and modify everyday interactions and environments to foster success and well-being (Dunn, 2007).

A wealth of information in the form of journal articles, books, workshops, and Internet resources is available to assist occupational therapists in evaluation of and intervention for sensory processing disorders, especially at Tier 3 (individualized) and Tier 2 (targeted). It is not the intent of this chapter to review this information. Instead, thoughts on how to apply an understanding of sensory processing to Tier 1 (universal) are provided. For example, attention to the importance of education (Dunn, 2007) and environmental modifications (Champagne, 2008; Vogel, 2008)

Box 3.4. Creative Arts Group Program—MasterPiece Kids

In July 2004, Cleveland Clinic Children's Hospital for Rehabilitation received a grant to develop a creative arts program for children with disabilities and their typically developing peers. An interdisciplinary group of professionals, including an occupational therapist, recreation therapist, teacher, and the head of volunteer services, developed a program titled MasterPiece Kids, targeting two groups of youth: (1) those ages 6–10 years and (2) those older than age 11. Sessions range from 4 to 6 weeks long and are held after school for 2 hours. Two different art experiences are offered during each weekly session. Local artists are involved in each session and represent a variety of creative expression, including music, dance, drumming, pottery, creative writing, puppetry, and baking. Children respond best to instructors who combine structure with flexibility. Participating children are happy and eager to try every new activity. It is gratifying to offer all kinds of creative arts opportunities for all children with and without disabilities.

—Susan Gara Mastromonaco, OTR/L

is growing to enhance an understanding of and respect for sensory differences and to create environments that support a sense of comfort and emotional well-being. Table 3.2 provides examples of sensory processing promotion, prevention, and intervention strategies and resources, and Box 3.5 lists examples of environmental modifications for working with clients with autism.

Applying knowledge at each tier requires the use of a broad range of strategies, including direct (individual or group interventions) and indirect (in-service education, consultation with teachers and families, environmental modifications).

Positive Behavioral Interventions and Supports

Behavior management has traditionally focused on changing the behaviors of children demonstrating problems (Mu & Gabriel, 2001). Recent approaches, however, have focused more broadly on promoting positive behavior by considering the combined influence of multiple systems (person, classroom, school, family, and community; Sugai et al., 2000). PBIS recognizes that several relevant factors can influence behavior, including those existing within the person and those reflected in the interaction between the child and the environment (Safran & Oswald, 2003). "[PBIS] interventions are designed to be proactive, to prevent problem behavior by altering a situation before problems escalate, and to concurrently teach appropriate alternatives" (Carr et al., 1999, as cited in Safran & Oswald, 2003, p. 361).

Recently, PBIS has been applied broadly as a behaviorally based systems approach to enhance the capacity of schools, families, and communities to design effective school environments based on research-validated practices (U.S. Department of Education, Office of Special Education Programs [OSEP] Technical Assistance Center on Positive Behavioral Interventions and Supports, 2010). *Schoolwide positive behavioral intervention and support (SWPBS)* systems support all students along a continuum of need based on the three-tiered PBIS prevention model of universal (all students, about 80%), targeted (students at risk for behavior problems, about 15%), and intensive (students with chronic or intense problem behavior, about 5%; Kutash, Duchnowski, & Lynn, 2006; Figure 3.2) interventions. Occupational therapists must consider how to embed their services within each level of intervention. The Technical Assistance Center on Positive Behavioral Interventions and Supports, established by OSEP, part of the U.S. Department of Education, provides

Table 3.2. Application of Sensory Processing Within a Public Health Model

Tier	Emphasis	Examples of Resources
Tier 3: Intensive, individualized • Children and youth with identified sensory processing challenges	• Evaluate individuals: Identify patterns of sensory processing (overresponsive, underresponsive) and impact on participation. • Use interventions on the basis of individualized need and setting: In schools, interventions are generally embedded within school environment (classroom, cafeteria). Example: Develop a sensory diet for the child. • Educate to enhance understanding about the meaning of behavior from a sensory perspective.	Assessments (examples, not an inclusive list): • *Sensory Processing Measure* (Miller-Kuhanek, Henry, Glennon, Parham, & Ecker, 2008) • *Sensory Profile* (Dunn, 1999). Sensory and environmental modifications applied in mental health: • Sensory Modulation Program; restraint reduction (Tina Champagne); www.ot-innovations.com • Sensory Connection Program (Karen M. Moore); www.sensoryconnectionprogram.com.
Tier 2: Selective • Small group • Targeted	• Screen at-risk children and youth for possible sensory processing challenges (e.g., autism spectrum disorder, anxiety disorders, those experiencing prodromal symptoms). • Modify environments (e.g., classroom, cafeteria, playground, home) to meet a range of sensory needs.	Evaluation: Observation in natural context; interviews of parents and teachers Intervention resources: • *The Alert Program: How Does Your Engine Run?* (Williams & Shellenberger, 1996) • *The Tool Chest: For Teachers, Parents and Students* (Henry, 2001).
Tier 1: Universal • Whole school • Community	• Educate children, youth, families, and professionals about sensory processing, impact on behavior, and accommodations. • Evaluate environments for design qualities to promote social participation and learning.	• In-services or presentations to children and youth, teachers and other school staff, and parent groups. • Serve on committees addressing school and community environmental design to address sensory variables in cafeteria, play areas, hallways, and classrooms.

capacity-building information and technical assistance for identifying, adapting, and sustaining effective schoolwide disciplinary practices.

Schoolwide PBIS Interventions

SWPBS, or universal, interventions are proactively designed to create positive school environments for all students, including the majority who do not frequently present behavior problems but who would benefit from incentives that motivate them to follow the school rules (Cartledge, 2003). Both the prevention of behavior problems and the teaching of prosocial behaviors are emphasized for the entire school (Freeman et al., 2006). Because implementation requires several changes at a systems level to ensure successful administrative involvement, ongoing support is essential.

Other key features of SWPBS include (1) clearly defined and communicated behavior expectations written in positive terms (e.g., be respectful of yourself and others); (2) specific strategies for teaching appropriate behaviors; (3) consistent application of procedures for correcting misbehavior, including consequences; (4) acknowledgment of appropriate behaviors; and (5) a support plan to meet the needs of students with chronic, challenging behaviors. Most school staff, typically about 80%, must agree to implement the intervention and training, and support must be provided on an ongoing basis (Kutash et al., 2006). Schools reporting

Box 3.5. Environmental Modifications for Working With Clients With Autism

- Adaptable (adjustable furnishings to re-create spaces, e.g., rolling shelving units)
- Nonthreatening (materials and furniture that are soft and inviting)
- Nondistracting (free of clutter and nonessential visual materials, fewer fluorescent lights)
- Predictable (easy to navigate, clear signage)
- Controllable (opportunities for choice and alone time)
- Sensorimotor attuned (opportunities for enhanced sensory input)
- Safe (remove hazardous materials; offer quiet spaces)
- Noninstitutionalized (softer lighting, home furnishings, plants).

Source. Vogel (2008).

success in implementing SWPBS have identified the following benefits: increased student attendance, student and teacher self-reports of a more positive and calm environment, and reduction in the number of behavioral disruptions (OSEP Technical Assistance Center on Positive Behavioral Interventions and Support, 2010).

Like schoolwide management, effective classroom management must be based on clearly stated behavioral expectations and positive learning environments (Cartledge, 2003). *Classroom management* can be defined as "actions taken by the teacher to establish order, engage students, or elicit their cooperation" (Emmer & Stough, 2001, p. 103). Practical classroom strategies are described in Box 3.6. Occupational therapists can work collaboratively with teachers to implement such strategies to help promote positive behaviors in the classroom.

Applying PBIS in nonclassroom school settings is also important. Hallways, cafeterias, and playgrounds account for approximately 50% of all problem behaviors (Safran & Oswald, 2003). These areas typically lack routines and clear behavioral expectation. Precorrection, active supervision, and group contingencies have all been found to be beneficial, especially when applied in combination. *Precorrection* involves adult prompts reminding students about appropriate behavior before a particular transition (e.g., change of classes) or activity (e.g., recess, field trip). For example, a teacher might review school rules and appropriate social behaviors for the playground. *Active supervision* involves the dynamic presence of school personnel during nonclassroom activities and is associated with fewer problem behaviors. *Group contingencies* involve rewarding the whole group of students with special snacks or activities after positive behavior (Safran & Oswald, 2003).

Targeted Interventions in PBIS

Targeted interventions are designed to support students who have learning, behavior, or life experiences that place them at risk of engaging in problematic behavior (Freeman et al., 2006). Implementation at this level begins with a short functional behavioral assessment (FBA) completed by a small team of people who brainstorm with the student to identify the purpose of the problem behavior (Freeman et al., 2006; Kutash et al., 2006). This brainstorming is followed by the development of a support plan that may "include such interventions as teaching the student a functionally equivalent replacement behavior for the problem behavior or rearranging

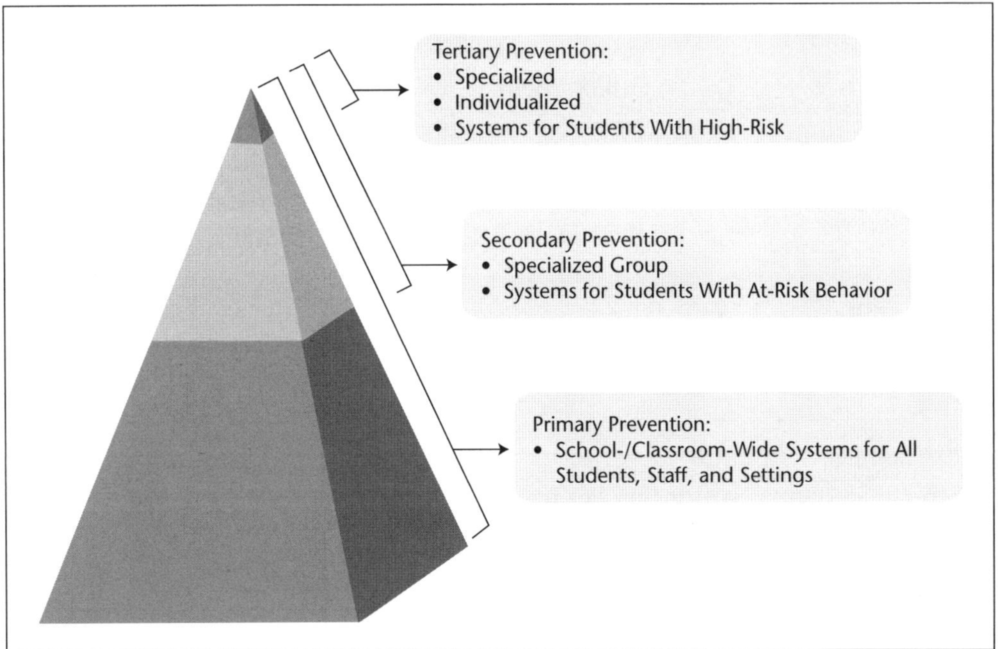

Figure 3.3. Continuum of schoolwide instructional and positive behavioral supports.

Source. From "What Is School-Wide Positive Behavioral Interventions and Supports." (2009). Retrieved July 7, 2009, from www.pbis.org/school/what_is_swpbs.aspx. Copyright © 2009 by PBIS.org. Used with permission.

Box 3.6. Practical Positive Behavioral Intervention and Support Classroom Strategies for Teachers

The following practical, proactive approaches are suggested for creating positive behavior in classrooms:

1. *Create a positive culture.* Creating a warm, positive culture that reinforces critical values such as respect and fairness helps students feel welcomed and successful. Teachers can help create a positive culture by genuinely communicating care and concern for students. Specifically, teachers might want to acknowledge students' birthdays and outstanding achievements, make an attempt to connect with each student daily, and end each day positively with students (Duhaney, 2003).
2. *Implement effective classroom instruction.* An important strategy is to make sure the curriculum is at the appropriate level for the student. Students often misbehave to avoid tasks that are too difficult. Another helpful approach is to give students a number of choices for meeting a particular curricular goal (e.g., writing a report, interviewing an expert on the subject). Choices allow students to make decisions and experience control. Teachers can also avoid misbehavior by anticipating events or stimuli that trigger misbehavior (e.g., time of day, types of learning activities). Specific instructional methods to increase student attending and response to academic material are being explored. Frequent pupil responding improves skill acquisition and application.
3. *Collaborate with students to establish classroom rules and consequences.* Students need to know exactly what the classroom rules are because these are often more specific than schoolwide rules. Rule making needs to involve a collaborative process between the teacher and students.
4. *Adjust behavioral interventions on the basis of the intensity and severity of student behavior.* To establish a positive classroom environment, the teacher may also consider ignoring mild disruptive behaviors (e.g., whispering, tapping a pencil). Instead of verbally reprimanding the student, it may be more effective to redirect him or her to the learning task.
5. *Seek ongoing teacher education and support.* General education teachers usually do not have the training and support needed to address challenging behaviors in students with or without disabilities. School administrators might want to consider providing educators with ongoing education and support in the form of weekly seminars or ongoing consultation.

Resource 3.1. Behavior Management

Mu, K., & Gabriel, L. (2001). Strategies to cope with severe challenging behavior. *OT Practice, 6*(2), 12–17.

Trott, M. (2002). *Oh behave! Sensory processing and behavioral strategies: A practical guide for clinicians, teachers and parents.* San Antonio, TX: Therapy Skill Builders.

the environment to reduce the probability of the problem behavior occurring" (Kutash et al., 2006, p. 30). Students with similar needs may be provided an intervention program designed to support a small group of students and thus promote the efficient use of resources and time. An example includes participation in a social skills group in which specific behaviors are taught, modeled, and used by the group members (Kutash et al., 2006). At this level, occupational therapists can collaborate with teachers, speech pathologists, or social workers to develop and co-facilitate such selective interventions. Resource 3.1 lists useful behavior management resources.

Individualized Interventions in PBIS

When targeted interventions do not meet the needs of an individual student, intensive interventions are developed to address behaviors that are highly disruptive or dangerous or that prevent learning (Freeman, et al., 2006). The process of FBA and behavioral intervention planning is more timely and complex at this level. FBA serves as the cornerstone for developing effective behavior support plans (Sugai et al., 2000).

> FBA is a person-centered, problem-solving process that involves collecting data to measure student behavior; determining why a student engages in a particular behavior; and identifying the instructional, social, affective, environmental, and contextual variables that appear to lead to and maintain the behavior. (Duhaney, 2003, p. 268)

An understanding of behavioral analysis and behavior management provides a foundation for this process. An outcome of the FBA should be a hypothesis statement that includes (1) an operational definition of the problem behavior, (2) descriptions of the antecedent events that predict the behavior, and (3) descriptions of consequences that help maintain the behavior. This information is used to develop behavior support plans (BSPs) that describe intervention in four areas: (1) setting event strategies, (2) antecedent strategies, (3) consequence strategies, and (4) behavioral teaching strategies (Sugai et al., 2000). Tools for conducting FBAs and BSPs are available at www.PBIS.org.

At the intensive level, the student's team typically includes family members, school professionals, and community members who meet regularly to develop, implement, and monitor an individualized support plan. Occupational therapists have many opportunities to observe student behaviors in a variety of school contexts (classroom, hallways, cafeterias, and playgrounds) and, thus, can contribute to both the FBA and the BSP processes.

Social and Emotional Learning

SEL was developed as a conceptual framework in 1994 to focus on children's emotional needs and address the fragmented programs meant to address those needs (Greenberg et al., 2003). *SEL* is defined as a process for helping children develop critical skills for life effectiveness—developing positive relationships, behaving ethically, and handling challenging situations effectively (Collaborative for Academic, Social, and Emotional Learning [CASEL], 2010).

Programs that foster SEL help children recognize feelings, control impulses, and acquire important social skills for developing and maintaining healthy relationships in life (Goleman, 1995). Emotional learning lessons should be given in small doses and delivered regularly over a sustained period of time. Experiences that are repeated allow the new skills to become "neural habits to apply in times of duress, frustration, and hurt" (Goleman, 1995, p. 263).

Elias et al. (1997) suggested that children need to develop skills in emotion, thinking, and behavior in the following four domains: (1) life skills and social competencies; (2) health promotion and problem prevention skills; (3) coping skills and social support for transitions and crises; and (4) positive, contributory service. Programming needs to help children recognize their emotions, think about their feelings and how one should act, and regulate their behavior on the basis of thoughtful decision making (Elias et al., 1997). In other words, emotional and social skills must be developed to prevent feelings from "hijacking" thoughts and actions (Goleman, 1995). The five major skill areas viewed as essential are (1) self-awareness, (2) self-management, (3) social awareness, (4) relationship skills, and (5) responsible decision making (CASEL, 2010; Box 3.7).

A growing body of research findings has demonstrated that SEL programs are effective in school and after-school settings for students with and without behavioral and emotional problems. A meta-analysis of 317 studies involving 424,303 SEL program participants indicated improvements in social–emotional skills, connection to school, academic performance, attitudes about self and others, and positive social behavior and reductions in conduct problems and emotional distress (Payton et al., 2008). As a national leader in the field, CASEL has focused on the development

Box 3.7. Five Core Social and Emotional Learning Skills and Competencies

1. *Self-awareness:* Accurately assessing one's feelings, interests, values, and strengths; maintaining a well-grounded sense of self-confidence
2. *Self-management:* Regulating one's emotions to handle stress, control impulses, and persevere in overcoming obstacles; setting and monitoring progress toward personal and academic goals; expressing emotions appropriately
3. *Social awareness:* Being able to take the perspective of and empathize with others; recognizing and appreciating individual and group similarities and differences; recognizing and using family, school, and community resources
4. *Relationship skills:* Establishing and maintaining healthy and rewarding relationships on the basis of cooperation; resisting inappropriate social pressure; preventing, managing, and resolving interpersonal conflict; seeking help when needed
5. *Responsible decision making:* Making decisions [on the basis of] consideration of ethical standards, safety concerns, appropriate social norms, respect for others, and likely consequences of various actions; applying decision-making skills to academic and social situations; contributing to the well-being of one's school and community.

Source. From "What Is SEL? Skills and Competencies," by Collaborative for Academic, Social, and Emotional Learning (CASEL), 2010. Copyright © 2010 by CASEL. Retrieved August 3, 2010, from www.casel.org/basics/skills.php. Used with permission.

of high-quality, evidence-based SEL as a necessary part of preschool through high school education. In a relatively short amount of time, significant progress has been made in accomplishing this goal. For example, in 2003, the Illinois Children's Mental Health Act was passed, ensuring that social and emotional development becomes an integral component of every child's education. Shortly thereafter, in 2004, SEL standards were developed along with a plan to incorporate them into each district's educational program in Illinois. A special edition of *Safe and Sound: An Education Leader's Guide to Evidence-Based Social and Emotional Learning (SEL) Programs* (CASEL, 2003) for Illinois schools is being used to prepare teachers and other personnel to implement the standards. Although Illinois was the first to adopt and implement SEL standards, others have followed. The CASEL Web site (www.casel.org) provides a comprehensive review of SEL programs, standards, research initiatives, and training materials and publications.

With research to support its effectiveness, SEL has grown significantly in its application throughout the United States in both school and after-school settings. As such, it is important for occupational therapists to

- Become knowledgeable about SEL and its implementation (e.g., read CASEL training materials);
- Determine whether the local school district or state has adopted SEL standards or an SEL curriculum, obtain information about such initiatives, and assist in implementation;
- Identify school committees that may address SEL programming and volunteer to become a member; and
- Embed SEL strategies into occupational therapy services (group, individual, and consultative).

Although multiple ways to promote SEL and embed strategies within occupational therapy exist, being vigilant to opportunities to become a part of SEL initiatives in school or community settings is essential. Box 3.8 provides a vignette demonstrating how one occupational therapist became involved in the school district's SEL initiative.

Cognitive–Behavioral Therapy

CBT is a relatively short-term, focused approach that teaches people how to modify their thought patterns to change troublesome feelings and behavior. The emphasis is on helping the person identify cognitive distortions (inaccurate beliefs), learn effective self-help skills, and practice them in daily life.

CBT has been used with children and youth demonstrating mental health problems including anxiety, depression, panic, posttraumatic stress disorder (PTSD), and obsessive–compulsive disorder. CBT is used most extensively with children experiencing anxiety disorders (Ginsburg & Kingery, 2007). Comorbidity of anxiety disorders with other conditions, including attention deficit hyperactivity disorder, oppositional defiant disorder, and autism spectrum disorder, is common and results in CBT being used with those populations as well (Monga, Young, & Owens, 2009).

CBT is one of the most extensively researched forms of psychotherapy in part because of its ongoing adaptation for an increasingly wide range of mental health

Box 3.8. An Occupational Therapist's Contribution to Schoolwide Social and Emotional Learning Programming

The large urban school district in which I am employed and the community it serves responded to a tragic act of violence in one of its premier high schools by conducting a full, districtwide appraisal of conditions for learning and programming that addressed safety and mental health services in the school setting. I became aware of the resulting recommendations and preliminary implementation plan through an e-mail sent to update faculty and staff. I requested more information from the chief academic officer in my district, indicating that I was in the process of completing my doctoral project, which focused on social and emotional learning (SEL) and its impact on social acceptance and participation of students with autism in general education settings.

I was quickly invited to become a member of the District Action Committee, made up primarily of administrators and leaders of the Teachers' and Staff Unions. This collaborative group's charge was to identify barriers to implementation and problem-solve "doable" solutions. I also volunteered to participate on the Evidence-Based Practice/Programs Task Force to address SEL with school district staff and community mental health agencies. The task force's charge was to review SEL learning curricula and recommend curricula that would best meet the diverse needs of our large urban school district and the unique challenges our students and families face.

As a staff occupational therapist, I have recognized over the past 21 years that students with special needs respond best to inclusion settings in which the teacher and classroom personnel consistently provide instruction in and reinforcement of social–emotional competencies. My scholarly research and experience as a school-based therapist provided a unique perspective from which to appraise curricula and learning materials to identify curricula that would be readily accessible to both general and special education students. My training and background provided a good foundation to identify key elements needed to support buy-in and sustainability of the Tier 1 SEL learning interventions across the district.

I am proud to be an active part of this comprehensive initiative to improve conditions for learning. It is satisfying when general and special educators report their excitement about the SEL curriculum we have adopted and the positive responses of their students. This collaborative work of community and school leaders in my school setting has resulted in a model for improving academic achievement that recognizes that Tier 1 and Tier 2 interventions must include both academic and social–emotional conditions for learning. As occupational therapists, I believe we bring a special understanding and perspective to how the social–emotional environment affects positive participation and performance in the school setting.

—Robin M. Kirschenbaum, OTD, OTR/L

problems and age groups, including children and youth. A meta-analysis of CBT with 16 disorders found that it is highly effective for many adult and childhood disorders, including depression, anxiety, panic disorder with or without agoraphobia, social phobia, and PTSD (Butler, Chapman, Forman, & Beck, 2006). CBT is the most effective psychosocial treatment evaluated for anxiety disorders in children, with response rates (defined as no longer meeting diagnostic criteria for the primary anxiety disorder) ranging from 60% to 80% (Ginsburg & Kingery, 2007). In addition, CBT has been shown to reduce symptoms of autism and anxiety in children with autism spectrum disorder (Sze & Wood, 2007; Wood et al., 2009).

Although CBT is primarily provided within an individual counseling framework, strategies are also typically taught to parents and other significant adults to promote carryover in home and school. Application of CBT at the universal, targeted, and intensive levels within school contexts has also been reported (Christner, Forrest, Morley, & Weinstein, 2007). A selection of programs using CBT strategies and applied at the universal and targeted levels are presented in Box 3.9. Occupational therapists need to be knowledgeable about specific CBT strategies to assist in carryover and strengthen its effectiveness. Major CBT strategies include psychoeducation,

Box 3.9. Examples of School Programs Using Cognitive–Behavioral Therapy Strategies

Universal Strategies

I Can Problem Solve Program (Shure, 2001)

- Targets violence prevention and general problem solving for children ages 4 to 12
- Implemented in classroom by teacher with parent follow-through
- Lessons focus on applying social problem-solving skills and creating alternative solutions to resolve conflicts using games and dialogue
- *Findings:* Increase in prosocial behaviors, well-being, resiliency, and academic concentration, as well as a decrease in stress, labels, multiple problems, and high-risk behaviors.

Promoting Alternative Thinking Strategies (PATHS; Kusche & Greenberg, 1994)

- Implemented within the classroom
- Focuses on emotional development, self-regulation, social interaction, and social problem-solving skills
- Has been applied in both urban and rural elementary school settings
- *Findings:* Increased knowledge about feelings and decreased self-reports of depression.

Targeted Strategies

Anger and Aggression: Coping Power Program (Lochman & Wells, 2003)

- The Coping Power Program is an evidence-based program designed to improve social–cognitive skills in aggressive youth.
- Lessons are structured and organized and focus on specific skills that are easily taught and practiced within a school environment, such as anger management interventions, goal setting, emotional awareness, relaxation training, social skills training, problem solving, and handling peer pressure.

Anxiety/Stress: Coping Koala Program (Tomb & Hunter, 2004)

- This group program's goal is to help children modify their frame of mind (cognitions) and experience of anxiety-producing events by learning coping mechanisms.
- Sessions provide participants with skills to help handle their fears through cognitive, behavioral, and physiological coping techniques.

affective education, cognitive restructuring, relaxation training, and exposure and contingency management (Ginsburg & Kingery, 2007; Table 3.3).

Summary

This chapter has presented information and resources on a selection of approaches relevant to occupational therapy services that focus on mental health promotion, prevention, and intervention with children and youth. Approaches traditional to occupational therapy practice (i.e., occupation based, sensory processing) were described, and several contemporary approaches relevant to mental health promotion and intervention and applicable to occupational therapy (developmental psychopathology, structured leisure participation, Art for Health, PBIS, SEL, and CBT) were introduced. Knowledge of those approaches, combined with an appreciation of their application within occupational therapy, will help occupational therapists articulate their role and practice in ways that reflect a commitment to mental health promotion for all children and youth. Occupational therapists working in schools may benefit from the materials described in Resource 3.2.

Resource 3.2. SchoolMentalHealth.org

SchoolMentalHealth.org (www.schoolmentalhealth.org) offers school mental health resources for clinicians, educators, administrators, parents/caregivers, families, and students.

- Refer to "Resources for Clinicians" for fact sheets and other resources on interventions specific to various conditions.
- The *Quick Guide to Clinical Techniques for Common Child and Adolescent Mental Health Problems* (Stephan & Marciante, 2007) provides information on the application of cognitive–behavioral strategies, relaxation techniques, and other useful approaches.

Table 3.3. Cognitive–Behavioral Therapy Strategies

Strategy	Description
Psychoeducation: Helps to demystify therapy, empower child and family, and instill hope for a positive outcome	• Educate child and family about the disorder, including typical symptoms (thoughts and bodily reactions), causes (usually multidimensional), course of treatment, and major intervention strategies. • Serve as coach to the child. • Provide homework practice in between sessions.
Affective education: Helps children recognize their own and others' feelings and respond appropriately	• Teach a range of feeling words and the ability to recognize emotions through facial expressions, tone of voice, and body language. • Recognize own emotions and those of others (empathy). • Identify somatic clues related to uncomfortable emotions—anxiety (heart pounding, palms sweating, stomach ache, and shortness of breath), depression (fatigue, lack of energy), and anger (physical tension, heart pounding). • Identify activities that influence emotions (e.g., participation in a hobby or sport can result in feelings of enjoyment and well-being).
Cognitive restructuring (reframing): Helps child learn to use self-talk to change thinking and emotions	• Recognize faulty thinking and its impact on feelings. • Identify faulty or anxious thinking and recognize why it is not realistic. • Generate coping thoughts for a situation, write them down on a card, and keep them handy. • Use "thought-stopping" strategies; replace feared thinking with less threatening views, realistic thoughts, and positive affirmations.
Relaxation training: Helps reduce feelings of anxiety and promote successful interaction and participation	• Teach progressive muscle relaxation teaches the difference between tense and relaxed states by tightening and relaxing muscles. The child systematically tenses and relaxes body parts to learn how to make them relax. Yoga and meditation might also be used. • Teach *deep breathing:* diaphragmatic breathing to promote relaxation. Using a balloon as a metaphor, children are instructed to put one hand on their stomach and one hand on their chest and inhale through their nose (filling stomach/chest up like a balloon), hold for 3 seconds, and exhale while imagining that they are allowing all of the anxious feelings to leave their bodies. • Teach guided imagery.
Exposure to fears and contingency management	• Explain rationale for exposure to situations—that avoiding a situation over time strengthens the avoidant response and increases anxiety; avoidance prevents the development of coping skills and the ability to succeed and gain confidence. • Gradually introduce the feared event progressing from imagining the situation and role playing before the actual event. • Provide *contingency management,* which involves rewarding brave behavior with a favored activity or small item to increase the occurrence of the behavior.

Source. Ginsburg and Kingery (2007).

To work in unison with all school personnel, occupational therapists must be knowledgeable about schoolwide approaches emphasizing promotion and prevention (e.g., PBIS, SEL). Working within a public health framework challenges occupational therapists to move beyond individual interventions for children with identified disabilities and apply their knowledge to serve all children (universal) and those at risk (targeted) in schools and the community. Such a shift in thinking calls for leadership and creative action.

References

American Occupational Therapy Association. (2008). *Addressing sensory integration across the lifespan through occupational therapy.* Bethesda, MD: Author.

Argyle, E., & Bolton, G. (2005). Art in the community for potentially vulnerable mental health groups. *Health Education, 105,* 340–354.

Barber, B. L., Stone, M. R., Hunt, J. E., & Eccles, J. S. (2005). Benefits of activity participation: The roles of identify affirmation and peer group norm sharing. In J. Mahoney, R. Larson, & J. Eccles (Eds.), *Organized activities as contexts of development: Extracurricular activities, after-school and community programs* (pp. 185–210). Mahwah, NJ: Lawrence Erlbaum.

Bazyk, S. (2005). Exploring the development of meaningful work for children and youth in Western contexts. *WORK, 24,* 11–20.

Bazyk, S., LaGuardia, T., Connors, K., Graves, S., & Howlett, B. (2010). *The meaning of long-term participation in dance for females with and without disabilities.* Manuscript submitted for publication.

Butler, A. C., Chapman, J. E., Forman, E. M., & Beck, A. T. (2006). The empirical status of cognitive–behavioral therapy: A review of meta-analyses. *Clinical Psychology Review, 26,* 17–31.

Cartledge, G. (2003). School-wide positive behavior management: A state improvement grant (SIG) partnership. *Special Insert on School-Wide Positive Behavior Management, 2,* 1–10.

Catalano, R. F., Hawkins, J. D., Berglund, M. L., Pollard, J. A., & Arthur, M. W. (2002). Prevention science and positive youth development: Competitive or cooperative frameworks? *Journal of Adolescent Health, 31,* 230–239.

Champagne, T. (2008). *Sensory rooms in mental health.* Retrieved January 15, 2010, from www.ot-innovations.com/content/view/49/46/

Christner, R. W., Forrest, E., Morley, J., & Weinstein, E. (2007). Taking cognitive–behavior therapy to school: A school-based mental health approach. *Journal of Contemporary Psychotherapy, 37,* 175–183.

Cole, M., & Tufano, R. (2008). *Applied theories in occupational therapy: A practical approach.* Thorofare, NJ: Slack.

Collaborative for Academic, Social, and Emotional Learning. (2003). *Safe and sound: An educational leader's guide to evidence-based social and emotional learning (SEL) programs.* Chicago: Author.

Collaborative for Academic, Social, and Emotional Learning. (2010). *What is SEL? Skills and competencies.* Retrieved August 3, 2010, from www.casel.org/basics/skills.php

Csikszentmihalyi, M. (1993). Activity and happiness: Towards a science of occupation. *Occupational Science: Australia, 1,* 38–42.

Dixon, E. (2006). *The meaning of an occupational therapy work group for children with multiple disabilities: A phenomenological study.* Unpublished master's project, Cleveland State University.

Duhaney, L. M. (2003). A practical approach to managing the behaviors of students with ADD. *Intervention in School and Clinic, 38,* 267–279.

Dunn, W. (1999). *The Sensory Profile manual.* San Antonio, TX: Psychological Corporation.

Dunn, W. (2007). Supporting children to participate successfully in everyday life by using sensory processing knowledge. *Infants and Young Children, 20,* 84–101.

Dworkin, J. (2003). Adolescents' accounts of growth experiences in youth activities. *Journal of Youth and Adolescence, 32,* 17–26.

Dworkin, J. B., Larson, R., & Hansen, D. (2003). Adolescents' accounts of growth experiences in youth activities. *Journal of Youth and Adolescence, 32,* 17–26.

Eccles, J. S., & Gootman, J. A. (Eds.). (2002). *Community programs to promote youth development.* Washington, DC: National Academies Press.

Elias, M. J., Zins, J. D., Weissberg, R. P., Frey, K. S., Greenberg, M. T., Haynes, N. M., et al. (1997). *Promoting social and emotional learning: Guidelines for educators.* Alexandria, VA: Association for Supervision and Curriculum.

Emmer, E. T., & Stough, L. M. (2001). Classroom management: A critical part of educational psychology, with implications for teacher education. *Educational Psychologist, 36,* 103–112.

Freeman, R., Eber, L., Anderson, C., Irvin, L., Bounds, M., Dunlap, G., et al. (2006). Building inclusive school cultures using school-wide PBS: Designing effective individual support systems for students with significant disabilities. *Research and Practice for Persons With Severe Disabilities, 31,* 4–17.

French, D., & Hainsworth, J. (2001). "There aren't any buses and the swimming pool is always cold!": Obstacles and opportunities in the provision of sport for disabled people. *Managing Leisure, 6,* 35–49.

Ginsburg, G. S., & Kingery, J. N. (2007). Evidence-based practice for childhood anxiety disorders. *Journal of Contemporary Psychotherapy, 37,* 123–132.

Goleman, D. (1995). *Emotional intelligence: Why it can matter more than IQ.* New York: Bantam Books.

Greenberg, M. T., Weissberg, R. P., O'Brian, M., Zins, J. E., Fredericks, L., Resnik, H., et al. (2003). Enhancing school-based prevention and youth development through coordinated social, emotional, and academic learning. *American Psychologist, 58,* 466–474.

Hansen, D., Larson, R., & Dworkin, J. B. (2003). What adolescents learn in organized youth activities: A survey of self-reported developmental experiences. *Journal of Research on Adolescence, 13,* 25–55.

Henry, D. (2001). *The tool chest: For teachers, parents and students.* Glendale, AZ: Henry OT.

Illinois Children's Mental Health Act of 2003, Pub. Act 93–0495.

Jackson, L. L., & Arbesman, M. (2005). *Occupational therapy practice guidelines for children with behavioral and psychosocial needs.* Bethesda, MD: AOTA Press.

Jacobs, K. (1994). Getting ready for work. *Rehabilitation Management, 7,* 120–121.

Kessler, R. C., Berglund, P., Demler, O., Jin, R., Merinkangas, K. R., et al. (2005). Lifetime prevalence and age-of-onset distributions of *DSM–IV* disorders in the National Comorbidity Survey replication. *Archives of General Psychiatry, 62,* 593–602.

Kleiber, D. (1999). *Leisure experience and human development: A dialectical approach.* New York: Basic Books.

Kusche, C. A., & Greenberg, M. T. (1994). *The PATHS (Promoting Alternative Thinking Strategies) curriculum.* Seattle, WA: Developmental Research & Programs.

Kutash, K., Duchnowski, A. J., & Lynn, N. (2006). *School-based mental health: An empirical guide for decision-makers.* Tampa: University of South Florida, Louis de la Parte Florida Mental Health Institute, Research and Training Center for Children's Mental Health.

Larson, R. W. (2000). Toward a psychology of positive youth development. *American Psychologist, 55,* 170–183.

Law, M., Finkelman, S., Hurley, P., Rosenbaum, P., King, S., et al. (2004). Participation of children with physical disabilities: Relationships with diagnosis, physical function, and demographic variables. *Scandinavian Journal of Occupational Therapy, 11,* 156–162.

Lochman, J. E., & Wells, K. C. (2003). Effectiveness of the Coping Power program and of classroom intervention with aggressive children: Outcomes at a 1-year follow-up. *Behavior Therapy, 34,* 493–515.

Macnaughton, J., White, M., & Stacy, R. (2005). Researching the benefits of arts in health. *Health Education, 105,* 332–339.

Mahoney, J. L., Harris, A. L., & Eccles, J. S. (2008). *The over-scheduling myth* (Research-to-Results Brief, Pub. No. 2008–12). Washington, DC: Child Trends. Retrieved June 28, 2009, from www.childtrends.org/Files//Child_Trends-2008_02_27_Myth.pdf

Mahoney, J. L., Larson, R. W., Eccles, J. S., & Lord, H. (2005). Organized activities as development contexts for children and adolescents. In J. Mahoney, R. Larson, & J. Eccles (Eds.), *Organized activities as contexts of development: Extracurricular activities, after-school and community programs* (pp. 3–23). Mahwah, NJ: Lawrence Erlbaum.

Mahoney, J. L., & Stattin, H. (2000). Leisure activities and adolescent antisocial behavior: The role of structure and social context. *Journal of Adolescence, 23,* 113–127.

Masten, A. S. (2006). Developmental psychology: Pathways to the future. *International Journal of Behavioral Development, 30,* 47–54.

Masten, A. S., Roisman, G. I., Long, J. D., Burt, K. B., Obradovic, J., Riley, J. R., et al. (2005). Developmental cascades: Linking academic achievement and externalizing and internalizing symptoms over 20 years. *Developmental Psychology, 41*(5), 733–746.

Miller-Kuhanek, H., Henry, D., Glennon, T., Parham, L. D., & Ecker, C. (2008). *The Sensory Processing Measure.* Los Angeles: Western Psychological Services.

McLaughlin, M. (2000). *Community counts: How youth organizations matter for youth development.* Washington, DC: Public Education Network.

Monga, S., Young, A., & Owens, M. (2009). Evaluating a cognitive behavioral therapy group program for anxious five to seven year old children: A pilot study. *Depression and Anxiety, 26,* 243–250.

Morse, T. E., & Schuster, J. W. (2000). Teaching elementary students with moderate intellectual disabilities how to shop for groceries. *Exceptional Children, 66,* 273–288.

Mu, K., & Gabriel, L. (2001). Strategies to cope with severe challenging behavior. *OT Practice, 6*(2), 12–17.

National Research Council, & Institute of Medicine. (2009). *Preventing mental, emotional, and behavioral disorders among young people: Progress and possibilities.* Washington, DC: National Academies Press.

Passmore, A. (1998). Does leisure have an association with creating cultural patterns of work? *Journal of Occupational Science, 5,* 161–165.

Payton, J., Weissberg, R. P., Durlak, J. A., Dymnicki, A. B., Taylor, R. D., Schellinger, K. B., et al. (2008). *The positive impact of social and emotional learning for kindergarten to eighth-grade students: Findings from three scientific reviews.* Chicago: Collaborative for Academic, Social, and Emotional Learning.

Safran, S. P., & Oswald, K. (2003). Positive behavior supports: Can schools reshape disciplinary practices? *Exceptional Children, 69,* 361–373.

Seligman, M. E. P. (2002). *Authentic happiness.* New York: Free Press.

Shure, M. B. (2001). I Can Problem Solve (ICPS): An interpersonal cognitive problem solving program for children. In L. A. Reddy & S. Pfeiffer (Eds.), *Innovative mental health programs for children: Programs that work* (pp. 2–14). Binghamton, NY: Haworth Press.

Stephan, S. H., & Marciante, W. (2007). *Quick guide to clinical techniques for common child and adolescent mental health problems.* Baltimore: University of Maryland, Center for School Mental Health Analysis and Action.

Sugai, G., Horner, R. H., Dunlap, G., Hieneman, M., Lewis, T., Nelson, C. M., et al. (2000). Applying positive behavioral support and functional behavioral assessment in schools. *Journal of Positive Behavior Intervention, 2,* 1–25.

Sze, K. M., & Wood, J. J. (2007). Cognitive behavioral treatment of comorbid anxiety disorders and social difficulties in children with high-functioning autism: A case report. *Journal of Contemporary Psychotherapy, 37,* 133–143.

Tomb, M., & Hunter, L. (2004). Prevention of anxiety in children and adolescents in a school setting: The role of school-based practitioners. *Children and Schools, 26,* 2.

Trott, M. (2002). *Oh behave! Sensory processing and behavioral strategies: A practical guide for clinicians, teachers and parents.* San Antonio, TX: Therapy Skill Builders.

U.S. Department of Education, OSEP Technical Assistance Center on Positive Behavioral Interventions and Supports. (2010). *What is school-wide positive behavioral interventions and supports?* Retrieved January 23, 2010, from www.pbis.org/school/what_is_swpbs.aspx

Vogel, C. L. (2008, May–June). Classroom design for living and learning with autism. *Autism: Asperger's Digest Magazine,* pp. 31–33. Retrieved January 5, 2010, from www.autismdigest.com/Portals/0/docs/Classroom(2)-AADMay08.pdf

Williams, M. S., & Shellenberger, S. (1996). *"How does your engine run?": A leader's guide to the Alert Program for self-regulation.* Albuquerque, NM: TherapyWorks.

Wood, J., Drahota, A., Sze, K., VanDyke, M., Decker, K., et al. (2009). Brief report: Effects of cognitive behavioral therapy on parent-reported autism symptoms in school-age children with high-functioning autism. *Journal of Autism and Developmental Disorders, 39,* 1608–1612.

CHAPTER 4

Pathways to Positive Development: Childhood Participation in Everyday Places and Activities

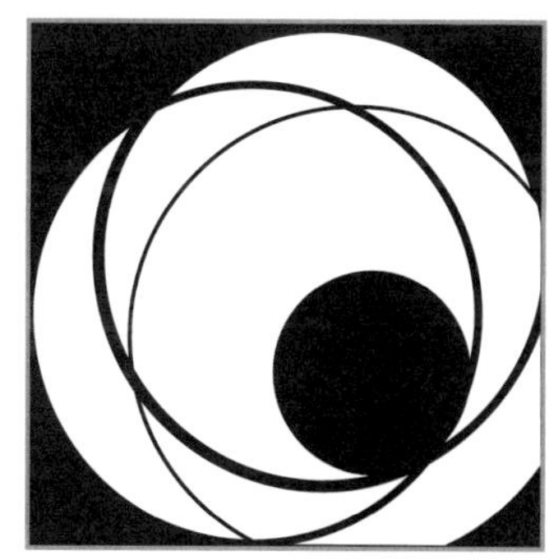

Theresa M. Petrenchik, PhD, OTR/L, and Gillian A. King, PhD

Learning Objectives

After reading this material and completing the examination, readers will be able to

- Recognize the interrelationships between childhood participation and the contexts in which it occurs;
- Identify current trends in environmental perspectives within occupational therapy;
- Differentiate the concepts of environment and place;
- Describe key attributes of child- and youth-friendly places; and
- Recognize the relationships between environmental qualities and growth-enhancing experiences.

The topics of participation, environments, and positive development are broad and complex, each with its own web of subtle nuances and critical distinctions. Only recently have scholars across a range of disciplines begun the work of integrating these subjects by articulating theories of positive development and studying its promotion through child and youth participation in everyday places and activities.

This chapter explores participation, environments, and positive development from a psychosocial, developmental perspective. It includes a focused discussion of environments and participation and describes attributes and processes of positive participation in child-friendly environments. The range of potential person–environment issues to be discussed is limited by giving attention to aspects of child–environment–activity relations that science and practical wisdom suggest are important for supporting positive development through child and youth participation in out-of-school activities. The concept of *participation,* defined in the *International Classification of Functioning, Disability and Health* (*ICF;* World Health

Organization [WHO], 2001, p. 14) as "involvement in life situations," is refined and discussed in terms of its composite parts, activity *performance* and *involvement*. Finally, the chapter also introduces two distinct but related conceptual frameworks. The first depicts key attributes of child- and youth-friendly places, and the second presents a developmental health model of the relationships between environmental qualities and growth-enhancing experiences.

Integrated View of Positive Development, Participation, and Environments

The extent to which participation in everyday activities and places contributes to positive psychological and social–emotional development can be understood only relationally—that is, when childhood participation is viewed as a contextually bound child-in-environment experience that is measured against the requirements of immediate and imminent developmental tasks in combination with personal attributions of meaning. Attention to subjective attributions of meaning is essential because participation is inherently storied. A portion of its significance is rooted in personal interpretations that are influenced by personal and shared memories of the past, experiences of the present, and individual and societal expectations of the future (Freysinger, 2006). Understanding the process of participation as a contributor to positive development, including successful transitions from childhood to adolescence to healthy adulthood, requires attention to the ways in which the child and environment jointly define one another through activity participation and engagement.

Just as a child's anatomy and physiology are interrelated and interdependent, so too are the integrated structures (environments) and processes (actions and experiences) that make up fused systems of person–environment relations (Lerner, Jacobs, & Wertlieb, 2005). Like the steady forces of wind and water interacting with rock canyon walls, experiences of participation over time carve, shape, and are influenced by identity development, character formation, and self-confidence, all of which contribute positively or negatively to feelings of belonging and connection (Connell, Gambone, & Smith, 2000; Lerner, Taylor, & Von Eye, 2002). The fruits of positive participation, which include the development of competencies, confidence, character, social connections, and making meaningful contributions to others and society (Pittman, Tolman, & Yohalem, 2005), form the bedrock of positive life course development (Eccles & Gootman, 2002; Peterson, 2004).

Positive Development

Positive development, an adaptive process of attaining a healthy sense of personhood (Csikszentmihalyi & Rathunde, 1998), is evident in patterns of behaviors that, over time, contribute positively to self, family, community, and civil society (Lerner et al., 2002). Those behaviors include the acquisition of attitudes, values, and skills that youth will need to lead a happy, healthy, successful adult life (Eccles & Gootman, 2002). Positive development is fertilized by ongoing participation in safe, developmentally supportive life situations in which children and youth enjoy supportive relationships with adults and peers, have meaningful opportunities for involvement and membership, and participate actively in challenging and engaging activities

(Connell et al., 2000). Developmentally, children and youth have a need for participation in places and activities that afford them varying degrees of privacy and social engagement, acceptance and belonging, appropriate challenges, and a balance between adult guidance and self-determination.

Role of Participation

Children's participation in everyday activities and places is a process and an outcome of development. It is a stream of person-in-environment transactions made up of an interrelated series of actions and experiences (Wapner & Demick, 1998). Participation both shapes and is shaped by development, which transpires through interactions of child and environment. When it is viewed in this way, holistically and contexually, childhood participation provides us with a snapshot of development in action. The sounds of childhood participation—shrieks of laughter, tearful sobs, and shouts of discovery, accomplishment, and frustration—help convey the tales of children's lives—their daily joys and sorrows, triumphs and challenges, and rituals of meaning.

Child and youth participation can be thought of as significant arrangements of activities and social interactions, together with their individual and collective meanings, that make up life situations and experiences. Like songs in a music album, participation is themed. Just as individual songs in an album can be connected by a central unifying theme (i.e., love songs), *participation* consists of collections of themed activities with recognizable patterns (i.e., team sports, after-school activities). Participation, in the form of *activity mosaics* (i.e., arrangements of recreational, social, artistic, work, educational activities), can serve as an indicator of whether a child or youth is moving along a pathway of positive development. In other words, patterns of activity participation in everyday environments over time represent trajectories or pathways of development.

Many pathways of participation lead to happy, well-adjusted children and youth (Weisner, 2005). Consequently, occupational therapists are interested in identifying the hallmarks of positive participation, which include freedom of expression and choice; social interaction with adults, friends, and peers in a variety of settings; and opportunities to test and develop personal abilities through appropriate levels of challenge and stimulation. Positive participation also invites personal and shared inquiry, exploration, creativity, and communication. It provides children with a critical sense of safety and opportunities for self-expression, and it fosters a sense of connectedness and belonging (Eccles & Gootman, 2002; Lerner & Benson, 2003; Mahoney, Larson, & Eccles, 2005; Peterson, 2004). In contrast, the hallmarks of unhealthy participation are life situations and settings that result in feelings of social exclusion, oppression, helplessness, or worthlessness; that promote chronic insecurity, anxiety, or fear; and that contribute to negative attitudes, destructive behaviors, or both.

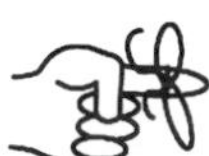

Remember this. . . .
Positive participation in developmentally favorable environments provides children with a critical sense of safety and opportunities for self-expression, and it fosters a sense of connectedness and belonging.

Viewing participation through a developmental lens means that the forms, meanings of, and opportunities for participation change over time, including the people, places, and objects of which participation is made. On any given day, patterns of childhood participation and their associated meanings mirror the shifting tides of development that underpin a child's evolving competencies, motivational beliefs, values, goals, activity interests, and choices (Eccles & Wigfield, 2002). Participation, with all of its composite parts, provides a window through which to view and ultimately understand a child's personality and temperament, talents and abilities, relational style, and personal preferences (Fidler & Fidler, 1978), including his or her sense of identity as an individual, as a member of groups, and as a member of society (Ellemers, Spears, & Doosje, 2002).

Role of Environments

The environmental surroundings in which children and youth live, learn, and play are powerful shapers of life course mental health and well-being (Halfon & Hochstein, 2002; Keating, 2000; Keating & Hertzman, 1999; National Research Council [NRC] & Institute of Medicine [IOM], 2004). In an ideal world, environments provide children with an essential sense of stability and continuity of experience (Bronfenbrenner, 1979, 1999; Searles, 1960). They are safe settings in which to take risks, face challenges, and develop interpersonal relationships. Optimally, environments offer children and youth places of peace and solace during times of stress and interpersonal conflict. Over time, interactions with and manipulation of nonhuman objects and structures allow children and youth to discover a sense of personal power and to develop a mature sense of personhood in relationship to society and the natural world (Searles, 1960).

Differences in the quality of children's social and physical environments produce important variations in activity participation and life experiences, which in turn influence children's physical and mental health, well-being, and competence (Keating & Hertzman, 1999). Identity development; appraisals of self-efficacy and self-worth (Bandura, 1997a); and feelings of competence, connection, and belonging (Masten, 2001) influence and are influenced by environments that contribute to the quality of children's daily life experiences, and they set the conditions for both positive and negative developmental outcomes.

Three Strands in a Braid

Participation, human environments, and child development are like three strands in a braid. The relationship among them—their interweaving—merits occupational therapists' attention and challenges them to develop conceptual frameworks and empirical methods suited to capturing their relational significance and intricacies. Included in this challenge are the elaboration and refinement of descriptions and indicators of environmental qualities relevant to positive participation. Research to identify and describe the processes and mechanisms responsible for the developmental health benefits of childhood participation in everyday environments is also needed. Surveys of *time use* (activities performed) and descriptions of the qualities of *activity settings* (where activities occur) provide incomplete explanations of participation when they lack participants' appraisals of the personal significance of observed activities and settings. What is needed is attention to *softly assembled systems* (Thelen & Smith, 1997) of participation—interwoven strands of actions, settings, and subjective experiences—from which patterns of participation emerge, transpire, and transform.

Environmental Perspectives in Occupational Therapy

The topic of environments has received increasing attention in the occupational therapy literature over the past 2 decades. Most of the published work on the topic has considered environments in a broad sense and offers descriptions of the physical, sociocultural, spiritual, temporal, and virtual aspects of a person's surroundings (American Occupational Therapy Association [AOTA], 2008; Law, 1991; Townsend et al., 1997). Despite these contributions, the occupational therapy literature on environments is relatively limited and focuses primarily on physical environments as they relate to occupational performance, independent living, daily functioning, accessibility, and safety (Lampinen & Tham, 2003; Vik, Lilja, & Nygard, 2007). Relatively little attention has been given to social aspects of the environment (Nyman & Lund, 2007) or to children's environments, particularly those outside of school settings.

Recent literature on child and youth participation has expanded the discussion of environments by beginning to articulate the general characteristics of positive participatory environments. These characteristics include opportunities for making choices (Lawlor, 2003; Wiseman, Davis, & Polatajko, 2005), for having fun (Bazyk & Bazyk, 2009), to feel successful, to do things independently, and to be with others (Heah, Case, McGuire, & Law, 2007). Opportunities to develop and strengthen positive social connections with friends and peers through participation in a variety of activities, both structured and unstructured, is also considered an important aspect of positive participatory environments (Imms, 2008; King et al., 2010; Law, Petrenchik, Ziviani, & King, 2006; Poulsen, Ziviani, Cuskelly, & Smith, 2007; Tanta, Deitz, White, & Billingsley, 2005). Fidler's (1999) work expands this list to include environments that encourage autonomy, individualization, affiliation, volition, consensual validation, predictability, self-efficacy, adventure, accommodation, and reflection.

Two trends, both noteworthy, are evident in the occupational therapy literature on environments. The first is a tendency to address social and physical environments as separate and often undifferentiated contexts. The second is considering environments from a strictly functional or performance-oriented perspective. Although the partitioning of physical and social environments is handy from a measurement standpoint, it contributes to an oversimplified understanding of both and obscures the fact that physical and social environments tend to be mutually defining (Wapner & Demick, 1998). In reality, "the physical environment simultaneously symbolizes, makes concrete, and conditions the social environment" (Levy-Leboyer, 1982, p. 15). Serious attention to this interrelationship, which is critical to understanding the motivation for participation in activities and its associated meaning, rarely occurs in the profession's literature on environments.

The "soft" influence of a physical setting on participation is often evident in the meaning it acquires from social aspects of the setting. For example, a church, temple, or mosque is more than a building to worshipers who enter that sacred place to gather together in prayer. A theater stage is transformed into mythic Carnegie Hall through shared meanings and memories of past performances and performers. Stepping onto a field of green grass takes on special symbolic significance when a child does so as a member of a Little League baseball team. The meaning deepens further when the child, dressed in his or hers team's baseball uniform, has a visible disability.

In each instance, "the physical environment . . . is as much a social phenomenon as it is a physical one" (Proshansky, Ittelson, & Rivlin, 1976, p. 5). These holistic person-in-environment experiences, which involve more than routine encounters with environmental barriers and supports, shape the actions and experiences occurring within a particular context. The meaning, value, and symbolic significance that a child or youth associates with an environment strongly influence his or her preference for that place (Chawla, 1992; Korpela, 2002) and the activities and social interactions it invites.

A second trend in the literature is an overriding concern with the functionality of environments. Because environments are typically regarded as containers for action, settings are viewed in terms of practical operations: activities they allow, performance barriers they present, and opportunities they afford. The emphasis here is on the *doing* aspects of living, which is implicit in the terms *activity setting* and *occupational performance*. The watchword here is *performance,* the environmental considerations of which are addressed pragmatically in terms of what they afford relative to areas of occupation (AOTA, 2008), activity engagement (Dunn, Brown, & McGuigan, 1994), occupational performance (Law et al., 1996), and lifestyle performance (Fidler & Velde, 1999).

Functionally, the environment is regarded as an external force, or set of forces, acting on a person in three basic ways: (1) as structural enablers of or barriers to participation in specific activity settings (Hemmingsson & Borell, 2002; Imms, 2008; Law, Petrenchik, King, & Hurley, 2007; Lawlor, Mihaylov, Welsh, Jarvis, & Colver, 2006; Letts, Rigby, & Stewart, 2003; Stark & Sanford, 2005), (2) as performance-facilitating or -inhibiting conditions (Mancini, Coster, Trombly, & Heeren, 2000; Schenker, Coster, & Parush, 2006), and (3) as sources of external demand or press in the form of societal expectations, life demands, and situational stressors (Hagedorn, 1995; Rigby & Letts, 2003). Considering environments functionally, or pragmatically, encourages a focus on the doing or performance aspects of occupation.

Others in the field of occupational therapy (Fidler & Velde, 1999; Gitlin, Corcoran, & Leinmiller-Eckhardt, 1995; Hasselkus, 2002) have emphasized the importance of simultaneously considering both the functional and the experiential aspects of environments. Such a perspective broadens occupational therapy's understanding of environmental significance by explicitly considering the role of the meaning-making mind in shaping environmental perceptions and experiences. Meaning making occurs in the mind, the language of which is symbols, metaphors, analogies, and codes of meaning (Cirlot, 1971).

Meaning results from a complex mixture of thoughts, memories, beliefs, values, goals, emotional state, and needs (Jung, 1956). It arises from interactions of factual life circumstances and storied experiences. For example, the internal symbolic representation of a space gives it a specific meaning: A house becomes a home, a fort made of tree branches and leaves becomes a secret clubhouse, and a church becomes a sanctuary. Likewise, internal symbolic representations of actions transform strings of discrete tasks and activities into meaningful ceremonies, daily rituals, and rites of passage. It is clear, then, that everyday environments are more than containers for action; they are lifescapes that require an integrated focus on the doing and the experiential aspects of occupation.

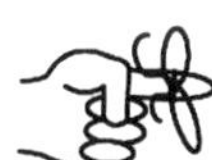

Remember this. . . .
Everyday environments are more than containers for action; they are lifescapes that require an integrated focus on the doing and the experiential aspects of occupation.

Conceptually, lifescapes are woven together from the threads of objective reality, symbolic relationships (Fidler, 1999); story making (Clark, Ennevor, & Richardson, 1996); and the doing, being, and becoming aspects of people as occupationally inclined beings (Wilcock, 2006). *Lifescapes* are melting pots in which the observable aspects of environmental context meld with subjective appraisals of action and experience to form a person's storied participation in life situations. *Storied participation,* the ways in which involvement in life situations is interpreted and experienced by the participators, is a linchpin connecting meaning making with mental health and well-being (Coatsworth, Palen, & Sharp, 2006; Eyles & Williams, 2008; McGuire, 1983).

New Directions: Supporting Participation in Everyday Places and Activities

Supporting meaningful participation in life is the overarching objective of occupational therapy intervention (AOTA, 2008). A focus on optimizing participation in life situations, which occurs in everyday places, differs significantly from a focus on improving functional behavior and activity performance in contrived activity settings. Addressing the latter has historically involved attention to the execution of tasks at the level of body function and structure (Rosenbaum & Stewart, 2007). The professional challenge ahead becomes apparent when one considers that activity performance is not synonymous with participation (WHO, 2001), just as changes in body function and structure do not necessarily translate into improvements in participation or quality of life (Albrecht & Devlieger, 1999; Kaplan, 2002).

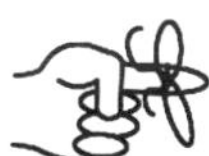

Remember this. . . .
Activity performance is not synonymous with participation, just as changes in body function and structure do not necessarily translate into improvements in participation or quality of life.

The *ICF* defines *participation* as "involvement in life situations" (WHO, 2001, p. 14), which includes the concepts of performance and involvement. Within the *ICF,* participation is not necessarily equated with performance, and a distinction is made between performance and involvement. *Involvement* encompasses the experiences of taking part, being included or engaged in a life area, being accepted, and having access to needed resources (WHO, 2001). It is a construct consisting of both observable characteristics (i.e., taking part) and subjective qualities (i.e., a sense of belonging). Such distinctions matter because they invite the development of more sophisticated yardsticks against which to measure intervention approaches and outcomes.

The *ICF* also encourages attention to both the observable actions and the subjective experiences of participation as important health constituents. Using the *ICF* as a guiding health framework promotes balanced attention between maximizing functional performance and optimizing child and youth participation in life situations. The latter emphasizes activity participation and social involvement and thereby establishes social inclusion as an important health outcome (WHO, 2001).

Differentiating Environment and Place

The terms *environment* and *context* are routinely used to refer to the settings and surroundings in which life situations and daily activities occur. These terms tend to ignore the psychological and social aspects of place-specific experience. They are value-neutral terms, neither positive nor negative, and devoid of meaning. For this reason, we substitute the term *place* for *environment* and begin by introducing its characteristics.

The concept of *place,* which builds on Barker's (1968) notion of behavior settings, incorporates the idea that environments simultaneously serve a function, motivate a person's participation, and are subject to real-time assessments of significance (or meaning) by the participant (Cassidy, 1997). Place differs from conceptualizations of activity settings by including, more directly, the understanding and expectations that participants have of the place they inhabit, together with the qualities and perceptual properties of that setting (Canter, 1977). It is subjective experience that links, in part, place with health and quality of life (Eyles & Williams, 2008).

Canter (1997) defined *place* as "focused units of environmental experience within which activities and physical forms are amalgamated," and he asserted that "places cannot be specified independently of the people who are experiencing them" (p. 111). Places are defined by a combination of their physical characteristics, the activities performed there, and the significance that settings have for people. This place-making process occurs whenever a setting or space acquires meaning through person–environment interactions in those surroundings (Canter, 2000). In other words, environments become places when they acquire personal or group meaning and thereby come to represent "organized worlds of meaning" (Tuan, 1977, p. 179). Reflection 4.1 provides readers with an opportunity to apply these concepts

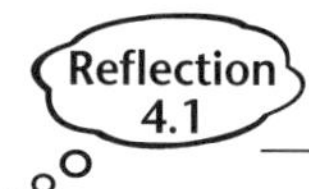

Try to Remember

In "The Ecology of Imagination in Childhood," Edith Cobb (1969) observed that children have a desire to make a world in which they are able to find a place to discover a self. In other words, children have a place-making impulse and the need to participate in world-making and world-shaping behaviors (Cobb, 1969). They need opportunities to create, shape, organize, and "own" places in which they can become themselves, either alone or in the company of a few special friends (Sobel, 2002). These places can be secret forts, a culvert in an overgrown lot, a dusty attic crawl space, or even a simple stairwell.

> Growing up in a large family and living in a small home did not allow for much alone time. My favorite place was the large attic stairs located in the front closet and behind a row of winter coats. It had an overhead light. I would go there to draw and to be alone. I loved to draw. I still remember the attic steps as a haven of sorts. My visual image of it is clear. It was not an environment that anyone would describe as attractive, but for me, it was wonderful. It became a "meaningful place" for me over time. It provided me with a sense of peace, quiet, and restoration.
>
> —Susan Bazyk, PhD, OTR/L, FAOTA

Exercise: Try to remember a special childhood place that you created for yourself. Hold that image in your mind, and reflect on the meaning of that place in your life. What "magic" did that place hold for you?

Practice considerations: Weaving considerations of place into interventions requires occupational therapists to look beyond the physical and social spaces a child occupies to discover from children themselves the meaning these spaces hold for them.

Place-Based Participation

Places such as a relative's home, a favorite hangout, or a secret fort can evoke strong emotions in children and adolescents. Places have psychological significance and can encourage a sense of emotional attachment that contributes to the development of place preferences and attachments (Altman & Low, 1992; Holloway & Valentine, 2000; Korpela, 2002; Sobel, 2002). Place attachment and preferences develop through person–place bonding that occurs during repeated interactions in a particular place (Altman & Low, 1992; Chawla, 1992). The distinctions between activity preferences and place preferences can blur, and at times they are two sides of the same coin. For example, certain activities lend themselves to particular settings (e.g., skateboarding, dancing, watching TV), just as certain places (e.g., water parks, gymnasiums, forests) invite specific types of activities and forms of participation (e.g., sports vs. the arts). Place preferences and activity preferences are synergistic, and together they contribute to mutually reinforcing patterns of activity participation.

Favorite places, which children and youth value, like, or consider important (Korpela, 2002), can play a significant role in sensory modulation and emotional self-regulation, as well as in the management of boundaries between solitude and social interaction. They can also have restorative effects during periods of stress or difficulty. Natural environments, compared with built environments, seem especially important for reducing emotions such as fear, anger, and sadness; for improving attentional behavior; and for fostering imagination and creativity (Dunkley, 2009; Louv, 2005; Nabhan & Trimble, 1994). Natural places are also important for nurturing restorative feelings such as fascination, being away, coherence, and compatibility (Korpela, 2002). Readers can use the examples in Reflection 4.2 to help think about ways to begin to include natural settings in their interventions.

Place experiences can be developmentally supportive or inhibiting, and they play a role in shaping and reinforcing the development of motivational beliefs, values, goals, and activity interests and choices (Eccles & Wigfield, 2002). Over time, these choices and related experiences become the cobblestones of children's preferred and acquired pathways of social participation and activity engagement. These pathways of participation serve to reinforce, both positively and negatively, a child's or youth's developing sense of self-identity, self-efficacy, and self-worth (Bandura, 1997b; Bandura & Locke, 2003). Places that contribute positively to a child's or youth's development are considered child friendly.

Child-friendly places provide children and youth with balanced opportunities for seclusion, engagement, skill development, and creative expression (Chawla, 1992). They also encourage exploration, encourage the development of competencies (Hertzman, 2002), and provide a living space in which children and youth can engage in the ongoing task of differentiating self from others (Becker, 1992). They are physically safe, emotionally secure, and psychologically enabling (WHO, 1999). Child-friendly environments encourage a sense of relatedness, engage the senses, excite interests, spark the imagination, and nurture both the doing and the being aspects of personhood. They offer a range of developmentally suitable choices that involve various types and levels of structure, effort, and stimulation, thereby both

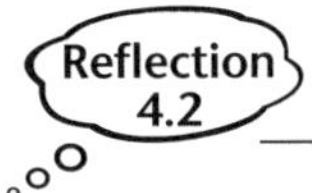

Nature as Healer

Time spent in natural settings often has a restorative effect for children. The theory is that natural environments hold a strong fascination for children. Because fascination involves involuntary attention, the directed attention required for structured activities is allowed to rest. Green spaces are considered restorative environments because they are stress reducing and calming and tend to have a sensory organizing effect for children. They also capture children's imagination and allow them to be swept up into an exquisite medley of sensory experiences.

Here is description of a striking natural encounter in childhood as recalled by Howard Thurman in his autobiography *With Head and Heart* (1980):

> When the storms blew, the branches of the large oak tree in our backyard would snap and fall. But the topmost branches of the oak tree would sway, giving way just enough to save themselves from snapping loose. I needed the strength of that tree, and like it, I wanted to hold my ground. Eventually, I discovered that the oak tree and I had a unique relationship. I could sit, my back against its trunk, and feel the same peace that would come to me in my bed at night. I could reach down in the quiet places of my spirit, take out my bruises and my joys, unfold them and talk about them. I could talk aloud to the oak tree and know that I was understood. It too, was a part of my reality, like the woods, and the night, and the pounding surf, my earliest companions, giving me space. (p. 103)

Practice considerations: Think about how you might begin to expand your interventions to include experiences in natural settings. An example of such a setting is the Spiral Gardens, an integrated outdoor art, garden, and play program that has been operating since 1984 as part of Bloorview Kids Rehab in Toronto, Ontario. Spiral Gardens is based on the simple idea that the natural world is a healing context for children with and without disabilities. The objectives of the program are to explore self- and collective expression through a variety of art media, to nurture children's relationship to nature through tending an organic garden, and to foster an inclusive community that gives attention to the whole person. The staff include artists from a variety of disciplines (musicians, puppeteers, dramatists, storytellers, art and music therapists) as well as educators, clowns, students, gardeners, and activity facilitators.

For more information, visit www.bloorview.ca/programsandservices/communityprograms/centreforthearts/spiralgarden.php

challenging and supporting development. They stimulate intellectual and emotional engagement and invite living and discovery by being adaptable and flexible.

Key Attributes of Child- and Youth-Friendly Places

Everyday participation, and the significance it holds for a person, group, community, or society, is as much a product of the places and people involved as it is a function of the activities performed. Places that foster growth-enhancing participation include, in various time–place–person-specific combinations, the attributes of safety and comfort, affordances, social cohesion, and meaningful activities and experiences (Figure 4.1). These attributes, and the relational patterns of organization within and across them, exist in dynamic relationship with one another. They both shape and are shaped by one another.

Metaphorically, places can be thought of as the axle on which the wheels of participation and development turn. When destructive environmental interference,

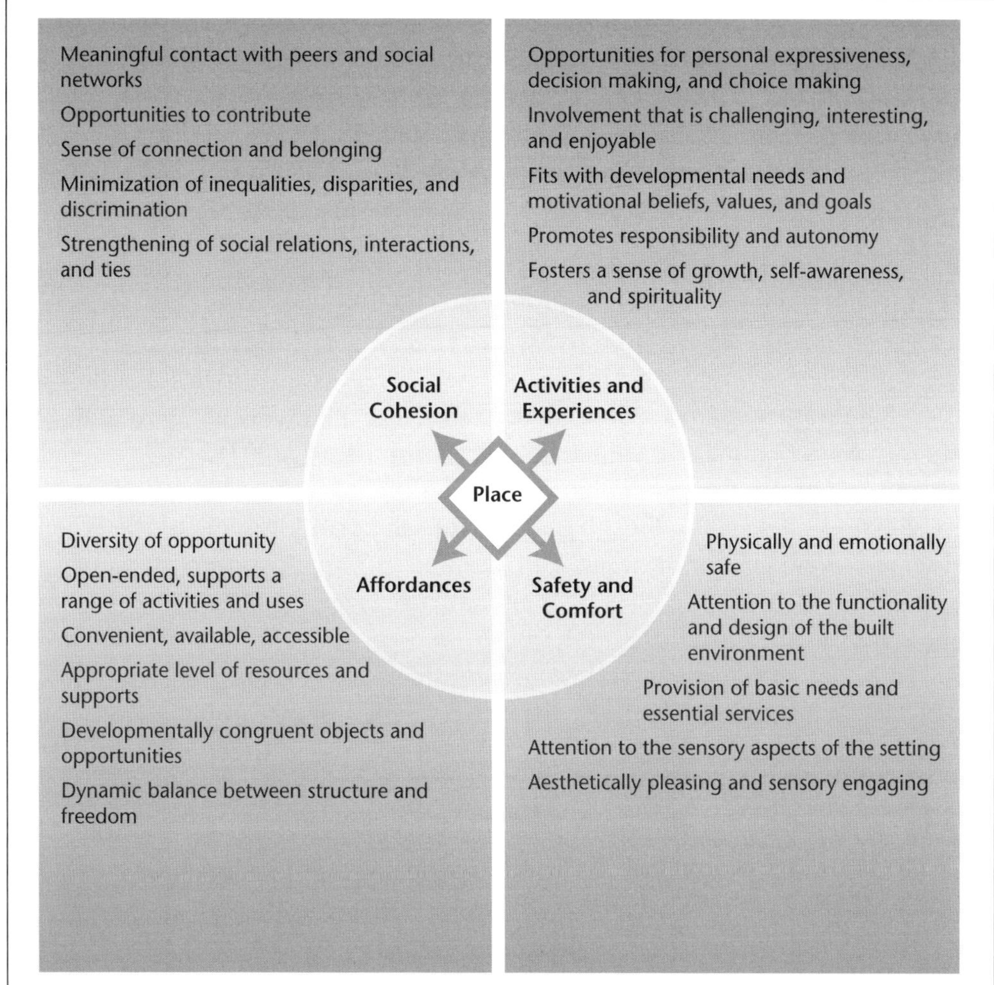

Figure 4.1. Attributes of child- and youth-friendly places. Items in the inner circle are key place attributes; items listed outside the circle are properties of those attributes. The arrows represent the interactions among the attributes and properties of developmentally favorable places.

such as chronic poverty and deprivation, throws the system into a state of imbalance (i.e., stressors overwhelm adaptive coping capacity), the wheels of participation and development can fall out of alignment, resulting in patterns of participation that undermine positive development. The balance among key attributes, rather than the absence or presence of a particular property of an attribute, shapes the quality of the places in which children and youth participate. This dynamic balance is represented by the arrows in Figure 4.1.

Comfort and Safety

The comfort and safety of places has received considerable attention in numerous bodies of literature, including child health and geography, environmental design, environmental psychology, and adverse childhood experiences and trauma. We have limited the potential range of topics to be discussed by addressing the general properties of place-based comfort and safety.

Comfort is defined as contented well-being or as a satisfying or enjoyable experience (Agnes, 2000), the conditions of which include the functionality of the built environment, aesthetics (i.e., attractiveness, use of color), object relations (i.e., tools, toys, resources), spatial arrangements of people and objects, and sensory aspects of the environment (i.e., sound and noise levels, odors, visual distractions, crowding).

Children and youth vary greatly in their responses to the sensory characteristics of daily environments. The work of Winnie Dunn (1997, 2001) has contributed much to occupational therapists' understanding of these differences and to the ways in which the sensory aspects of everyday environments can affect a child's or youth's behavior, attention, and activity performance. Teaching children and youth to recognize their own self-regulation strategies in response to environmental stimuli is an important step in enabling them to structure their daily environments and routines in ways that maximize their comfort (Dunn, 1997, 2001).

Safety is a multidimensional construct and includes physical and emotional safety. *Physical safety* is the most basic form of safety, and it refers to the absence of violence; avoidance of unnecessary risks; and minimal exposure to dangerous circumstances, people, and objects. It encompasses considerations such as cleanliness, exposure to environmental toxins, and provision of appropriate adult supervision. *Emotional safety,* sometimes considered *social safety* (Bloom, 2005), refers to a person's sense of safety with other people. An emotionally safe setting provides children and youth with the freedom to express themselves and their thoughts, feelings, and opinions without fear of retaliation, judgment, rejection, or condemnation.

Safety is not synonymous with an overly protective environment that is devoid of any risk or environmental flux. The phrase the *more stable the environment, the better* is an oversimplification because too much stability, in the forms of high structure and low stimulation or high structure and low diversity, may be as problematic as too little stability. Also, living and participating in a stable, developmentally supportive environment is very different from similar experiences in a stable, developmentally inhibiting environment (Wachs, 1999). So environmental stability is a relative term, not an all-or-none phenomenon, and it includes varying amounts of calculated risk and unpredictability.

Affordances

The term *affordance,* as conceptualized by Gibson (1979), represents the action possibilities within an environment. Affordances are functionally significant properties of the environment that offer, or afford, something to a person (Heft, 1997). For example, a graspable object affords throwing and an empty room affords solitude. Affordances are task, person, and environment specific, meaning that what a person considers possible in a setting is dependent on the intentional action of a particular person in a specific setting. For Gibson, affordances are functional and observable (they exist or not), they support action, and they operate independently of a person's experience, knowledge, culture, or perceptual abilities. Norman (1988) countered this stance by arguing that affordances can be perceived or observed and that they are influenced by a person's experience, knowledge, culture, and perceptual abilities. Similar to Norman, our view of affordances includes a person's subjective perceptions of action possibilities in the objective environment.

As a place attribute, affordances include the diversity of opportunities available in a setting, the balance among structured and unstructured activities, and the participatory properties of the setting (i.e., convenience, availability, accessibility, range of supports and resources). Affordance encompasses the property of adaptability, which involves balancing the need for structure and openness in activities and settings. Adaptable settings are intentional. They are purposefully designed to encourage structured interactions, and they do so in ways that allow children to exercise personal power by encouraging them to modify their settings and activities in ways that accommodate their own developmental and activity-related needs.

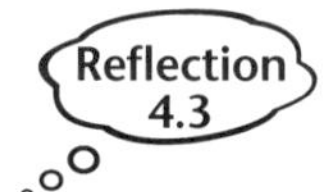

Groups as Positive Places of Shared Meaning and Social Identity

Community-based programs are social systems and contexts that have the power to either enhance or diminish a developing child's sense of personal and social identity. An example of an identity-enhancing social context is the Special Gifts Theater (SGT) created in 2000 by Susan B. Field. SGT is a community-based creative drama and arts program for children and teens with disabilities. Since its inception, SGT has created 19 productions, each involving approximately 55 children and youth with special needs (Ciukaj, Suarez-Balcazar, & Field, 2009). Over time, SGT has become an organized world of meaning and a place of positive shared social identities for children with disabilities and their families. Not only does SGT enable participants' personal growth, it also works to break down stereotypes about disabilities within the community at large.

For more information, visit www.specialgiftstheatre.com.

Social Cohesion

Social cohesion is the attitudinal, behavioral, and communal glue that brings people in society together through relationships with people, families, and organizations (Mattessich, Monsey, & Roy, 1997). As a key attribute of child- and youth-friendly places, social cohesion is a complex, multifaceted construct that differs depending on whether one is referring to cities, neighborhoods, places, or a particular social group (Turok, Kearns, Flint, McKenzie, & Abbotts, 2006).

In this section, we focus on four basic tenets of place-level social cohesion: passive relationships, active relationships, inclusion, and equality (Turok et al., 2006). *Passive social relationships* refers to tolerance and respect for other people. Such qualities are important for fostering a sense of personal safety and security. *Active relationships* refers to positive social interactions and dynamic networks between children, youth, and families and their local communities. These webs of connections are potential resources for places because they offer people and organizations mutual support, information, and trust (Turok et al., 2006).

Active relationships also provide children with opportunities to strengthen or develop supportive social relationships with competent, caring adults and chances to form strong social bonds and friendships. Within the intimate bondings of significant relationships, children and youth experience the freedom, safety, and acceptance necessary to express themselves fully and to openly explore thoughts, ideas, meanings, and new activities. Intimate relationships provide children and youth with occasions to experience the joys of companionship and to know themselves more fully (Moustakas, 1995). Readers can use the ideas presented in Reflection 4.3 to help think about ways to put these concepts into practice.

Social inclusion and equality are also elements of place-level social cohesion. *Social inclusion* is the extent to which children and youth are integrated into the daily rhythm of mainstream activities and community life, including the institutions and settings in which these occur. It includes a child's or youth's sense of belonging and the strength of the shared experiences, identities, and values between peers and adults of different backgrounds and abilities. Last, *social equality* refers to the degree of equity in access to opportunities and material circumstances, such as health or quality of life or future life chances (Turok et al., 2006).

Activities and Experiences

Ongoing participation in personally relevant and developmentally nutritive activities is central to a child's or youth's physical and psychosocial development (Halfon & Hochstein, 2002; Keating & Hertzman, 1999). However, not all activity participation contributes equally to a child's or youth's sense of happiness, fulfillment, or identity formation (Coatsworth et al., 2006). For example, some activities are more self-defining than others, meaning they are more strongly representative of whom the child or youth is or would like to become (Coatsworth et al., 2005). Other activities, such as passive leisure pursuits (e.g., television viewing), are not as influential in contributing to a child's or youth's sense of meaning, purpose, and direction in life (Waterman, 1993). Still, common pastimes such as playing cards and video games, which are not necessarily identity forming (Coatsworth et al., 2006), can provide flow experiences, which are indicative of high intrinsic motivation and a sense of personal control (Nakamura & Csikszentmihalyi, 2002). Research has suggested (Coatsworth et al., 2006; Eyles & Williams, 2008) that the subjective experience of activity participation mediates, in part, the relationship between activities and well-being. Places, therefore, that invite and support engagement in personally relevant activities and experiences serve an important function by providing place-based opportunities for positive developmental experiences to occur.

What, then, are the properties of positive place-based activities and experiences? They include opportunities for personal expressiveness (Waterman, 1993), decision making, and choice (Dunst, Bruder, et al., 2001). They include activity involvement that is challenging, interesting, and enjoyable (Hunter & Csikszentmihalyi, 2003) and that fits with a youngster's developmental needs, motivational beliefs, values, and goals (Eccles & Wigfield, 2002). Positive place-based activities and experiences support involvement and membership in ways that promote personal responsibility and autonomy and foster a sense of growth, self-awareness, and spirituality (Lerner & Benson, 2003). Readers can use the resources presented in Reflection 4.4 to help explore ways to incorporate these concepts into practice.

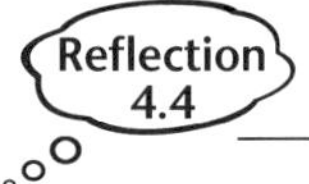

A Clinic in the Trees

How might you expand your practice to include activity-based therapy in children's everyday environments? This expansion may perhaps take the form of collaborations with an existing after-school program or the development of a summer day camp for children with special needs. Here are two program examples for you to consider:

- The Occupational Therapy Sensory Integration Summer Day Camp is a full-day summer camp for children who receive occupational therapy for sensory integration issues, including children with Asperger syndrome, with attention deficit hyperactivity disorder, and on the autism spectrum, ages 5 to 11. The camp Web site reads, "Every day begins at the playground. The playground looks like an OT clinic in the trees. There are multiple zip lines, rope swings, tire swings, slide tubes, platforms, and cargo nets . . . all built into the trees of a beautiful wooded area." Camp activities include music therapy, dance therapy, yoga, fishing, hiking, biking, water activities, and other movement-based activities.
- The Outdoor Sensory Adventures program is an adjunct to treatment for children receiving therapy for sensory integration issues. The aim is to provide children with opportunities to develop skills and abilities in challenging outdoor settings while carefully considering their sensory processing concerns and motor-planning difficulties. Outdoor adventures are designed to provide children with challenging yet successful outdoor experiences.

For more information, visit http://claywhite.us/osa.html

Engaging Versus Marginalizing Environments

Environments are experienced differently by different children and youth, and they have varying effects on children's sense of engagement or marginalization. *Psychological engagement* refers to a sense of absorption in an activity, setting, or both. *Marginalization* is the social process of being relegated to an unimportant or powerless position within a society or group. For example, children and youth with disabilities may be materially and socially marginalized as the result of inaccessible built environments, stigmatizing attitudes, and social arrangements that limit their engagement and inclusion in many aspects of life (Gibson, Young, Upshur, & McKeever, 2007). Many of these children and youth feel extremely isolated by physical barriers and exclusionary behaviors and attitudes (Baker & Donelly, 2001; Davis & Watson, 2001). Even when they are physically included in an activity setting, many are not engaged in activities in a meaningful way (King, Petrenchik, Law, & Hurley, 2009; Perlman, 2007).

Social inclusion implies opportunity for meaningful engagement in activity, which occurs when an individual derives a sense of fulfillment from activity, feels connected to others (a sense of belonging), or derives understanding of the self or his or her abilities (King, 2004; Raphael, Brown, Renwick, & Rootman, 1996). Processes of relationship (support) and opportunities are implied in the concept of inclusion, as well as in a psychosocial and spiritual perspective concerned with the meaning of activity engagement.

Not all environments or settings are equal in terms of inviting or encouraging children and youth to become actively engaged. Some environments foster a sense of place, and others do not (Wilson, 1997). When a setting provides limited opportunities for engagement and inclusion, children's potential for meaningful participation is also limited. Occupational therapists need to understand the nature of the conditions that make some children and youth engaged and happy with the places in which they live and play while others feel marginalized from their communities (Chawla, 2002a). Therapists also need to understand the processes underlying place experiences that encourage children to actively engage (Wilson, 1997) and grow into fully realized people (Lynch, 1981).

Environmental Transactions and Growth-Enhancing Experiences

Relatively little is known about the ways in which the developmental benefits of participation accrue or are realized (Ben-Arieh & Ofir, 2002). Little work has been done to differentiate the processes or experiences by which positive changes occur (Eccles & Templeton, 2002). To facilitate understanding and guide future research, we have developed a Developmental Health Model that considers the nature of the relationships among environmental qualities and growth-enhancing experiences (Figure 4.2). This conceptual model has been informed by various literatures, including research on environmental qualities, the developmental benefits of activity participation, and quality of experience. The model links environmental qualities of potential importance to psychological engagement and to developmental benefits, through processes of choice (intrinsic motivation), support, and opportunity (King et al., 2009).

Figure 4.2 depicts constructs considered to be important in the derivation of positive benefits from activity participation, embedded within contextual features of

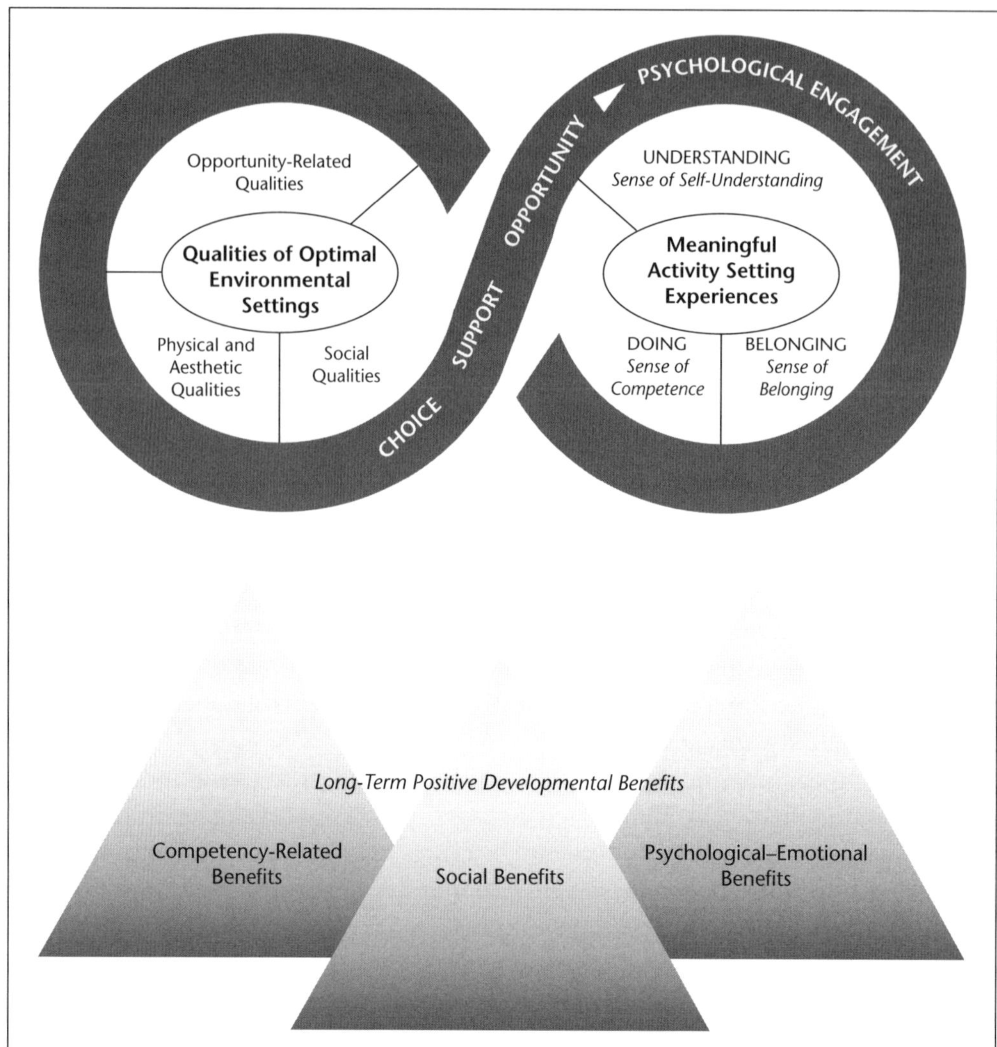

Figure 4.2. A developmental health model of the relationships between environmental qualities and growth-enhancing experiences. The left side of the model incorporates the primary qualities of optimal environmental settings, and the right side of the model represents aspects of psychological engagement (King et al., 2009), which includes meaningful activity-specific experiences that arise through the operation of three opportunity-related mechanisms: doing, belonging, and understanding (King, 2004).

optimal environments (Eccles & Templeton, 2002). These qualities provide opportunities for growth-enhancing or positive developmental experiences to occur and include physical safety, comfort, and an appropriate degree of structure; positive physical and aesthetic qualities (e.g., freedom of movement, lack of noise); positive social qualities (e.g., presence of supportive people); and positive aspects of place (e.g., opportunities for seclusion, exploration, belonging, skill development, creative expression; Chawla, 2002b; NRC & IOM, 2004).

The right side of the model is based on work by King (2004; King et al., 2009). *Psychological engagement in activity* refers to a sense of absorption characterized by deep concentration and involvement, arising through processes of choice (intrinsic motivation), support, and opportunity. The perception of choice is considered to be crucial for there to be intrinsic motivation to engage in an available activity. The processes of intrinsic motivation, combined with opportunities and supports afforded by the activity setting (Greeno, 1998), lead to psychological engagement.

Meaningful activity-specific experiences, then, arise through the operation of three opportunity-related mechanisms (i.e., doing, belonging, understanding; King, 2004). These mechanisms reflect engagement with the activity (leading to a sense of competence when the activity is challenging yet commensurate with skills), engagement with co-participants (leading to a sense of belonging), and connection of the activity to the self (leading to a sense of self-awareness and self-understanding). Longer-term positive developmental benefits include competency-related benefits (i.e., skill development, physical benefits, academic–educational benefits); social benefits (relationship-based benefits, civic benefits); and psychological–emotional benefits (i.e., enhanced self-efficacy and self-confidence, heightened self-worth, heightened sense of identity and self-concept).

This model is informed by research on the benefits of participation in organized, out-of-school activities for typically developing children and youth, which indicates that organized activities are especially important and potent contexts for development, with wide-ranging benefits that include social skills, self-esteem, and the formation of self-concept and identity (Beauvais, 2001; Eccles & Barber, 1999); self-efficacy and self-determination (Catalano, Berglund, Ryan, Lonczak, & Hawkins, 1999); enhanced competencies, such as initiative (Larson, 2000); and enhanced academic, physical, social, psychological, and civic development outcomes (Mahoney, Harris, & Eccles, 2006; Mahoney, Larson, Eccles, & Lord, 2005; Peck, Roeser, Zarrett, & Eccles, 2008).

The model is also informed by work in occupational therapy indicating that expending effort and being committed to an activity leads to identity building, sense of purpose, and meaning in life (Christiansen, 1999). Moreover, research on the learning opportunities afforded by natural environments has indicated the importance of (1) children's interests, choice, and environmental adaptations and supports; (2) learning opportunities afforded to young children with disabilities in family, community, and preschool activity settings (Dunst, Bruder, et al., 2001; Dunst, Trivette, Humphries, Raab, & Roper, 2001); (3) activity settings that provide natural opportunities for children to learn social roles, cultural goals and values, and socially adaptive skills (Childress, 2004; Dunst, Trivette, et al., 2001; Humphry, 2002); and (4) interest-based participation in everyday family and community activities (Raab, 2005). Last, research on the quality of experience has indicated the importance of a person-centered approach for determining the value of leisure (Brown, Frankel, & Fennell, 1991; Lloyd & Auld, 2002) and points to a relationship between structured leisure activities and optimal experience, or *flow* (Csikszentmihalyi, 1997; Delle Fave & Bassi, 2003; Delle Fave & Massimini, 2003).

Many literatures support the idea that meaning in everyday life results from active engagements or commitments to goals that help people feel connected, mobilize their activities and efforts, and contribute to their understanding of themselves and the world (King, 2004). Participation in everyday places offers children opportunities that go beyond competence development by allowing them to experience a sense of belonging to a group or community and to develop a sense of who they are as individuals, which are essential to mental health.

Summary

This chapter provided an integrated view of positive development, participation, and environments. It included a discussion of participation in everyday places and activities as pathways to positive development, and it emphasized the importance of viewing participation developmentally, contextually, and thematically. Positive development has been defined as positive behaviors that meet the developmental tasks of developing competence, confidence, character, and connections and making contributions. Youth's overall patterns of participation and behaviors are important for determining which direction their developmental pathway is taking—toward vulnerability and illness or toward positive development.

It is not enough to consider environments in strictly functional terms—as barriers to and enablers of participation that are devoid of personal attributions of meaning. What is needed is a view of environments as intertwined aspects of mutually defining physical and social settings, imbued with subjective perceptions of meaning, that influence and are influenced by participation. The meaning of participation is derived in part from the forms and qualities of these integrated settings and from the sense a child or youth makes of the actions and experiences that emerge, transpire, and regenerate within them. This conceptualization makes room for the symbolic meaning of participation, and it counterbalances the idea that activity performance is synonymous with participation with a weightier understanding of participation as braided strands of storied, place-based actions and experiences that are ripe with personal and shared meanings.

Participation in everyday places offers children opportunities for competence development, and it allows them to experience a sense of belonging to a group or community and to develop a sense of who they are as individuals. Places that offer safety and comfort, environmental affordances, social cohesion, and a range of activities and experiences support a child's development by providing opportunities for doing, for belonging, and for understanding themselves and others. Ideally, the meaning that children and youth make of their direct engagements with people, places, and activities helps them feel connected to one another and to a larger life purpose, motivates and organizes their activities and efforts, and contributes to their understanding of themselves and the world.

References

Agnes, M. (Ed.). (2000). *Webster's new world college dictionary.* Foster City, CA: IDG Books Worldwide.

Albrecht, G. L., & Devlieger, P. J. (1999). The disability paradox: High quality of life against all odds. *Social Science and Medicine, 48,* 977–988.

Altman, I., & Low, S. M. (1992). *Place attachment.* New York: Plenum Press.

American Occupational Therapy Association. (2008). Occupational therapy practice framework: Domain and process (2nd ed.). *American Journal of Occupational Therapy, 62,* 625–683.

Baker, K., & Donelly, M. (2001). The social experiences of children with disability and the influence of the environment: A framework for intervention. *Disability and Society, 16,* 71–85.

Bandura, A. (1997a). Developmental analysis of self-efficacy. In A. Bandura (Ed.), *The exercise of control* (pp. 162–211). New York: W. H. Freeman.

Bandura, A. (1997b). *Self-efficacy: The exercise of control.* New York: W. H. Freeman.

Bandura, A., & Locke, E. A. (2003). Negative self-efficacy and goal effects revisited. *Journal of Applied Psychology, 88*(1), 87–99.

Barker, R. (1968). *Ecological psychology: Concepts and methods for studying the environment of human behavior.* Stanford, CA: Stanford University Press.

Bazyk, S., & Bazyk, J. (2009). Meaning of occupation-based groups for low-income urban youths attending after-school care. *American Journal of Occupational Therapy, 63,* 69–80.

Beauvais, C. (2001). *Literature review on learning through recreation.* Ottawa, ON: Canadian Policy Research Networks.

Becker, C. (1992). *Living and relating: An introduction to phenomenology.* Newbury Park, CA: Sage.

Ben-Arieh, A., & Ofir, A. (2002). Time for (more) time-use studies: Studying the daily activities of children. *Childhood, 9*(2), 225–248.

Bloom, S. L. (2005). Introduction to special section. Creating sanctuary for kids: Helping children to heal from violence. *Therapeutic Community, 26*(1), 57–63.

Bronfenbrenner, U. (1979). *The ecology of human development: Experiments by nature and design.* Cambridge, MA: Harvard University Press.

Bronfenbrenner, U. (1999). Environments in developmental perspective: Theoretical and operational models. In S. L. Friedman & T. D. Wachs (Eds.), *Measuring environment across the life span: Emerging methods and concepts* (pp. 3–30). Washington, DC: American Psychological Association.

Brown, B. G., Frankel, G., & Fennell, M. (1991). Happiness through leisure: The impact of type of leisure activity, age, gender and leisure satisfaction on psychological wellbeing. *Journal of Applied Recreational Research, 16,* 368–392.

Canter, D. (1977). *The psychology of place.* New York: St. Martin's Press.

Canter, D. (1997). The facets of place. In G. T. Moore & R. W. Marans (Eds.), *Advances in environment, behavior, and design. Volume 4: Towards the integration of theory, methods, research and utilization* (pp. 109–148). New York: Plenum.

Canter, D. (2000) Seven assumptions for an investigative environmental psychology. In S. Wapner, J. Demick, T. Yamamoto, & H. Minami (Eds.), *Theoretical perspectives in environment–behavior research: Underlying assumptions, research problems, and methodologies* (pp. 191–206). New York: Plenum

Cassidy, T. (1997). *Environmental psychology: Behaviour and experience in context.* London: Psychology Press.

Catalano, R. F., Berglund, M. L., Ryan, J. A. M., Lonczak, H. S., & Hawkins, J. D. (1999). *Positive youth development in the United States: Research findings on evaluations of the positive youth development programs.* New York: Carnegie Corporation.

Chawla, L. (1992). Childhood place attachments. In I. Altman & S. Low (Eds.), *Place attachment* (pp. 63–86). New York: Plenum Press.

Chawla, L. (Ed.). (2002a). *Growing up in an urbanising world.* London: Earthscan.

Chawla, L. (2002b). Toward better cities for children and youth. In L. Chawla (Ed.), *Growing up in an urbanising world* (pp. 219–241). London: Earthscan.

Childress, D. C. (2004). Special instruction and natural environments: Best practices in early intervention. *Infants and Young Children, 17*(2), 162–170.

Christiansen, C. H. (1999). Defining lives: Occupation as identity: An essay on competence, coherence, and the creation of meaning (Eleanor Clarke Slagle Lecture). *American Journal of Occupational Therapy, 53,* 547–558.

Cirlot, J. E. (1971). Introduction. In *A dictonary of symbols* (2nd ed., pp. xi–lv). New York: Philosophical Library.

Ciukaj, M., Suarez-Balcazar, Y., & Field, S. B. (2009). Incorporating creative drama into the lives of children with disabilities. *OT Practice, 14,* 19–23.

Clark, F., Ennevor, B. L., & Richardson, P. L. (1996). A grounded theory of techniques for occupational storytelling and occupational story making. In R. Zemke & F. Clark (Eds.), *Occupational science: The evolving discipline* (pp. 373–392). Philadelphia: F. A. Davis.

Coatsworth, J. D., Palen, L., & Sharp, E. H. (2006). Self-defining activities, expressive identity, adolescent wellness. *Applied Developmental Science, 10*(3), 157–170.

Coatsworth, J. D., Sharp, E. H., Palen, L., Darling, N., Cumsille, P., & Marta, M. (2005). Exploring adolescent self-defining leisure activities and identity experiences across three countries. *International Journal of Behavioral Development, 29,* 361–370.

Cobb, E. (1969). The ecology of imagination in childhood. In P. Shepard & D. McKinley (Eds.), *The subversive science* (pp. 122–132). Boston: Houghton Mifflin.

Connell, J. P., Gambone, M. A., & Smith, T. J. (2000). Youth development in community settings: Challeges to our field and our approach. In *Youth development: Issues, challenges and directions* (pp. 281–300). Philadelphia: Public/Private Ventures.

Csikszentmihalyi, M. (1997). *Finding flow: The psychology of engagement with everyday life.* New York: Basic Books.

Csikszentmihalyi, M., & Rathunde, K. (1998). The development of the person: An experiential perspective on the ontogenesis of psychological complexity. In R. M. Lerner (Ed.), *Handbook of child psychology. Theoretical models of human development* (5th ed., Vol. 1, pp. 635–684). New York: John Wiley.

Davis, J. M., & Watson, N. (2001). Where are the children's experiences? Analyzing social and cultural exclusion in "special" and "mainstream" schools. *Disability and Society, 16*(5), 671–687.

Delle Fave, A., & Bassi, M. (2003). Italian adolescents and leisure: The role of engagement and optimal experience. In S. Verma & R. Larson (Eds.), *Examining adolescent leisure time across cultures: Developmental opportunities and risks.* (New Directions in Child and Adolescent Development Series, Vol. 99, pp. 79–94). San Francisco: Jossey Bass.

Delle Fave, A., & Massimini, F. (2003). Optimal experience in work and leisure among teachers and physicians: Individual and bio-cultural implications. *Leisure Studies, 22*(4), 323–342.

Dunkley, C. M. (2009). A therapeutic taskscape: Theorizing place-making, discipline and care at a camp for troubled youth. *Health Place, 15*(1), 88–96.

Dunn, W. W. (1997). The impact of sensory processing abilities on the daily lives of young children and families: A conceptual model. *Infants and Young Children, 9*(4), 23–25.

Dunn, W. W. (2001). The sensations of everyday life: Empirical, theoretical, and pragmatic considerations. *American Journal of Occupational Therapy, 55,* 608–620.

Dunn, W., Brown, C., & McGuigan, A. (1994). Ecology of human performance: A framework for considering the effects of context. *American Journal of Occupational Therapy, 48,* 595–607.

Dunst, C. J., Bruder, M. B., Trivette, C. M., Hamby, D., Raab, M., & McLean, M. (2001). Characteristics and consequences of everyday natural learning opportunities. *Topics for Early Childhood Special Education, 21*(2), 68–92.

Dunst, C. J., Trivette, C. M., Humphries, T., Raab, M., & Roper, N. (2001). Contrasting approaches to natural learning environment interventions. *Infants and Young Children, 14*(2), 48–63.

Eccles, J. S., & Barber, B. L. (1999). Student council, volunteering, basketball, or marching band: What kind of extracurricular involvement matters? *Journal of Adolescent Research, 14*(1), 10–43.

Eccles, J., & Gootman, J. A. (Eds.). (2002). *Community programs to promote youth development.* Washington, DC: National Academies Press.

Eccles, J. S., & Templeton, J. (2002). Extracurricular and other after-school activities for youth. *Review of Research in Education, 26,* 113–180.

Eccles, J. S., & Wigfield, A. (2002). Motivational beliefs, values, and goals. *Annual Review of Psychology, 53*(1), 109–132.

Ellemers, N., Spears, R., & Doosje, B. (2002). Self and social identity. *Annual Review of Psychology, 53*(1), 161–186.

Eyles, J., & Williams, A. (Eds.). (2008). *Sense of place, health and quality of life.* Hampshire, England: Ashgate.

Fidler, G. S. (1999). Messages of the environment. In G. S. Fidler & B. P. Velde (Eds.), *Activities: Reality and symbol* (pp. 154–162). Thorofare, NJ: Slack.

Fidler, G. S., & Fidler, J. W. (1978). Doing and becoming: Purposeful action and self-actualization. *American Journal of Occupational Therapy, 32,* 14–22.

Fidler, G. S., & Velde, B. P. (Eds.). (1999). *Activities: Reality and symbol.* Thorofare, NJ: Slack.

Freysinger, V. J. (2006). Play in the context of life-span human development In D. P. Fromberg & D. Bergen (Eds.), *Play from birth to twelve and beyond: Contexts, perspectives, and meanings* (2nd ed., pp. 53–62). New York: Routledge.

Gibson, B. E., Young, N. L., Upshur, R. E. G., & McKeever, P. (2007). Men on the margin: A Bourdieusian examination of living into adulthood with muscular dystrophy. *Social Science and Medicine, 65,* 505–517.

Gibson, J. J. (1979). *The ecological approach to visual perception.* Boston: Houghton Mifflin.

Gitlin, L. N., Corcoran, M., & Leinmiller-Eckhardt, S. (1995). Understanding the family perspective: An ethnographic framework for providing occupational therapy in the home. *American Journal of Occupational Therapy, 49,* 802–809.

Greeno, J. G. (1998). The situativity of knowing, learning, and research. *American Psychologist, 53*(1), 5–26.

Hagedorn, R. (1995). *Occupational therapy: Perspectives and processes.* Edinburgh: Churchill Livingstone.

Halfon, N., & Hochstein, M. (2002). Life course health development: An integrated framework for developing health, policy, and research. *Milbank Quarterly, 80*(3), 433–479.

Hasselkus, B. R. (2002). Space and place: Sources of meaning in occupation. In B. Hasselkus (Ed.), *The meaning of everyday occupation* (pp. 26–38). Thorofare, NJ: Slack.

Heah, T., Case, T., McGuire, B., & Law, M. (2007). Successful participation: The lived experience among children with disabilities. *Canadian Journal of Occupational Therapy, 74,* 38–47.

Heft, H. (1997). The relevance of Gibson's ecological approach for environment–behavior studies. In G. T. Moore & R. W. Marans (Eds.), *Advances in environment, behavior, and design* (Vol. 4, pp. 71–108). New York: Plenum.

Hemmingsson, H., & Borell, L. (2002). Environmental barriers in mainstream schools. *Child Care and Health Development, 28*(1), 57–63.

Hertzman, C. (2002). *Leave no child behind: Social exclusion and child development.* Toronto: Laidlaw Foundation.

Holloway, S. L., & Valentine, G. (2000). Children's geographies and the new social studies of childhood. In S. L. Holloway & G. Valentine (Eds.), *Children's geographies: Playing, living, learning* (pp. 1–28). London: Routledge.

Humphry, R. (2002). Young children's occupations: Explicating the dynamics of developmental processes. *American Journal of Occupational Therapy, 56,* 171–179.

Hunter, J. P., & Csikszentmihalyi, M. (2003). The positive psychology of interested adolescents. *Journal of Youth and Adolescence, 32*(1), 27–35.

Imms, C. (2008). Children with cerebral palsy participate: A review of the literature. *Disability and Rehabilitation, 30*(24), 1867–1884.

Jung, C. G. (1956). *Symbols of transformation: Collected Works of C. G. Jung* (Vol. 5). London: Princeton University Press.

Kaplan, R. M. (2002). Quality of life: An outcomes perspective. *Archives of Physical Medicine and Rehabilitation, 83*(Suppl. 2), S44–S50.

Keating, D. P. (2000). Social capital and developmental health: Making the connection. *Developmental and Behavioral Pediatrics, 21*(1), 50–52.

Keating, D. P., & Hertzman, C. (Eds.). (1999). *Developmental health and the wealth of nations: Social, biological, and educational dynamics.* New York: Guilford Press.

King, G. A. (2004). The meaning of life experiences: Application of a meta-model to rehabilitation sciences and services. *American Journal of Orthopsychiatry, 74*(1), 72–88.

King, G., Petrenchik, T., DeWit, D., McDougall, J., Hurley, P., & Law, M. (2010). Out-of-school time activity participation profiles of children with physical disabilities: A cluster analysis. *Child: Care, Health, Development, 36,* 726–741.

King, G., Petrenchik, T., Law, M., & Hurley, P. (2009). The enjoyment of formal and informal recreation and leisure activities: A comparison of school-aged children with and without physical disabilities. *International Journal of Disability, Development, and Education, 56*(2), 109–130.

Korpela, K. (2002). Children's environment. In R. B. Bechtel & A. Churchman (Eds.), *Handbook of environmental psychology* (pp. 363–393). New York: John Wiley.

Lampinen J., & Tham K. (2003). Interaction with the physical environment in everyday occupation after stroke: A phenomenological study of persons with visuospatial agnosia. *Scandinavian Journal of Occupational Therapy, 10*(4), 147–156.

Larson, R. W. (2000). Toward a psychology of positive youth development. *American Psychologist, 55*(1), 170–183.

Law, M. (1991). The environment: A focus for occupational therapy. *Canadian Journal of Occupational Therapy, 58,* 171–179.

Law, M., Cooper, B., Strong, S., Stewart, D., Ribgy, P., & Letts, L. (1996). The person–environment–occupation model: A transactive approach to occupational performance. *Canadian Journal of Occupational Therapy, 63*(1), 9–23.

Law, M., Petrenchik, T., King, G., & Hurley, P. (2007). Perceived barriers to recreational, community, and school participation for children and youth with physical disabilities. *Archives of Physical Medicine and Rehabilitation, 88,* 1636–1642.

Law, M., Petrenchik, T., Ziviani, J., & King, G. (2006). Participation of children in school and community. In S. Rodger & J. Ziviani (Eds.), *Occupational therapy with children: Understanding children's occupations and enabling participation.* Oxford, England: Blackwell.

Lawlor, K., Mihaylov, S. I., Welsh, B., Jarvis, S., & Colver, A. (2006). A qualitative study of the physical, social and attitudinal environments influencing the participation of children with cerebral palsy in northeast England. *Pediatric Rehabilitation, 9,* 219–228.

Lawlor, M. C. (2003). The significance of being occupied: The social construction of childhood occupations. *American Journal of Occupational Therapy, 57,* 424–434.

Lerner, R. M., & Benson, P. I. (Eds.). (2003). *Developmental assests and asset-building communities.* New York: Kluwer Academic.

Lerner, R. M., Jacobs, F., & Wertlieb, D. (Eds.). (2005). *Applied developmental science: An advanced textbook.* Thousand Oaks, CA: Sage.

Lerner, R. M., Taylor, C. S., & Von Eye, A. (Eds.). (2002). *Pathways to positive development among diverse youth: New direction for youth development* (Vol. 95). San Francisco: Jossey-Bass.

Letts, L., Rigby, P., & Stewart, D. (Eds.). (2003). *Using environments to enable occupational performance.* Thorofare, NJ: Slack.

Levy-Leboyer, C. (1982). *Psychology and environment.* Thousand Oaks, CA: Sage.

Lloyd, K. M., & Auld, C. J. (2002). The role of leisure in determining quality of life: Issues of content and measurement. *Social Indicators Research, 57,* 43–71.

Louv, R. (2005). *Last child in the woods : Saving our children from nature-deficit disorder.* Chapel Hill, NC: Algonquin Books of Chapel Hill.

Lynch, K. (1981). *A theory of good city form.* Cambridge, MA: MIT Press.

Mahoney, J. L., Harris, A. L., & Eccles, J. S. (2006). Organized activity participation, positive youth development, and the over-scheduling hypothesis. *Social Policy Report, 20*(4), 1–31.

Mahoney, J. L., Larson, R. W., & Eccles, J. S. (Eds.). (2005). *Organized activities as contexts of development: Extracurricular activities, after-school and community programs.* Mahwah, NJ: Lawrence Erlbaum.

Mahoney, J. L., Larson, R. W., Eccles, J. S., & Lord, H. (2005). Organized activities as developmental contexts for children and adolescents. In J. L. Mahoney, R. W. Larson, & J. S. Eccles (Eds.), *Organized activities as contexts of development: Extracurricular activities, after-school and community programs* (pp. 3–22). Mahwah, NJ: Lawrence Erlbaum.

Mancini, M. C., Coster, W., Trombly, C., & Heeren, T. (2000). Predicting elementary school participation in children with disabilities. *Archives of Physical Medicine and Rehabilitation, 81,* 339–347.

Masten, A. S. (2001). Ordinary magic: Resilience processes in development. *American Psychologist, 56,* 227–238.

Mattessich, P., Monsey, B., & Roy, C. (1997). *Community building: What makes it work—A review of factors influencing successful community building.* Saint Paul, MN: Amherst H. Wilder Foundation.

McGuire, M. (1983). Words of power: Personal empowerment and healing. *Culture, Medicine, and Psychiatry, 7*(3), 221–240.

Moustakas, C. (1995). *Being-in, being-for, being-with.* Northvale, NJ: Jason Aronson.

Nabhan, G. P., & Trimble, S. (1994). *The geography of childhood: Why children need wild places.* Boston: Beacon Press.

Nakamura, J., & Csikszentmihalyi, M. (2002). The concept of flow. In S. J. Lopez & C. R. Snyder (Eds.), *Handbook of positive psychology* (pp. 89–105). London: Oxford University Press.

National Research Council, & Institute of Medicine. (2004). *Children's health, the nation's wealth: Assessing and improving child health.* Washington, DC: National Academies Press.

Norman, D. A. (1988). *The psychology of everyday things.* New York: Basic Books.

Nyman, A., & Lund, M. L. (2007). Influences of the social environment on engagement in occupations: The experience of persons with rheumatoid arthritis. *Scandinavian Journal of Occupational Therapy, 14*(1), 63–72.

Peck, S. C., Roeser, R. W., Zarrett, N., & Eccles, J. S. (2008). Exploring the roles of extracurricular activity quantity and quality in the educational resilience of vulnerable adolescents: Variable- and pattern-centered approaches. *Journal of Social Issues, 64*(1), 135–156.

Perlman, D. (2007). The best of times, the worst of times: The place of close relationships in psychology and our daily lives. *Canadian Psychology, 48*(1), 7–18.

Peterson, C. (Ed.). (2004, January). Positive development: Realizing the potential of youth. *Annals of the American Academy of Political and Social Science, 591,* 6–12.

Pittman, K., Tolman, J., & Yohalem, N. (2005). Developing a comprehensive agenda for the out-of-school hours: Lessons and challenges across cities. In J. Mahoney, R. Larson, & J. Eccles (Eds.), *Organized activities as contexts of development: Extracurricular activities, after-school and community programs* (pp. 375–397). Mahwah, NJ: Lawrence Erlbaum.

Poulsen, A. A., Ziviani, J. M., Cuskelly, M., & Smith, R. (2007). Boys with developmental coordination disorder: Loneliness and team sports participation. *American Journal of Occupational Therapy, 61,* 451–563.

Proshansky, H. M., Ittelson, W. H., & Rivlin, L. G. (1976). *Environmental psychology: People and their physical settings* (2nd ed.). Oxford, England: Holt, Rinehart & Winston.

Raab, M. (2005). Interest-based child participation in everyday learning activities. *CASEinPoint, 1*(2).

Raphael, D., Brown, I., Renwick, R., & Rootman, I. (1996). Assessing the quality of life of persons with developmental disabilities: Description of a new model, measuring instruments, and initial findings. *International Journal of Disability, Development and Education, 43*(1), 25–42.

Rigby, L., & Letts, L. (2003). Environmnet and occupational performance: Theoretical considerations. In L. Letts, P. Rigby, & D. Stewart (Eds.), (2003). *Using environments to enable occupational performance* (pp. 17–32). Thorofare, NJ: Slack

Rosenbaum, P., & Stewart, D. (2007). Perspectives on transitions: Rethinking services for children and youth with developmental disabilities. *Archive of Physical Medicine and Rehabilitation, 88*(8), 1080–1082.

Schenker, R., Coster, W., & Parush, S. (2006). Personal assistance, adaptations, and participation in students with cerebral palsy mainstreamed in elementary schools. *Disability and Rehabilitation, 28,* 1061–1069.

Searles, H. F. (1960). *The non-human environment in normal development and in schizophrenia.* New York: International Universities Press

Sobel, D. (2002). *Children's special places: Exploring the role of forts, dens, and bush houses in middle childhood.* Tucson, AZ: Zephyr Press.

Stark, S. L., & Sanford, J. A. (2005). Environmental enablers and their impact on occupational performance. In C. H. Christiansen, C. M. Baum, & J. Bass-Haugen (Eds.), *Occupational therapy: Performance, participation, and well-being* (3rd ed., pp. 300–336). Thorofare, NJ: Slack.

Tanta, K. J., Deitz, J. C., White, O., & Billingsley, F. (2005). The effects of peer-play level on initiations and responses of preschool children with delayed play skills. *American Journal of Occupational Therapy, 59,* 437–445.

Thelen, E., & Smith, L. B. (1997). Dynamic systems theories. In R. M. Lerner (Ed.), *Handbook of child psychology: Vol. 1. Theoretical models of human development* (5th ed., pp. 563–633). New York: Wiley.

Thurman, H. (1980). *With head and heart: The autobiography of Howard Thurman.* New York: Harcourt.

Townsend, E., Stanton, S., Law, M., Polatajko, H., Baptiste, S., Thompson-Franson, T., et al. (1997). *Enabling occupation: An occupational therapy perspective.* Ottawa, Ontario: Canadian Association of Occupational Therapists.

Tuan, Y. F. (1977). *Space and place: The perspective of experience.* Minneapolis: University of Minnesota.

Turok, I., Kearns, A., Flint, J., McKenzie, C., & Abbotts, J. (2006). *State of English cities: Social cohesion.* Retrieved July 10, 2009, from www.communities.gov.uk/documents/citiesandregions/pdf/154184.pdf

Vik, K., Lilja, M., & Nygard, L. (2007). The influence of the environment on participation subsequent to rehabilitation as experienced by elderly people in Norway. *Scandinavian Journal of Occupational Therapy, 14*(2), 86–95.

Wachs, T. D. (1999). Celebrating complexity: Conceptulization and assessment of the environment. In S. L. Friedman & T. D. Wachs (Eds.), *Measuring environment across the life span: Emerging methods and concepts* (pp. 357–392). Washington, DC: American Psychological Association.

Wapner, S., & Demick, J. (1998). Developmental analysis: A holistic, developmental, systems-oriented perspective. In R. M. Lerner (Ed.), *Handbook of child psychology: Theoretical models of human development* (5th ed., Vol. 1, pp. 761–806). New York: John Wiley.

Waterman, A. S. (1993). Finding something to do or someone to be: A eudaimonist's perspective on identity formation In J. Kroger (Ed.), *Discussion on ego identity* (pp. 147–167). Hillsdale, NJ: Lawrence Erlbaum.

Weisner, T. S. (Ed.). (2005). *Discovering successful pathways in children's development: Mixed methods in the study of childhood and family life.* Chicago: University of Chicago Press.

Wilcock, A. A. (2006). *An occupational perspective of health* (2nd ed.). Thorofare, NJ: Slack.

Wilson, R. (1997). A sense of place. *Early Childhood Education Journal, 24*(3), 191–194.

Wiseman, J. O., Davis, J. A., & Polatajko, H. J. (2005). Occupational development: Toward an understanding of children's doing. *Journal of Occupational Science, 12,* 26–35.

World Health Organization. (1999). *Creating an environment for emotional and social well-being.* (WHO information series on school health, Document 10). Retrieved July 1, 2009, from www.who.int/school_youth_health/media/en/sch_childfriendly_03.pdf

World Health Organization. (2001). *International classification of functioning, disability and health.* Geneva: Author.

CHAPTER 5

Development and Implementation of Groups to Foster Social Participation and Mental Health

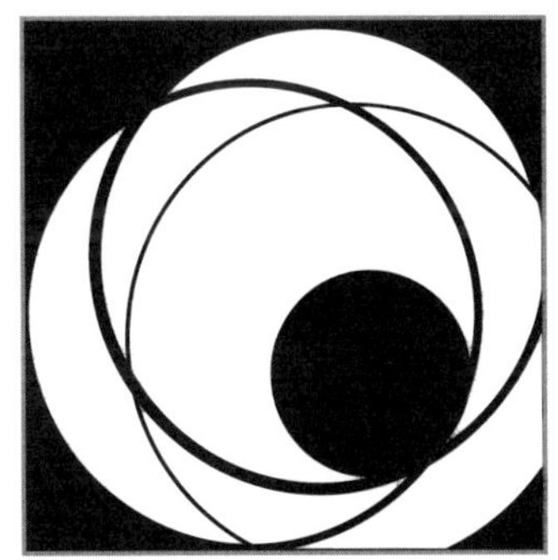

Laurette Olson, PhD, OTR/L

Learning Objectives

After reading this material and completing the examination, readers will be able to

- Recognize the curative factors of therapeutic groups;
- Delineate occupation-based groups from therapeutic groups offered by other professionals and describe their unique benefits;
- Identify factors critical to fostering group process;
- Recognize the stages of group development and when cohesiveness is likely to occur;
- Identify the benefits of group planning, routines, adapting activities, and reflecting on group sessions; and
- Identify examples of family-based occupational therapy groups.

Several compelling reasons exist for all occupational therapists to develop skills in leading occupation-based groups. Social interaction and participation are a central part of most human occupations. Most skills have little meaning if they are not useful in family, school, work, or community activities. Although solitary activity is important throughout the lifespan for developing one's sense of self, it is most often preparation for or a retreat from group participation in the occupations of one's life. In addition to the need for engaging with others for survival, healthy children and adults have a need and a hunger for the companionship of others. Positive social bonds and relationships provide children and adults alike with feelings of safety and security in spite of the demands, stresses, and uncertainty of life. The presence and support of others help a person maintain emotional regulation in the face of challenges. In general, human relationships are at the center of most occupations and give meaning to them. Consequently, group interventions should be a key element of any occupation-based intervention program.

Although some skills are best learned with the individual instruction and facilitation of an occupational therapist, many skills must be further developed or practiced in a social environment. Skills that are not developed or practiced in a social environment may limit clients' full use of skills gained in occupational therapy. Group interventions provide a microcosm of the everyday human experience of using skills with or in the presence of others. Participating in group tasks increases the demands on one's attentional skills and capacities for social problem solving. The presence of and engagement with peers in a group can enhance a person's functioning through the increased number of opportunities for learning and social support.

Dramatic shifts in U.S. public policy for public education give added impetus for pediatric occupational therapists and all related service personnel to make group interventions a central part of their intervention methods. *Response to intervention* (RtI; American Occupational Therapy Association, 2007; Cahill, 2007; Howard, 2009), a three-tiered approach to addressing children's educational needs in general education, requires that educators carefully monitor the academic progress of all children and implement evidence-based interventions when children do not make expected gains. This requirement has shifted the focus of related service personnel from attending to the needs of at-risk or failing students to considering the progress of all children. Beginning interventions occur in classrooms in large-group and small-group formats. Professionals monitor children's learning, proactively identify additional needs of some children, and implement progressively more specialized interventions until all students make sufficient progress. Although RtI makes high demands on professionals for outcomes and for collaboration, it also provides new productive opportunities for service provision. Professionals can now collaborate with teachers to support all children. Related service personnel such as occupational therapists do not need to wait until children fail before becoming part of children's educational team and committed to mental health promotion.

It is now recognized that for children's positive educational participation and outcomes, professionals must address the social and emotional development of all students in addition to academic interventions (Coolahan, Fantuzzo, Mendez, & McDermott, 2000; Raver, 2002; Zins, Weissberg, Wang, & Walberg, 2004). Educational professionals are redefining their social–emotional interventions to align with the RtI model (Clark & Brennan, 2009; Van Velsor, 2009). Occupational therapists have much to add to the collaborative group work occurring in public education to develop all children's skills for social participation in schools, community, and families.

This chapter focuses on defining the value of and critical factors to be considered in developing occupation-based groups to support children's social participation. It also provides examples of groups. Although spontaneous groups often happen when multiple therapists treat individual children in the same space, the chapter does not address those situations. Although such spontaneously occurring groups serve important needs for children, they are typically not purposefully defined or developed as group intervention. Each therapist remains focused on intervening with the particular child for whom he or she provides individual service.

Value of Groups

Therapeutic groups are active and interactive and unfold over time. Group leaders optimally create positive group climates in which members develop common ground, mutual trust, and the ability to support and collaborate with each other. Therapeutic groups are different from *group instruction settings,* in which members are focused on the instructor and the content to be learned. Although relationships may be acknowledged in group instruction, they are not central to the change process, as they are in therapeutic groups.

Yalom (1995) identified the following *curative factors* present in therapeutic groups that support growth and healing:

- Opportunities for imparting information
- Experiencing hope and a sense of universality of the human condition
- Altruism
- Family reenactment
- Imitating the behavior of others
- Interpersonal learning
- Developing techniques for socialization, cohesion, and catharsis.

Those curative factors have been recognized, studied, and supported by research and clinical practice in a variety of fields and with clients of all ages (Falk-Kessler, Momich, & Perel, 1991; Kivlighan & Holmes, 1991; Shechtman, 2007). Having peers who experience similar concerns and struggles provides a sense of universality, and observing others confront challenges can provide a sense of hope and opportunity for learning (Gettinger & Guetschow, 1998; Mishna & Muskat, 2004). Groups are interactive, and members have the opportunity to experiment with different ways of interacting with each other and to share and receive feedback about the effectiveness of their socialization strategies. Members also have opportunities to help one another at various points in a group's process. Having the opportunity to help another has a positive impact on one's self-efficacy and self-perception.

Research related to the positive development of children and youth has strongly supported the use of family and peer group interventions in all professions. After completing a longitudinal study of children's coping from birth through adolescence, Murphy (1962) concluded that the most critical factor in children's development of the capacity to confront challenges in their everyday activities was their mother's enjoyment of the children. Larson (2007) and Larson, Hansen, and Walker (2005) highlighted the power of youth groups for developing teamwork, civic responsibility, self-determination, and initiative. Although those studies referred to community groups, they are very applicable to occupational therapists seeking to develop effective occupation-based group interventions. These researchers' work has suggested that youth are most likely to develop these key skills for successful occupational functioning in group settings in which youth are confronted with opportunities to work with other youth in authentically solving real-life problems together. The essence of occupational therapy intervention is developing clients' strengths and supporting their positive development for life roles and activities.

Occupation-based groups provide unique services that meet children's developmental needs. They also enhance and complement the work done by other professionals. Although a social worker or psychologist may use a group to assess social or emotional deficits interfering with children's physical or mental health at home or school or to help children share their intrapsychic concerns related to family and peer challenges, an occupational therapist provides a group environment in which families or children learn and practice performance skills and patterns in meaningful, occupationally related activities. Occupation-based groups for supporting children's social participation in school, home, and community contexts have been broadly described in the occupational therapy literature (Barnes, Vogel, Beck, Schoenfeld, & Owen, 2008; Bazyk & Bazyk, 2009; Olson, 2010; Olson, Heaney, & Soppas-Hoffman, 1989; Schultz, 2003).

Defining Occupation-Based Groups

Occupation-based groups provide a setting in which children have the opportunity to explore and participate in meaningful activities related to their life roles, including student, friend, community member, and family member. In these groups, children develop skills, productive habits, and performance patterns that will support their ability to successfully cope with the social and task demands in their daily occupations.

A leader of an occupation-based group considers ways to make necessary occupational tasks meaningful to group participants. Because emotion is powerful in engaging or disengaging people from occupation-based activities, the therapist assesses group members' emotional response to the group tasks. People are attracted to particular activities in response to their own developmental or emotional needs at a particular time (Olson, 1997). This attraction increases attention and motivation for participation. Positive emotion also enhances a person's sense of self-efficacy, which in turn supports engagement in activities. Negative emotion reduces one's feelings of self-efficacy and results in decreased activity engagement (Bandura, Caprara, Barbaranelli, Gerbino, & Pastorelli, 2003). A therapist works to enhance group members' positive mood in relation to the occupation-based tasks before them.

Occupation-based groups are ideal environments for children to develop *self-efficacy*—a belief in their own abilities to succeed in particular occupation-based tasks—because they provide opportunity to incorporate all four pathways that Bandura (1995) identified. He stated that mastery experiences, vicarious experiences, social persuasion, and physiological and emotional state regulation are key to a person's developing self-efficacy. Research has suggested that self-regulation capacities are the central underpinning for social competence (Augustyniak, Brooks, Rinaldo, Bogner, & Hodges, 2009; Posner & Rothbart, 2000). Some occupation-based groups are specifically focused on developing skills for self-regulation (Williams & Shellenberger, 1996); others include such activities at the beginning of group sessions to prepare members for engagement (Olson, Colangelo, & Shaw, 2009).

Sabel (2007) suggested that yoga be considered as a preparatory activity before occupation-based tasks. Mollo (2008) made a connection between the heavy work, deep breathing, and demands for increased attention in yoga and an occupational therapist's focus on promoting sensory modulation. The studies of Peck, Kehle, Bray, and Theodore (2005) and Stueck and Gloeckner (2005) supported the use of yoga in promoting children's attention and self-regulation.

Mastery experiences are at the basis of developing skills for occupational participation. Occupation-based groups provide the opportunity to learn through observing others' strategies and task performance. A leader can also create an environment in which children are persuaded by feedback from others that they are competent.

Occupation-based groups best fit under the general categories of psychoeducational groups and task groups. In a *psychoeducational group,* a leader first teaches members new skills or strategies for managing specific life and developmental challenges. Leaders share information and then provide opportunities to practice skills within the safety of the group. Group members then explore how the skills are relevant to their lives beyond the group and work to transfer the skills to their everyday occupations. Delucia-Waack (2006) described how a leader might develop and lead psychoeducational groups for children and adolescents. When pediatric occupational therapists apply psychoeducational group approaches, they most often use them in small-group settings over a series of sessions. The most common psychoeducational groups that occupational therapists lead are ones for teaching parents or children skills for sensory modulation (Barnes et al., 2008; Williams & Shellenberger, 1996). Williamson and Dorman (2002) also demonstrated the use of some psychoeducational methods for teaching children skills needed for social participation. Occupational therapists may use a psychoeducational group as preparation for children's participation in a task-oriented group or may integrate psychoeducational group methods into an occupation-based group design as did Williamson and Dorman (2002).

In *task groups,* leaders engage members in working on individual or group tasks. Members have the opportunity to build the social skills and cognitive and physical skills required for task participation. In a school-based setting, occupational therapists may lead groups in which children create games to build physical or academic skills while building skills for social participation. In one after-school program in which the author worked, for example, an occupational therapy student used children's interest in learning and creating new marble games as a vehicle for creating a group to enhance children's social competence. To successfully design and play new marble games, the boys needed to share ideas, listen to one another, work together to explore activity ideas, and resolve social and activity challenges. Two other occupational therapy students engaged third-grade boys in developing their task and coping skills through the building and flying of increasingly complex paper airplanes. Both groups used the power of a group approach to intervention by creating a group structure and process that allowed members to experience many of the curative factors of groups discussed earlier in this chapter.

Task groups have been a key method of occupational therapy intervention since the inception of occupational therapy (Howe & Schwartzberg, 2001; Mosey, 1986; Posthuma, 2002). Occupational therapy theorists and researchers have emphasized the importance of active doing for self-efficacy and for mental health. Within an occupational therapy task group, members change through the process of reflecting on their own task performance and in how they collaborate with others on a task. The profession has developed a theory and practice for task groups that is more complex than the definition of *task group practice* provided by the Association for Group Specialists: "a group specialization featuring the application of group dynamic principles and processes such as collaborative group problem solving, team building, program development consultation, and/or system change strategies" (Wilson, 1998, p. 181). Wilson (1998) also stated that it is not likely that task group work would enhance individual life competencies or enhance individual adaptation to life problems and that it is very unlikely that task groups would remediate individual mental, emotional, and or behavioral dysfunction. Many occupational therapy authors have described different strategies for leading task groups depending on the level of development and functioning of the group's members or the group's purpose (Cole, 2005; Howe & Schwartzberg, 2001; Mosey, 1986).

Olson et al. (2009) shared an analysis of a few school-based task groups in the middle stages of group development. Each group session lasted 30 minutes. Group sessions were videotaped so that the authors could analyze time use in addition to the flow of content and process of sessions. Time in each session was divided among planning and setup, activity implementation, and activity cleanup and reflection. Two groups were described in which four to five elementary school children planned how they would play together on sensorimotor equipment. Each session began with a brief orientation to the task, which was then followed by the leaders facilitating children's planning of how to set up equipment collaboratively. The children then negotiated turn taking and cooperative play before they played on the equipment. As the children played, the leaders continued to facilitate social problem solving. The children reflected on what occurred in the sessions as they put away the equipment at the end of the sessions. Although playtime was an essential part of each group session, children spent more of the group session planning what they would play and how they would play together than in actually playing. In successful group sessions, leaders carefully guided the children through successful planning. At times, leaders took on authoritative roles when children were stuck and not likely to resolve their differences. In this way, children always had the experience of successfully carrying out their mutually planned activity.

Recently, Van Velsor (2009) recommended that school counselors consider task groups in the repertoire of services that they provide in public education. She suggested that they collaborate with teachers in leading children's task groups so that important academic tasks are accomplished while children learn important social–emotional skills for teamwork. She highlighted that in this way, group leaders have the opportunity to guide students in managing their own behavior and to teach them productive ways to interact with others in their everyday activities and environment. Her recommendations are important for all related service personnel to consider, and they resonate with accepted occupation-based group practice.

Additional examples of occupation-based groups are described in Boxes 5.1, 5.2, and 5.3. The examples are derived from the author's experiences in supervising graduate occupational therapy students in leading occupation-based groups for children and adolescents in an urban after-school program that serves children and families in a low-income community as well as after-school and evening groups in residential treatment centers for children and youth diagnosed with psychiatric disorders.

Box 5.1. Group Protocol for an After-School Occupation-Based Group

Group Name

Community Builders

Purpose

To increase children's understanding of community and simple ways that members make a positive difference and to design a collective project to make a difference in their school community.

Goals

Members will

1. Recognize the importance of community;
2. Explore how small groups of children have contributed to their school;
3. Choose a community project that they can do together;
4. Demonstrate behaviors indicative of teamwork in completing the community project; and
5. Demonstrate initiative individually and collectively in the process of carrying out their group project.

Method

Over the course of 8 sessions and through discussion, Internet exploration, and the creation of collages, the leaders will engage a group of 5 children in understanding how children have positively affected their community. The leaders will then guide children in designing and implementing their own project within their capabilities and group resources and time allotment.

—Based on the work of Ridvan Foxhall, OTS, and Bettina Franco, OTS

Box 5.2. Healthy Chefs

Learning about healthy eating and how to prepare healthy meals promotes health and meets occupation-based needs of many children and youth. Below is an example of part of a protocol that Mercy College graduate occupational therapy students have led for children and youth at residential treatment centers serving youth with psychiatric disorders.

Healthy Chefs: A girls' group at a residential facility for children with psychiatric disorders.

Purpose

In this psychoeducational cooking group, members will learn about healthy eating and menu planning and how to prepare nutritious, quick snacks or desserts. They will also have the opportunity to practice teamwork with their cottage mates.

Goals

Members will

1. Identify healthy foods that group members also enjoy;
2. Learn how to make favorite snacks and desserts healthier by substituting healthy ingredients for high-calorie, low-nutrition ingredients; and
3. Share responsibilities in meal preparation.

Method

Psychoeducational group methods will be used to teach members about healthy eating. Leaders will prepare easy-to-read handouts with key information about the nutrition–cooking topic and possible recipes of the week. Leaders will lead a short discussion about the topic at the start of each session; members will participate in brief games and activities related to the topic to foster engagement and learning. Members will then choose one of the recipes listed in the handout. They will work together to prepare the chosen snack, appetizer, or dessert.

Box 5.3. The Community Makeover: A Group for Young Adolescent Boys at a Residential Center for Youth With Psychiatric Disorders

Below is a portion of the group protocol developed by two Mercy College graduate occupational therapy students (Waiming Cheung, now a school-based occupational therapist in New York City, and Glenn Yedowitz, now an occupational therapist in a children's hospital in Westchester County in New York) designed to facilitate a group of adolescent boys in developing capacities for positive and productive engagement with each other. The protocol is followed by excerpts from the content and process notes of this group (see Boxes 5.5 and 5.6). The excerpts illustrate the type of interactions that a group leader might experience with a group of adolescent boys in the transitional and middle stages of group development. The excerpts, written by Cheung, are provided to help readers better understand and appreciate the nature of the stages of group development and how they affect the function of an occupation-based group.

Purpose

To facilitate group members' working together to beautify their common living space. To promote adolescents' ownership and pride in their mutual living space.

Goals

Members will develop skills for teamwork, group problem solving, and successful task completion, including sustained attention to a task, organization, and frustration tolerance.

Method

Members will participate in a series of group activities designed first to help them identify common physical factors in a community room that would support their feeling comfortable and relaxed and support their participation in activities in the room. Members will choose and carry out room decoration projects with the guidance of the group leaders.

Considering Group Process and Group Development in Occupation-Based Groups

In addition to considering what content and what teaching–learning strategies are most likely to be effective for skill development with the particular group of children, a leader must have competency in applying theory and research related to therapeutic group process. The latter is often overlooked in favor of an emphasis on group content. How a leader structures, manages, and guides members' interactions with each other can enhance or hinder a group member's ability to learn skills or to successfully complete tasks. When a leader does not consider how to mobilize group process to support all members engaging in the group, he or she may be inadvertently drawn into using a group format to provide individual interventions for group members. The power of group process to support learning and development is thus lost; at best, the intervention for each child is weak compared with an individual intervention. Leaders are also more likely to be distracted from the group content and process by individual members' demands for attention, thus compromising the group experience for all members.

To successfully mobilize group process in the interest of group members' experiencing the curative factors of groups, group leaders must create a positive group climate. A *group climate* is the emotional environment among group members and leaders. It is the comfort level among members and the openness of members to the group experience. After analyzing studies of children's groups, Kivlighan and Tarrant (2001) found that a critical factor in whether group members experience positive therapeutic outcomes from a group is whether leaders build warm and supportive group climates.

Building a positive group climate requires that group leaders be cognizant of the stages of group development so that they prepare content that is consistent with group members' readiness to participate in the group and guide group members' interactions in ways that engage them with one another. Groups, like any dynamic, living entity, develop over time and through stages (Shechtman, 2007). Each stage has developmental challenges related to social participation that need to be mastered; with each success, groups become more complex and more able to meet members' emotional and learning needs. If a group is unsuccessful in mastering the social participation challenges as it develops, then the group becomes stuck and unproductive. Children's developmental levels related to social participation affect how complex the demands for group interaction can be at any stage and how a group develops over the course of time.

Stages of Groups

The stages of groups have been given different names by different theorists, but they can be generally classified as beginning, transition, middle, and ending stages (Jacobs, Masson, & Harvill, 2009). The stages reflect group members' collective emotional experience as they develop from individual members who are unsure and uncomfortable forming as a group to members who are united in working together toward their group goals. In occupation-based groups, activities and tasks facilitate members identifying their commonalities and differences in the process of a group developing its identity. They also provide common ground for learning key strategies for social participation, including turn taking, compromise, and negotiation.

Tuckman (1965) named the stages of groups *forming, storming, norming,* and *performing.* In the forming stages, members orient to the group and other members and figure out the group's purpose. Members may be unsure about remaining in the group; hence, Bion (1959) named this stage *flight.* Beginning stage activities focus on members getting to know and becoming comfortable with other members and the leader. Activities orient members to the group's purpose and highlight the group's norms, rules, and structure to promote positive habits and routines for the group members' interactions. The leader monitors the intensity of the activity and the emotions provoked by participating in a particular group activity as members have not yet developed trust in the leader or one another. An example of establishing group rules is described in Box 5.4.

In the transition stage of a group's development, members adjust to group norms introduced by leaders and establish norms particular to the group. *Norms* are the typical ways in which members behave in a group, and they may support or hinder interaction. Compared with rules, norms are typically unspoken. A leader should reflect on the developing norms of behavior within the group, reinforce norms that are supportive of the group's functioning, and work to extinguish developing norms that are counterproductive to the group's goals. The storming stage is also considered part of the transition stage. Members may experience some dissatisfaction or conflict as they get to know and work with other group members. Conflict is expected as members begin to behave with each other in authentic ways and express their

Box 5.4. Working With Children to Establish Group Rules

Below is an excerpt from the group process notes of two Mercy College graduate occupational therapy students. In it, they share their understanding of the impact of their having collaborated with the children participating in their occupation-based group in establishing group rules as a written agreement.

> Having the rules as a written agreement clearly written out on poster board and hanging it up during group sessions is working out well. Children remind each other of their agreement, and as leaders, we were pleased to hear them use words like *respectful,* which was on the poster. The process of painting their hands was fun for them. They especially enjoyed signing their names by using their hand stamps. We sensed pride and ownership among them when they signed their names.
>
> This is in contrast to the last session, in which all group members were speaking at once. We feel that by creating an official agreement about behavior in group, we have established ground rules that the children are open to following. The children were better at taking turns and allowing each other to complete their sentences.

—Ridvan Foxhall, OTS, and Bettina DiFranco, OTS

individual desires and needs relative to group's tasks. Optimally, group leaders guide group members to recognize the differences in their own needs and desires and those of other members and then to develop strategies for compromise and negotiation in the interest of working toward group goals. Leaders use their knowledge of group members' chronological and developmental ages to help members manage their differences and conflicting needs and desires. This stage of group development should be recognized as expected and an opportunity for growth for group members. Group leaders can become frustrated at this stage and prematurely assess a group as unsuccessful or group members as not being ready for a group experience.

Cohesiveness develops in the middle stage of a group—Tuckman's (1965) stage of performing or Bion's (1959) stage of uniting. Yalom (1995) defined *cohesiveness* as a member's experiencing interpersonal warmth and comfort and feeling that they belong, can trust, and are trusted. Members seek to be kind and supportive of one another. Competition is minimized in the interest of collaboration. Cohesion is measured by the degree of involvement of all group members in group activities and how accepted and supported individual members feel within the group (Harpine, 2008). Although all people have this need, children have a high need for acceptance by and belonging to a group and are particularly sensitive to rejection and disrespect.

Cohesion provides the critical element that allows groups to have their most potent and positive impact on members. Members are comfortable with the group structure and with each other, responsive to group norms and rules, and able to use a group for skill building and learning. Leaders should make full use of the opportunities for member growth at this stage by designing occupation-based group activities that challenge members' capabilities for success and that encourage members to explore new ways of thinking, interacting, and behaving.

Once goals have been achieved, leaders help group members end a particular group experience in a way that recognizes what members have achieved together. Leaders also help group members recognize the interpersonal bonds that have developed among members over the learning process, task process, or both. Children need closure to each group experience, even in environments in which the children may participate in a series of occupation-based groups with many of the same children over the course of one or more school years. Learning to give closure to group experiences in a positive way is an important life skill. For example, children who participated in a group designed to help them learn skills for playing with peers shared a special snack in their last group session while the leaders helped them reflect on the events of the group that were most meaningful to them. Leaders facilitated children's articulation of how they would apply the strategies used in the group to play interactions in the classroom and at recess. An example of group transition that occurred in a Community Makeover Group is depicted in Boxes 5.3, 5.5, and 5.6.

Group Leader Skills

Developing one's leadership skills is instrumental to a therapist achieving desired outcomes from a group intervention. Kivlighan and Tartrant (2001) found that a positive leadership style that included providing positive structure was associated with more cohesive and engaged child group climates. Members feel more positive about group leaders who structure discussion, solicit elaboration of material, and give feedback about group member behaviors.

Although Karver, Handelsman, Fields, and Bickman (2005) reported that little research has examined how therapists use themselves as intervention tools (i.e., therapeutic use of self), they identified some useful guidelines for group leaders to consider as they reflect on themselves as a therapeutic factor within a group. A leader's interpersonal skills influence how group members interact with each other; therefore, leaders should carefully reflect on their own skills and how they use or develop their own interpersonal skills. Therapists leading all groups should be knowledgeable and skillful in applying the person-centered therapist behaviors identified by psychologist Carl Rogers (1951), such as empathy, warmth, and active listening, because they are central for positive outcomes in all group approaches. These leadership behaviors are described and applied to group leadership in most textbooks about group development (Cole, 2005; Jacobs, Masson, & Harvill, 2009; Posthuma, 2002). To be credible and trusted, therapists need to work to present themselves clearly, understandably, confidently, and directly within group members' receptive language capabilities.

Planning Children's Occupation-Based Groups

Occupational therapists plan groups to meet different needs in a variety of school-based contexts. A therapist could develop a psychoeducational occupation-based group to increase children's awareness of their sensory preferences and needs and to guide them in exploring sensory-based strategies to support their remaining alert and attentive to their school-based tasks. Another therapist may collaborate with a school psychologist to develop a task group to address the social and task development needs of a group of children with dyspraxia. The leaders could design a group in which children are guided in the planning and building of a Halloween haunted house while providing them with the opportunity to learn how to work

Box 5.5. Community Makeover Group in Transition Stage of Group Development

Content

Group members decided where to hang shelves and then hung them throughout their community room.

Process

Numerous displays of hostility and conflicts occur among members. Some of the more vocal members tend to be argumentative and seem to disagree to preserve their comfort zones. The activity today of hanging shelves almost demands some sort of interaction among the people doing it. However, both teams of two members largely participated in this activity in a parallel manner. I rarely saw team members speak or engage each other. They did engage with me, and in some ways, I served as a conduit for members communicating with each other. One of the boys was initially reluctant to accept help from me because he seemed to feel that offerings of help from me made him childlike. He kept insisting that he knew what to do. Only when I allowed him the freedom to try and fail did he allow me to help him. One boy told me that his team member was having a hard time putting in a screw and suggested that he might need another screwdriver. That he vocalized this to me as opposed to directly speaking to his activity partner was interesting. Another disappointing aspect of the group activity this week was that the most proficient group member just got up and walked out of the group when he completed his part of the task. He didn't offer help or assistance to others at all. I am very troubled by group members' lack of social regard for each other. They live in the same cottage but just don't seem to think highly of each other.

At the end of the activity, group members focused on how the shelves were not exactly level and that the height of some shelves from the floor wasn't right. Although I realize that it is healthy to have high expectations and standards, I was a bit deflated by the boys' inability to celebrate their successes and to feel pride in their accomplishment. However, as I was leaving the cottage, I saw a group member tell another cottage member how our group had hung up shelves for everyone and made the room look better. Even group leaders need hope instillation.

Reflection on Leadership

At this point, I feel that I am an autocratic leader. I feel that at this early stage of group development, the group is always on the verge of being out of control. I think that this style of leadership is necessary for the functioning of the group at this time. I am flexible at times during the group and encourage democracy when possible. I am hoping that I will exert a lesser degree of control as the group develops.

I must work to be less at the center of the tasks. Today, I was very focused on completing the task at hand. I was so concerned about hanging the shelves in the allotted time that I lost sight of my goals for the group, which is to promote teamwork and problem solving. When one of the students was struggling with putting in a screw, instead of taking the time to guide the activity, I did the activity for him. I need to find the balance between completing the tasks and the boys gaining from the therapeutic process of working together on the group task. I also need to promote more communication and interaction among group members.

—Waiming Cheung, MS, OTR

collaboratively with one another. In a preschool setting, an occupational therapist and speech therapist may develop a sensorimotor play group in which children build foundational sensorimotor skills while also working with each other on their communication skills. Another therapist may have the opportunity to develop task groups to facilitate a group of children through the process of planning and carrying out productive recess activities. In yet another school, occupational therapists could develop after-school task groups to promote the play and leisure or independent living skill development of children with disabilities. Developing a group protocol and session plans will support group leaders' success in implementing any of these groups. When group leaders do not take the time to fully plan a group intervention, the curative factors of group process may not be optimally mobilized, and children are less likely to gain skills for social participation or optimally increase their sense

Box 5.6. Content and Process of the Community Makeover Group in the Middle Stage of Group Development

Content

Our activity was to have the boys decorate a lampshade that would be hung from the ceiling in the room that we are beautifying. Each boy was given a lampshade and then asked to sit around the group table and share paints, markers, magazines, scissors, and so forth.

Process

The group activity proceeded in a parallel manner. Last week, the boys were unable to share supplies; this week, they were able to work out how to share supplies. Although each boy had his own lampshade to decorate, group members made efforts to engage each other about their lampshade designs on numerous occasions throughout the group session. This session was the first in which the boys were focused on following through on the activity from start to finish. After completing the painting and decorating of their lampshades, two members showed initiative by volunteering to start cleaning up the table. The other boys followed in turn, and members cleaned up as a team. The leaders assigned responsibility for hanging up the lampshades; all members accepted their assigned responsibility. After we hung up the lampshades, all of the boys demonstrated pride in what we accomplished as a group. We then asked each boy to state something they liked, disliked, and had learned so far through participating in the group. For once, the boys stated things that they liked and didn't focus on their dislikes.

One major factor that changed the dynamics of the group was a new group member who demonstrated positive social skills. He was encouraging to the other boys and allowed a younger peer to help him with his project when the other boy got frustrated.

—*Waiming Cheung, MS, OTR*

of self-efficacy and interest in participating in occupation-based activities that have been challenging to them.

A *group protocol* is a written articulation of the rationale, goals, basic group plan, and structure. It outlines all the basic features of a group, including its name, time and place, rationale, goals, methods, procedures, and outcome criteria. Along with organizing the potential leaders' thinking about a group, a group protocol is also helpful in articulating the group purpose and plans to other stakeholders so that they can support the group's implementation.

The writing of a group protocol structures leaders in carefully thinking about their group format. Most often, an occupational therapist will choose to lead or colead a psychoeducational or task group. (These group approaches have previously been described.) A therapist may decide that a task group is optimal for a group of children but that psychoeducational methods are necessary in the early stages of the group so that children learn basic skills to support their group participation. When children have poor capacity for behavior regulation, a therapist may devote initial sessions or the beginning of each session to teaching children strategies for physical regulation that can be incorporated into the beginning stages of each group session. See Boxes 5.1, 5.2, and 5.3 for examples.

After writing a protocol, a leader should write the first few session plans. *Session plans* describe the specific goals, activities, and sequence of events for particular group sessions. As leaders outline sessions, they have an opportunity to visualize and preview how particular sessions may play out. Leaders estimate time, supplies, and equipment needed; room and material setup; the flow of activities; and goals for each part of the session. Occupational therapy textbooks devoted to group interventions provide full discussions of protocols and session plans, along with examples (Cole, 2005; Schwartzberg, Howe, & Barnes, 2008).

Although session plans provide a concrete road map for a session, it is important that leaders always expect the unexpected and consider that plans might need to shift as a result of the children's needs at the time of the group. A clearly articulated group protocol and session plan support leaders by having the planning issues for sessions resolved. Leaders can then focus their attention and energies on carefully observing children's reactions to the group activities and other members and making adjustments in how the session plan is carried out in response to their understanding of group needs at a particular moment in time during a group session.

Before the first group session, leaders should consider the rules and norms that they envision are necessary to provide positive structure for the children identified as potential group members. The optimal way to establish rules with a group of children is to collaborate with them and to outline rules in children's own words. In this way, members take ownership of the rules and work to enforce them collaboratively with the leader. It is best to have a vision of optimal rules before the group, so that leaders can guide children in identifying many of these rules for group behavior while also listening to children's ideas.

Building in Routines to Support Social Participation

All successful group structures include routines that help group members make transitions to group sessions and between activities within a session. Routines allow group members to anticipate what will occur, are comforting, and stress executive function capacities less. Having a routine way of walking to a group room or reorganizing a classroom space with children for a group session is helpful. A "group box" may contain special supplies for group sessions. The leader or a member retrieves the box, and then members organize materials on the group table. The start of a group could be the sound of a chime or bell indicating time for a relaxation activity before engaging in the particular session activities.

Applying Activity Analysis to Group Planning

A core skill of occupational therapy is the ability to analyze activities and people's performance from different perspectives. When applying a psychoeducational group approach, leaders first decide what skill will be taught in a particular session and the best teaching–learning strategy for introducing the skill and guiding children in understanding and practicing its components. For example, a leader may teach children about how breathing affects how physically active or tense people feel and then teach children how to control their own breathing. After the initial instruction, the leader should consider how to make use of the small-group process to support learning and practice of the skill. Children should not only ask questions of leaders but also be guided in sharing their ideas with each other and in helping each other practice the new skill.

In a task group, leaders analyze the steps of the activity and then break it down into meaningful subtasks for individual members or cooperative subgroups. If group members are ready for the challenge, leaders should consider how they will share the steps of the task with group members so that the leader can facilitate the members identifying the subtasks that need to be accomplished on the road to task completion. Leaders should reflect on how they will guide the group process to support group problem solving, because this process uncovers differences among members and can be hindered by children's underlying social or cognitive deficits. With the executive functioning, social, motor planning, and coordination deficits of group members in mind, therapists analyze activities so that they may quietly incorporate strategies to support the functioning of individual members in the interest of productive group interaction and participation.

Children sometimes need preparatory activities at the start of each group to help them focus on their peers' social cues, or they may require modeling or cueing from therapists to help them observe and translate social messages throughout a group session so that a harmonious group process is maintained. Winner (2002, 2005), a speech pathologist, has written helpful books with activities that teach older children and adolescents with autism spectrum disorder how to read and respond to social cues. If group members have significant difficulty with social communication, leaders should consider task complexity. A decision must be made about the degree and number of challenges with which group members can cope.

Processing Group Events With Children

In any task group session, remember that if its outcome is not processed with group members, the opportunity for learning and growth may be lost. A discussion with children after a group activity can be brief, but it is important that group members have time to review and evaluate what occurred during the session. Jackson (2002) described a simple structure for having a discussion with children after an activity. His steps to summarize the discussion are *what, so what, now what,* and *summarize. What* refers to engaging children in describing what they actually did in a session. In the *so-what* component of the discussion, leaders guide children in sharing their thoughts about what they learned and what the value the activity might have to them and to others. In the *now-what* component, children and leaders then consider how children might apply what they learned to their interactions in school and at home. Finally, in the *summarize* component, the leader summarizes or helps children summarize what they discussed in the final moments of a group session.

Reflecting on Group Sessions as a Leader

Throughout the process of leading a group from session to session, it is important for leaders to take time to consider what is happening in group sessions and how each group is developing. Reflection is a key group leader habit that supports positive group outcomes. It provides leaders with the space and time to consider what is going well so that those elements of a particular group are included or further developed in subsequent sessions. It also provides structure for leaders to consider environmental, task, or interpersonal group factors that may need to be adjusted to support children gaining what leaders originally planned for them to gain. Through the process of reflecting on group sessions, group leaders become more aware of their opportunities and choices in their interventions, and they become more directed and confident in their decision making.

As a group progresses, leaders should note the ratio between their focus on the content of the group and the process among group members. Both are important. If content is overemphasized, children's relationships with each other or the leader may not be maximized for social learning; if leaders overfocus on process, they may lose children's cooperation and interest. Children optimally participate in occupation-based groups for the opportunities to be involved in engaging, interesting, meaningful tasks and activities. Keep in mind that, similar to occupational activities in one's daily life, planning typically requires more time than does the implementation of an activity. As group leaders plan group sessions, they should engage children in the planning of activities, as developmentally appropriate. See Boxes 5.5 and 5.6 for examples of group leader reflections.

Family-Based Occupation-Based Groups

Occupation-based groups also provide an optimal environment for promoting parents' and children's engagement with each other for health promotion, for prevention in families at risk for occupational dysfunction, and for families that include a child with a disability.

All parents need support and an opportunity to learn how to optimally understand what their children need and how they might best meet their children's needs within the context of the needs of all family members and the family's particular cultural and socioeconomic setting. It has been suggested that intervention is best received at natural points of transition in a child's development (Hauser-Cram, Warfield, Shonkoff, & Krauss, 2001). It is a time when parents need to shift their parenting style in response to the changes in their children and in the environmental demands on their children and family. As a family adjusts to the birth and early development of a new baby, professionals have the opportunity to influence how parents understand their interactions with their infant and how they develop new habits, routines, and rituals to incorporate the infant into that family. As children enter peer groups and school, professionals have new opportunities to assist parents in thinking through how they might best respond and adjust family life in support of their children's changing needs. Adolescence and the youth's entry into middle school and high school again add new stresses and demands for adjustments in family interactions, routines, and rituals of daily living.

Occupational therapists can offer psychoeducational groups for parents that support their understanding of their children's sensorimotor development and how they might support this development within the context of daily parent–child co-occupations. An occupational therapist may provide a psychoeducational group program that helps parents think through how they might apply sensory modulation strategies for supporting all children's capacity to attend to and complete homework. A psychoeducational group's basic structure is enhanced by opportunities to practice occupationally related activities and obtain support in transferring those new behaviors and skills to a family's home environment. Occupational therapists have strong skills in understanding daily occupations and the influence of contexts on participation.

Olson, Martell, Nunez, and Rojas (2010) described the application of psychoeducational group methods to educating parents of children attending preschool classes at a Head Start program about their children's sensory processing developmental needs and how they might support their children's occupational participation at home and in school by considering their children's sensory diet. The group first allowed parents to learn and explore the concepts related to children's sensory diets with each other. Parents then had the opportunity to explore sensory diet activities and sensory play with their children within the group, which provided parents and children with the leaders' guidance and support and with peer models and support.

All communities have children whose emotional or sensory regulation is poorly developed and limits their productive occupational participation at home and in school and the community. Other children's motor awkwardness make it difficult for them to gain acceptance in peer groups and to fully explore play or participate in age-appropriate self-management activities at home. The socioeconomic stresses on some families may make it difficult for caregivers to focus sufficiently on their children's developmental needs. Occupational therapists can lead groups in school settings that support the occupational engagement of children at risk and their parents with each other. Olson et al. (1989) described a parent–child group that was embedded in a preschool setting and designed to engage parents of children at risk with their children in play. In the process, parents learned to shift their interaction style to support their children's engagement in joint activities.

A family that includes a child with a disability may have difficulty developing habits and routines that are supportive of the child while supporting other family members' functioning. Family occupation-based groups can offer children with disabilities and their families crucial opportunities to develop healthy habits, routines, and rituals that enhance the children's functioning and that of caregivers and siblings. Within the context of a family occupation-based group, families can learn how to adapt materials, task structure, or interactional approaches to include a child with disability in mutual family activities. A multifamily occupational-based group can provide parents and children with the camaraderie of other families experiencing similar challenges and the opportunity to learn from strategies applied by other families. Olson et al. (2010) described a model for developing parent–child groups for families with a child with disability. Refer to Box 5.7 for an example of parent–child groups and Box 5.8 for guidelines for parent–child activity groups.

Summary

Group interventions have long been a part of occupational therapy education and practice. This chapter has described the theory, practice, and research related to developing and leading occupation-based groups for children and adolescents. With the shifts in service delivery in public education, along with the increasing recognition of the central role of social–emotional learning in children's successful academic participation and performance, it is critical that occupational therapists consider how they might develop more occupation-based group interventions in school and community settings. If knowledge of group process and group development is integrated with the specialized content that pediatric occupational therapists offer in educational settings, occupational therapists will play central roles in collaborating with educators to integrate social–emotional interventions in public education for all children.

Box 5.7. Developing a Parent–Child Occupation-Based Group for an After-School Program

This example of a session plan for a family-based group was developed and implemented as part of a graduate "capstone" project in which three graduate occupational therapy students participated. Following the session plan, excerpts of the content and process notes are provided to illustrate how the session plan was implemented.

Group

Family Night

Session Title

Yoga for Self-Regulation

Rationale

Evidence has suggested that routine practice of simple yoga poses can increase children's physical regulation and ability to attend to tasks. Simple routines can easily be learned and incorporated into routines at home and in school. Practicing these routines is a way for parents and children to engage with each other in a positive, relaxing, and connected way. It is also supportive of the individual and collective functioning of all participating family members.

Session Goals

Parents and children will learn a few yoga poses to use before homework time to increase attention and focus.

Sequence of Activities for Session

1. Welcome parents and children to the group, and the leaders will help families find a spot in the room so that they can practice routines as a family (10 minutes).
2. Introduce the activity plan for the group and the rationale for incorporating yoga into daily family life (10 minutes).
3. Demonstrate and teach parents and children a few yoga poses for focusing attention, relaxation, and stress reduction (30 minutes).
4. Have group members move to the arts-and-crafts room. Leaders will lead table discussions about the yoga poses learned and how parents and children might use them in their daily lives (10 minutes).
5. Introduce the activity of making a poster of the yoga poses learned and practiced this evening (30 minutes).

Group Closure

Sharing of yoga posters; take pictures of families with their yoga posters as a memory of Family Night.

Excerpt From Yoga Practice Group Process

The more humorous and playful poses elicited some laughter from children and parents and thus acted as an ice breaker. Children intermittently asked their parents to help them lift their legs higher. Some children modeled for other children when they had difficulty with a pose. This modeling occurred spontaneously but was encouraged once it occurred because it increased group members' camaraderie. Music and aromatherapy lotions introduced in the session helped to set the tone during certain parts of the session.

Excerpt From Poster-Making Process

Parents and their children worked as teams parallel to other families. Roles were established in each family. For example, some children cut out pictures, and their parents glued them on the poster. In other families, all members simultaneously cut, pasted, and decorated their posters. The activity promoted conversation and laughter among certain families as they worked. Supplies were shared across families, and there were some interactions among different families. There were a few moments when some members of the group seemed hesitant about participating in the parent–child activity of making a yoga poster together and needed the guidance of a group leader to get started. They needed assistance in getting their materials organized or in figuring out how to get started on the project together. A few children lost interest over the course of the 30-minute activity and wandered around the room while their parents continued to work on the activity. A group leader redirected the children and helped them negotiate ways to reengage in the activity with their parents.

—Laurette Olson, PhD, OTR; Christina Francesconi, OTS; Kristina Mele, OTS; and Carola Gomes, OTS

Box 5.8. Guidelines for Parent–Child Activity Groups

These guidelines were developed by the author and are published in Olson (2006).

Purpose

To promote pleasurable and reciprocal interactions between parents and children in structured play.

Goals

1. Increase children's interest in and motivation for play by increasing their experience of their parents' interest and enjoyment of mutual play with them.
2. Increase parents' self-efficacy in managing and guiding their children's behavior in mutual activity.

Group Structure and Format

Parent–child activity groups are designed as task-oriented groups. Individual families work together on an open-ended construction project in the presence of other families. Group leaders introduce and guide families in making decisions and working together to create a project that is satisfying to its members in the process and in the end product.

Activity Characteristics

Open-ended projects that families can put their own stamp on; projects that are simple, are easy to understand, can be adjusted to each family's physical abilities and interactional style, and are within parents' capacities to engage and assist their child; and activities that inherently suggest the need for engagement of both parent and child.

Group Environment

Tables set up so that each parent–child dyad sits together and has space to manipulate materials together in front of them. Seating and table arrangement should make eye contact and interaction easy. Families are situated around a table so that they can easily observe and interact with other families as well.

The therapist should view the group space as a different environment in which parents' and children's routine ways of interacting can be shifted, and parents and children have the opportunity to explore new ways of being together and interacting through occupation-based activity.

Leader Role

1. Plan activities that are open ended and that can easily be graded to the interests and abilities of each parent–child dyad or triad.
2. Structure the group environment so that parents and children are focused and engaged in mutual activity.
3. Support positive engagement of parents and children with each other by assisting parents and children through the activity and interactional challenges.
4. Facilitate conversation and interaction across families sharing a table so that families have an opportunity to experience mutual support and have the opportunity to help and learn from one another.

References

American Occupational Therapy Association. (2007). *New resource: Response to intervention.* Retrieved January 11, 2010, from www.aota.org/Practitioners/PracticeAreas/Pediatrics/Highlights/40150.aspx

Augustyniak, K. M., Brooks, M., Rinaldo, V. J., Bogner, R., & Hodges, S. (2009). Emotional regulation: Considerations for school-based group interventions. *Journal for Specialists in Group Work, 34*(4), 326–350.

Bandura, A. (1995). Exercise of personal and collective efficacy in changing societies. In A. Bandura (Ed.), *Self-efficacy in changing societies* (pp. 1–45). New York: Cambridge University Press.

Bandura, A., Caprara, G. V., Barbaranelli, C., Gerbino, M., & Pastorelli, C. (2003). Role of affective self-regulatory efficacy on diverse spheres of functioning. *Child Development, 74*(3), 769–782.

Barnes, K. J., Vogel, K. A., Beck, A. J., Schoenfeld, H. B., & Owen, S. V. (2008). Self-regulation strategies of children with emotional disturbance. *Physical and Occupational Therapy in Pediatrics, 28*(4), 369–287.

Bayzk, S., & Bayzk, J. (2009). Meaning of occupation-based groups for low-income urban youth attending afterschool care. *American Journal of Occupational Therapy, 63,* 69–83.

Bion, W. R. (1959). *Experiences in groups.* New York: Basic Books.

Cahill, S. (2007). A perspective on response to intervention. *School System Special Interest Section Quarterly, 14*(3), 1–4.

Clark, M. A., & Brennan, J. C. (2009). School counselor inclusion: A collaborative model to provide academic and social–emotional support in classroom setting. *Journal of Counseling and Development, 87*(1), 6–11.

Cole, M. B. (2005). *Group dynamics in occupational therapy: The theoretical basis and practice application of group intervention* (3rd ed.). Thorofare, NJ: Slack.

Coolahan, K., Fantuzzo, J., Mendez, J., & McDermott, P. (2000). Preschool peer interactions and readiness to learn: Relationships between classroom peer play and learning behaviors and conduct. *Journal of Educational Psychology, 92,* 458–465.

DeLucia-Waack, J. L. (2006). *Leading psychoeducational groups for children and adolescents.* Thousand Oaks, CA: Sage.

Falk-Kessler, J., Momich, C., & Perel, S. (1991). Therapeutic factors in occupational therapy groups. *American Journal of Occupational Therapy, 45,* 59–66.

Gettinger, M., & Guetschow, K. W. (1998). Parent and parent/child groups for young children with disabilities. In K. C. Stoiber & T. R. Kratochwill (Eds.), *Handbook of group intervention for children and families* (pp. 345–360). Needham Heights, MA: Allyn & Bacon.

Harpine, E. C. (2008). *Group interventions in schools: Promoting mental health for at risk children and youth.* New York: Springer.

Hauser-Cram, P., Warfield, M. E., Shonkoff, J. P., & Krauss, M. W. (2001). Children with disabilities. *Monographs of the Society for Research in Child Development, 66*(3, Serial No. 266).

Howard, M. (2009). *RTI from all sides: What every teacher needs to know.* Portsmouth, NH: Heinemann.

Howe, M. C., & Schwartzberg, S. L. (2001). *A functional approach to group work in occupational therapy* (3rd ed.). Baltimore: Lippincott Williams & Wilkins.

Jackson, T. (2002). Why have a discussion? And four steps to a great discussion. In T. Jackson (Ed.), *Conducting group discussions with kids: A leader's guide for making activities meaningful* (pp. 7–24). Cedar City, UT: Active Learning Center.

Jacobs, E., Masson, R., & Harvill, R. (2009). *Group counseling: Strategies and skills* (6th ed.). Pacific Grove, CA: Brooks/Cole.

Karver, M. S., Handelsman, J. B., Fields, S., & Bickman, L. (2005). A theoretical model of common process factors in youth and family therapy. *Mental Health Services Research, 7*(1), 35–51.

Kivlighan, D. M., Jr., & Holmes, D. C. (1991). Endorsement of therapeutic factors as a function of stage of group development and participant interpersonal attitudes. *Journal of Counseling Psychology, 38,* 150–158.

Kivlighan, D. M., & Tarrant, J. M. (2001). Does group climate mediate the group leadership–group member outcome relationship? A test of Yalom's hypotheses about leadership priorities. *Group Dynamics: Theory, Research, and Practice, 5*(3), 220–234.

Larson, R. W. (2007). From "I" to "we": Development of the capacity for teamwork in youth programs. In R. K. Silbereisen & R. M. Lerner (Eds.), *Approaches to positive youth development* (pp. 277–292). Los Angeles: Sage.

Larson, R. W., Hansen, D., & Walker, K. (2005). Everybody's gotta give: Development of initiative and teamwork within a youth program. In J. L. Mahoney, R. W. Larson, & J. S. Eccles (Eds.), *Organized activities as contexts of development: Extracurricular activities, after-school and community programs* (pp. 159–183). Mahwah, NJ: Lawrence Erlbaum.

Mishna, F., & Muskat, B. (2004). I'm not the only one! Group therapy for older children and adolescents who have learning disabilities. *International Journal of Group Psychotherapy, 54*(4), 455–476.

Mollo, K. (2008). The use of Kripalu yoga to decrease sensory over-responsivity: A pilot study. *Sensory Integration Special Interest Section Quarterly, 31*(3), 1–4.

Mosey, A. C. (1986). *Psychosocial components of occupational therapy.* New York: Raven Press.

Murphy, L. (1962). *The widening world of childhood.* New York: Basic Books.

Olson, L. J. (1997). Sublimations of the grade school child. In J. D. Noshpitz, P. F. Kernberg, & J. R. Bemporad (Eds.), *Handbook of child and adolescent psychiatry. Volume 2: The grade school child: Development and syndromes* (pp. 107–113). New York: John Wiley.

Olson, L. J. (2006). Parent–child activity groups reconsidered. *Occupational Therapy in Mental Health, 22*(3/4), 103–119.

Olson, L. J. (2010). A frame of reference to enhance social participation. In P. Kramer & J. Hinojosa (Eds.), *Frames of reference for pediatric occupational therapy* (3rd ed., pp. 306–348). Baltimore: Lippincott Williams & Wilkins.

Olson, L., Colangelo, C., & Shaw, M. (2009, April). *Addressing children's social participation: Reflecting on the content and process of a few school-based occupational therapy groups*. Workshop presented at the AOTA Annual Conference & Expo, Houston, TX.

Olson, L., Heaney, C., & Soppas-Hoffman, B. (1989). Parent–child activity group treatment in preventative psychiatry. Jointly published in *Health Promotion and Preventative Programs: Models of Occupational Therapy Practice* and *Journal of Occupational Therapy in Health Care, 6*(1), 29–43.

Olson, L., Martell, C., Nunez, R., & Rojas, N. (2010, May). *Sensory processing, attention, emotional regulation and learning: All parents need to understand the connections—Working with Spanish-speaking parents in a Head Start program in the United States*. Poster session presented at the Congress of the World Federation of Occupational Therapy, Santiago, Chile.

Peck, H. L., Kehle, T. J., Bray, M. A., & Theodore, L. A. (2005). Yoga as an intervention for children with attentional problems. *School Psychology Review, 34*(3), 415–424.

Posner, M. I., & Rothbart, M. K. (2000). Developing mechanisms of self regulation. *Development and Psychopathology, 12,* 427–441.

Posthuma, B. W. (2002). *Small groups in counseling and therapy: Process and leadership* (4th ed.). Boston: Allyn & Bacon.

Raver, C. C. (2002). Emotions matter: Making the case for the role of young children's emotional development for early school readiness. *Social Policy Report, 16*(3), 3–19.

Rogers, C. (1951). *Client-centered therapy, its current practice, implications, and theory.* Boston: Houghton Mifflin.

Sabel, R. (2007). Restorative yoga: An integrative approach to promote occupational performance. *OT Practice, 12*(19), 16–21.

Schultz, S. (2003, September). Psychosocial occupational therapy in schools. *OT Practice,* CE1–CE7.

Schwartzberg, S. L., Howe, M. C., & Barnes, M. A. (2008). *Groups: Applying the functional model.* Philadelphia: F. A. Davis.

Shechtman, Z. (2007). How does group process research inform leaders of counseling and psychotherapy groups? *Group Dynamics: Theory, Research, and Practice, 11*(4), 293–304.

Stueck, M., & Gloeckner, N. (2005). Yoga for children in the mirror of the science: Working spectrum and practice fields of the training of relaxation with elements of yoga for children. *Early Child Development and Care, 175*(4), 371–377.

Tuckman, B. W. (1965). Developmental sequence in small groups. *Psychological Bulletin, 63,* 384–399.

Van Velsor, P. (2009). Task groups in the school setting: Promoting children's social and emotional learning. *Journal for Specialists in Group Work, 34*(3), 276–292.

Williams, M. S., & Shellenberger, S. (1996). *"How does your engine run?" A leader's guide to the Alert Program for Self-Regulation.* Albuquerque, NM: TherapyWorks.

Williamson, G. G., & Dorman W. J. (2002). *Promoting social competence.* San Antonio, TX: Therapy Skill Builders.

Wilson, R. F. (1998). Toward a standards-based classification of group offerings by Robert K. Conyne. *Journal of Specialists in Group Work, 23*(2), 177–184.

Winner, M. G. (2002). *Thinking about you, thinking about me.* San Jose, CA: Author.

Winner, M. G. (2005). *Think social! A social thinking curriculum for school-age students: For teaching social thinking and related social skills to students with high functioning autism, Asperger syndrome, PDD–NOS, ADHD, nonverbal learning disability, and for all others in the murky gray area of social thinking.* San Jose, CA: Author.

Yalom, I. D. (1995). *The theory and practice of group psychotherapy* (4th ed.). New York: Basic Books.

Zins, R. P., Weissberg, M. C., Wang, M., & Walberg, H. J. (Eds.). (2004). *Building academic success on social and emotional learning.* New York: Teachers College Press.

PART 2

Addressing the Mental Health Needs of Diverse Groups of Children and Youth

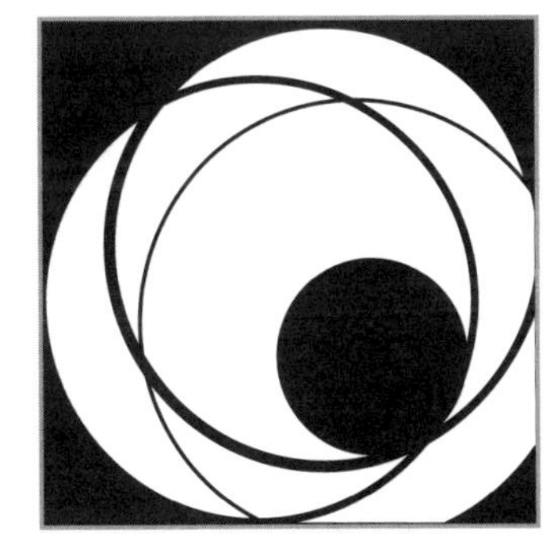

CHAPTER 6

Enduring Challenges and Situational Stressors During the School Years: Risk Reduction and Competence Enhancement

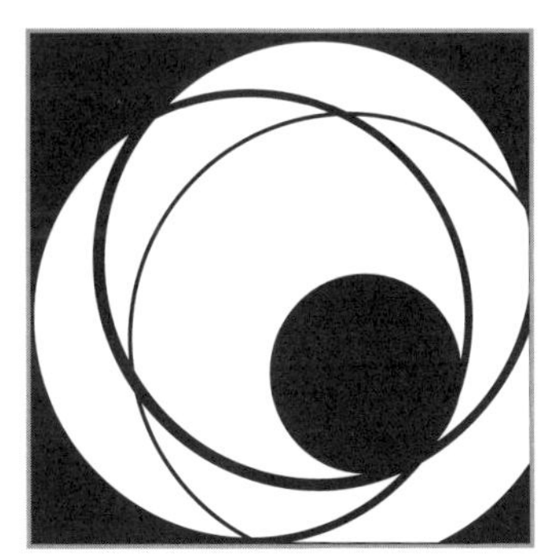

Susan Bazyk, PhD, OTR/L, FAOTA

Learning Objectives

After reading this material and completing the examination, readers will be able to

- Differentiate occupational deprivation and occupational justice, and identify the implications for occupational therapy practice;
- Delineate the physical and social environments of low-income youth entering the street versus nonstreet path;
- Recognize elements of the Occupational Therapy Groups for Healthy Occupations for Positive Emotions and the meaning of participation for low-income urban youth (Bazyk & Bazyk, 2009);
- Identify the mental health risks associated with being the victim, bully, or bystander;
- Delineate bullying prevention efforts espoused by positive behavioral intervention and supports and social and emotional learning;
- Identify how an occupational therapist could promote the development of key social behaviors important to the development of friends;
- Identify strategies for reducing weight bias and promoting weight tolerance;
- Recognize current obesity prevention efforts focusing on nutrition, physical activity, and environmental modifications; and
- Identify occupational therapy strategies for promoting healthy grieving.

Children with and without physical or emotional disabilities are likely, at some point in their lives, to struggle with situational stressors such as parental divorce, the death of a family member, poverty, friendship issues, bullying, or academic challenges, to name a few. During such times, character strengths, coping strategies, participation in enjoyable occupations, and environmental supports can serve as important buffers in the prevention of mental ill health (Catalano, Hawkins, Berglund, Pollard, & Arthur, 2002). While interacting with and observing children, occupational therapists must remain vigilant to the presence of possible stressors and advocate for and help develop services to counteract stressors and build competencies (e.g., grief support training for school personnel, participation in after-school clubs). Although addressing all situational stressors is impossible, this chapter is devoted to considering occupational therapy's role in reducing risks and promoting competencies in children and youth faced with poverty, bullying, obesity, loss, and participation in risky behaviors.

Poverty

> The task of a sound education, Plato argued 25 centuries ago, is to teach young people to find pleasure in the right things. If children enjoyed math, they would learn math. If they enjoyed helping friends, they would grow into helpful adults. If they enjoyed Shakespeare, they would not be content watching television programs. If they enjoyed life, they would take greater pains to protect it.
>
> —Csikszentmihalyi (1993, p. 39)

All humans need a range of occupations to create a balance among physical, mental, social, and relaxation needs (Wilcock, 1993), yet certain sociocultural changes may negatively influence participation in occupation. Occupational risk factors, such as poverty, lack of resources, or inequality of access, may lead to *occupational deprivation*—the inability to express one's occupational nature (Wilcock, 1998). Many physical and mental health problems can be attributed to these risk factors, including depression, anxiety, sleep disturbances, disease, obesity, and alcoholism. Occupational therapists can begin to address occupational deprivation by adopting an occupational perspective, acting at a broader social level, and embracing occupational justice (Townsend, 1999). *Occupational justice* emphasizes the "economic, political, and social forces that create equitable opportunity and the means to choose, organize, and perform occupations that people find useful or meaningful in their environment" (Townsend, 1999, p. 154). Occupational therapists are called to social action—to help all people engage in a diverse number of occupations to promote health and well-being. Actions supporting this philosophy can be used to promote mental health at each tier of a public health model: universal, targeted, and individualized.

"In an ideal world, all children would grow up in safe places surrounded by caring adults, with plenty of challenging opportunities to encourage their development" (Wilson, 1999, p. 1). However, many children—especially youth living in poverty—are living without one or more of these essential elements. Approximately 37% (27 million) of children in the United States live in low-income families, and 16% (more than 11 million) live in homes considered to be within the federal poverty level ($13,861 for a family of three; Crockett, 2003). Impoverished youth are less likely to have the family structure and economic security associated with positive outcomes. On the basis of the everyday risks of impoverished youth,

Box 6.1. Needs of Impoverished Children and Youth

- *Need for structured leisure occupations:* How children use their time may be an important indicator of their adaptation to the demands of low-income environments (Bruno, 1996). Engagement in a wide range of active leisure occupations is associated with higher academic achievement and social adjustment (Passmore, 1998). Impoverished children may not have the social or financial resources to be exposed to and to engage in a variety of structured leisure occupations. Involvement in nonlegitimate occupations, such as vandalism and gang activity, may become an attractive alternative to meet social–emotional, physical, and relaxation needs (Snyder, Clark, Masunaka-Noriega, & Young, 1998). If only passive or aggressive opportunities for action are available (e.g., hanging out, gang activity, violent computer games), the child will miss the opportunities to seek out and experience health-promoting challenges. Passive forms of leisure generally lack complexity, provide little or no challenge, and require no skills.
- *Need for social and emotional learning:* Although it is important to foster emotional intelligence in all children as a means of preventing social and emotional difficulties, impoverished youth have a heightened need for such programming given the inherent risks associated with their living situation (Nabors, Proescher, & DeSilva, 2001). Poverty, family distress, and community violence are all risks associated with living in inner-city neighborhoods that, in turn, place children at risk for delinquency, child abuse and neglect, and lower educational and occupational expectations (Mason & Chuang, 2001). Poverty can cause psychological distress among parents, which can negatively influence their behavior (McLoyd, 1990). Higher rates of internalizing (e.g., depression) and externalizing (e.g., aggression) psychological symptoms have been found in low-income youth (Grant et al., 2004). In addition, children living in dangerous neighborhoods may demonstrate symptoms that resemble posttraumatic stress disorder, such as sleep disturbances or aggressive outbursts. Programs that foster social–emotional learning help children recognize feelings, control impulses, and acquire important social skills for developing and maintaining healthy relationships in life (Goleman, 1995; Nabors et al., 2001).
- *Need for quality after-school care:* The need for quality after-school programs has grown considerably over the past 20 years (Garey, 2002). Economic changes have resulted in a significant increase in the number of parents working outside of the home. Risky teen behaviors (e.g., drinking, smoking, sex) most often occur between 3:00 p.m. and 6:00 p.m., causing professionals to explore the best ways for youth to fill after-school hours. Research has found that participation in after school programs reduces the likelihood of risky behaviors and promotes social and behavioral skills (e.g., peer friendships, conflict resolution; Hall, Israel, & Shortt, 2004; National Institute on Out-of-School Time, 2004). Quality after-school programs are thought to reduce negative behaviors in low-income children by providing (1) supervised, constructive activities that enhance the development of critical skills; (2) a safe environment during peak hours for juvenile crime; and (3) a structured program for reinforcing and enhancing academic skills.

the needs relevant to occupational therapy practice have been identified and are described in Box 6.1.

Although low-income urban youth face a combination of limited resources and increased exposure to everyday risks, Jarrett (1998) found that youth follow one of two major developmental pathways: (1) the street system or (2) a conventional, nonstreet system. Each path provides distinct developmental contexts and, thus, fosters the development of different skills. Essentially, the group of impoverished youth who become socialized into a conventional system do so by building on existing strengths (strong adult role models and careful monitoring; Jarrett, 1998). These children are taught critical values—the importance of hard work, discipline, and delayed gratification—by their parents and other adults. An expanded group of adults, including parents, extended family, neighbors, teachers, and related service providers, plays a prominent role in promoting the development of mainstream skills and behaviors. In addition, parents consciously veer children away from street influences by carefully monitoring their time, space, and friendships and actively promoting engagement in structured leisure. The "hidden curriculum" of sports and structured church groups nurtures discipline, cooperation, and teamwork (Jarrett, 1998).

In contrast, "children of less-competent parents are channeled, more by default than intent, into street-oriented developmental niches" (Jarrett, 1998, p. 6). Such parents have less emotional and physical energy to focus on their children and are less competent in promoting positive behaviors. As a result, these children are drawn to an adult and adolescent street culture characterized by an individualistic, competitive, and predatory influence in which peer relationships are valued for creating a sense of belonging and self-esteem. The children learn how to respond and cope with neighborhood violence by developing skills valued in street culture—bravery, fighting, daring, and a fluid ability to exchange verbal insults. In transition to adulthood, street children often become school dropouts, premature parents, welfare recipients, marginally employed, and struggling family members. Some may also become drug dealers or users and perpetrators or victims of violence (Jarrett, 1998). In sum, Jarrett's analysis illustrates the power of the environment—that is, that access to different types of social and institutional resources can determine the developmental pathway taken by youth living in poverty.

With this awareness, occupational therapists can be vigilant about the physical and social environments in which children live, go to school, and play and identify opportunities to provide a range of services designed to support participation in contexts and occupations likely to promote positive youth development. In schools, for example, this might involve assisting in the implementation of a program focusing on social and emotional learning (SEL), such as the Promoting Alternative Thinking Strategies (better known as *PATHS*) curriculum (Kusche & Greenberg, 1994) described in Box 3.9. Helping children and families access available community programs that promote the development of positive behaviors and leisure participation (e.g., church groups, library activities, youth clubs) is another strategy. In addition, advocating for and supporting public policy to support community recreation and sports programs in impoverished areas is a way to provide Tier 1(universal) indirect services. Identifying opportunities to embed direct services in after-school programs and community-based settings to foster participation in structured leisure activities and promote SEL for impoverished youth can help promote mental health and a sense of well-being (Bazyk & Bazyk, 2009). An occupation-based group program designed to do just that is described in Box 6.2.

Bullying and Friendship Issues

Bullying is considered one of the most common forms of violence in schools, and as such, most schools adopt programs to reduce bullying and create physically and emotionally safe contexts for learning (Collaborative for Academic, Social, and Emotional Learning [CASEL], 2009; Espelage & Swearer, 2003; Nansel et al., 2001). In addition, 41 states (as of January 2010) have passed antibullying laws, including clear prohibitions on bullying and legislative findings of its negative effects on school environments (see http://bullypolice.org).

What is bullying? Although many definitions have been proposed, the Center for the Study and Prevention of School Violence (2008) has described *bullying* as an act of intentional aggression carried out repeatedly over time and occurring within

Box 6.2. Occupational Therapy Groups for HOPE

The Occupational Therapy Groups for HOPE (Healthy Occupations for Positive Emotions) program, which is embedded in an after-school program in Cleveland, Ohio, was developed to address the occupation-based, social–emotional, and interaction needs of low-income urban youth.

HOPE Group Curriculum

The integration of knowledge about group process, meaningful occupation, social and emotional learning (SEL), and positive behavioral interventions and supports (PBIS) provided the foundation for the 8-week HOPE groups. Under the supervision of the project director (Susan Bazyk), two graduate occupational therapy students from Cleveland State University coplan and facilitate the weekly groups, each consisting of 8 to 10 children ranging in age from 8 to 15. Each year since 2004, approximately 70 to 100 children participate in the groups. After-school care providers also participate in the group activities to learn how to simultaneously engage children in meaningful occupations and attend to SEL.

- *Group process:* Research has suggested that children who demonstrate personal or social difficulties benefit more from small groups that provide a supportive environment and an opportunity to develop positive relationships with caring adults than those who receive individual interventions. The HOPE groups were designed to foster peer interaction and group process to promote change at both the individual and the group levels. Task-oriented groups enhance skill development in various occupations and improve interpersonal and intrapersonal learning.
- *Participation in meaningful occupation:* On the basis of the risk of occupational deprivation in impoverished youth, the HOPE groups focus on providing opportunities for participating in a meaningful range of structured leisure occupations (e.g., arts and crafts, games). The occupational therapy students select the activities on the basis of input from the children with the goal of encouraging the development of new leisure interests.
- *Social and emotional learning activities:* Social and emotional learning (SEL) activities are embedded into each of the task-oriented groups and focus on the development of social competencies (e.g., understanding the relationship among feelings, thoughts, and behaviors; empathy), friendship skills, conflict resolution skills, and anger management skills. The social–emotional aspects of the group session help children recognize their emotions, think about their feelings and how one should act, and regulate their behavior on the basis of thoughtful decision making. The SEL curriculum *Self-Science: The Emotional Intelligence Curriculum* by McCown, Jensen, Freedman, and Rideout (1998) is used as a guide. Strategies for teaching appropriate ways to express anger are adapted from *Volcano in My Tummy: Helping Children to Handle Anger* (Whitehouse & Pudney, 1996).
- *Positive behavioral interventions and supports:* PBIS promotes the use of proactive strategies to prevent problem behavior by altering a situation before problems escalate and concurrently teaching appropriate alternatives. Examples of PBIS strategies embedded during the HOPE groups included clearly communicating group rules and creating a warm and positive group environment.

Organization of the Group Sessions

Group sessions are structured into three segments: conversation time, project activity, and closure. Conversation time focuses on introducing the social–emotional theme for the session, setting the emotional tone, and promoting group cohesion. The occupation-based project activity is considered the heart of the group because it exposes the children to activities that may develop into long-term interests and allows them to practice the social–emotional skill introduced during conversation time. Examples of projects and activities include making greeting cards using rubber stamping, crocheting scarves, creating paper mâché masks, and doing yoga. The project activities focus on exposing children to a variety of structured leisure occupations to broaden their repertoire of interests and promote the development of hobbies. Closure involves revisiting the SEL theme and occupational reflection—an opportunity to think about the influence of activity on emotional and physical health.

Findings From a Qualitative Study: Becoming Hooked on Doing

Several findings, based on a phenomenological study exploring the meaning of the groups from the participants' perspective (Bazyk & Bazyk, 2009), have been identified regarding the children's responses to the HOPE groups. Using a combination of in-depth interviews and participant observations, Bazyk and Bazyk found that children perceive the groups to be fun (occupational meaning) because of engagement in novel and challenging projects and talking about feelings within a supportive group context (occupational form). Participation in creative leisure occupations that allow for choice transforms mood; children experience happiness and forget their problems (occupational function). The children enjoy the projects and activities and express wanting to do more. Children are often heard saying, "What are we going to do today?" or "I wish you could come every day." They become "hooked on doing" and experience firsthand the power of occupation—that participating in creative occupations fosters positive feelings. In addition, as the weeks pass, the children begin to interact as a cohesive group, sharing materials and praising each other's accomplishments. Many children also indicate that they enjoy being able to talk about their feelings.

Source. Bazyk and Bazyk (2009).

a relationship characterized by an imbalance of power. Three types of bullying have been identified (CASEL, 2009):

1. *Direct bullying:* Physical acts of aggression (hitting, pushing), verbal acts of aggression (taunting, name calling, malicious teasing), or both
2. *Indirect bullying:* Behavior characterized by one or more forms of relational aggression (peer exclusion, spreading rumors, manipulating friendships to hurt the victim)
3. *Cyberbullying:* Sending threatening or hurtful messages or images using an electronic device (cell phone, computer).

Boys tend to be involved in more direct acts of bullying, whereas girls are more likely to engage in indirect forms (Jenson & Dieterich, 2007). Because indirect and cyberbullying are less visible to external parties, it is often difficult for adults to detect and address such behavior (Nansel et al., 2001). In 2007, approximately 32% of students ages 12 to 18 reported being bullied within the past year; of this group, 63% were bullied 1 to 2 times over the year, 21% were bullied 1 to 2 times per month, 10% were bullied 1 to 2 times per week, and 7% were bullied almost daily (CASEL, 2009). Bullying tends to peak between age 11 and 13 and continues to decline throughout the high school grades (CASEL, 2009; Jenson & Dieterich, 2007).

Many mental health risks are associated with victims, bullies, and bystanders. Victims of bullying report symptoms of emotional distress, including low self-esteem, loneliness, depression, anxiety, and poor academic performance (Jenson & Dieterich, 2007). Children who bully often display a range of negative outcomes, including poor school adjustment, conduct problems, depression, and peer rejection. In addition, bystanders who witness bullying can experience feelings of fear, anger, guilt, and sadness (Batsche & Porter, 2006). Bystanders may also play a role by acting in ways to maintain bullying behavior by either responding positively (e.g., laughing, joining in) or by passively watching rather than intervening to help the victim. Although most discussions of bullying generally label people as either bully or victim, some researchers have suggested that bullying should be viewed along a continuum and as a group phenomenon that occurs in a social context (CASEL, 2009). For example, most students experience moments of both roles throughout their development—partaking in some form of bullying as well as being teased or harassed by peers (Espelage & Swearer, 2003).

Schoolwide Bullying Prevention Programs

Because bullying can affect the entire student body and school climate, existing research has supported universal school-based programs as opposed to involving only victims and bullies. Recent systematic reviews of bullying prevention programs (Swearer, Espelage, Love, & Kingsbury, 2008; Ttofi & Farrington, 2009; Vreeman & Carroll, 2007) identified effective whole-school approaches as consisting of a variety of strategies, such as teacher training, schoolwide rules, classroom curricula and management strategies, parent education, improved playground supervision, and peer involvement to combat bullying. Embedding bullying prevention within a schoolwide SEL and positive behavioral interventions and supports (PBIS) program has been proposed (CASEL, 2009; U.S. Department of Education, Office of Special

Education Programs [OSEP] Technical Assistance Center on PBIS, 2010). Bullying prevention in PBIS emphasizes remediation of problem behavior and prevention of further bullying. Two bullying prevention program manuals, one for elementary school and the other for middle school, are available from the OSEP Technical Assistance Center on PBIS Web site (Box 6.3). Bullying prevention within an SEL framework emphasizes the promotion of a positive school climate (warmth, respect) and positive student interactions (increasing SEL competencies). Students who have greater SEL competency are less likely to be aggressors, targets of bullying, or passive bystanders. Additionally, schools that create positive schoolwide environments are not conducive to bullying, making such behaviors less likely to occur or continue. A document describing an SEL and bullying prevention framework is available on the CASEL Web site (CASEL, 2009; Box 6.4). A combination of PBIS and SEL approaches appears to provide a comprehensive way to ensure the prevention of bullying and the promotion of skills emphasizing positive interaction.

Occupational therapists need to become aware of state and district policies and approaches for addressing bullying and actively support such efforts by embedding school and classroomwide strategies into occupational therapy intervention when possible. Special attention to the development of skills important for developing and sustaining friendships can easily be embedded in occupational therapy services.

Children with disabilities are often targets of bullying because of their differences (Heinrich, 2003). Those with special needs, such as children diagnosed with attention deficit disorder, oppositional defiant disorder, bipolar disorder, obsessive–compulsive disorder, nonverbal learning disability, Asperger syndrome, and learning disorders, may experience anxiety and depression and are typically more rejected by their peers. It is essential that adaptations and modifications be integrated into

Box 6.3. Bully Prevention in Positive Behavioral Interventions and Supports

Bully Prevention in Positive Behavioral Interventions and Supports (BP–PBIS) was designed to augment schoolwide PBIS by teaching all students behaviors that will reduce the probability of bullying. The program emphasizes prevention and remediation of the problem. BP–PBIS gives students the tools necessary to remove the social rewards maintaining inappropriate behavior, thereby decreasing the likelihood of problem behavior occurring in the future. The manuals provide clear methods and user-friendly worksheets for teaching this program to students and staff.

Students are taught a three-step response to problem behavior to prevent the reinforcement of bullying and to extinguish it. Separate sections apply the three steps to the problems of gossip, inappropriate remarks, and cyberbullying:

1. *Stop:* Teach students the schoolwide "stop signal" (verbal and physical action) for problem behavior, and practice when and how to use it appropriately.
2. *Walk:* Teach students to walk away when the problem behavior continues after the stop signal. Walking away removes the reinforcement for problem behavior.
3. *Talk:* Teach students to talk to an adult if the problem behavior continues after using stop and walk.

Staff (e.g., teachers, paraprofessionals, administrators) are taught a clear and simple method of responding to reports of problem behavior and delivering consequences.

See the *Bully Prevention Manuals* (available for free online at www.pbis.org) for a complete description of the program.

Source. Stiller, Ross, and Horner (n.d.-a, n.d.-b).

Box 6.4. Schoolwide Approaches: Applying a Social and Emotional Learning Framework to Bullying

- *Assessment:* To identify how often bullying occurs, the forms it takes (e.g., relational aggression, cyberbullying), where incidents occur, and how students and adults respond to such incidents.
- *Awareness and training:* All adults who oversee groups of children (staff and volunteers) need training to recognize and respond to bullying incidents. *Example: Eyes on Bullying: What Can You Do?* (Storey, Slaby, Adler, Minotti, & Katz, 2008).
- *Discipline policy:* The discipline policy should clearly indicate that bullying is not acceptable, specify the consequences for policy violations, and be consistently enforced.
- *Adult models of behavior:* All adults in the school need to model respectful and caring behavior toward students and one another and demonstrate social problem-solving skills.
- *Promoting positive peer interactions:* Promote opportunities for students to interact with one another in cooperative, positive, and inclusive ways to help generate cohesion and compassion among students and encourage them to apply the social and emotional learning (SEL) skills they have been taught.
- *Classroom climate:* Teachers need to establish respectful standards of ways to interact and take action when student norms support aggression. Teachers should model inclusive behaviors, making a special effort to reach out to peer-rejected and withdrawn students and to encourage students to be inclusive of their peers.
- *SEL curricula and activities:* Help children think about the harmful consequences of their bullying behaviors to others and how their own relationships may reduce these behaviors.
- *Interventions:* For children who are victimized, who witness bullying, or who regularly bully others, extended opportunities are needed to practice relevant SEL skills, such as anger management, assertive communication, and social problem-solving.
- *Parental involvement:* Because family interaction patterns can contribute to both bullying and victimization, it is important to help parents reflect on their own parenting styles and behavior and to provide them with specific guidance on handling conflicts at home.

Source. Collaborative for Academic, Social, and Emotional Learning (2009).

bullying prevention programs as necessary to successfully meet the requirements of children with special needs.

Promotion of Friendship Skills

Research has suggested that having high-quality friendships, or at least one best friend, can help prevent children from being a victim of bullying (CASEL, 2009). Friendships are also an important source of happiness (Demir, Zdemir, & Weitekamp, 2007). Friendship is a qualitative relationship that represents voluntary interdependence over time and involves varying degrees of companionship, affection, intimacy, and mutual assistance. Recent research has suggested that close friendships contribute to happiness above and beyond the influence of one's personality (Demir & Weitekamp, 2007). Additionally, the companionship and self-validation features of friendship were found to be the most important predictors of happiness. *Companionship* refers to doing things with friends—sharing in activities perceived as enjoyable or exciting. *Self-validation,* the second feature of friendship associated with happiness, refers to perceiving the friend as being supportive of one's self-image by listening, agreeing, reassuring, and encouraging (e.g., gives compliments, points out strengths; Demir & Weitekamp, 2007). In addition to the relationship between friendships and happiness, children who have friends tend to be more sociable, self-confident, cooperative, and emotionally supportive than those without friends (Wentzel, Baker, & Russell, 2009).

Resource 6.1. Friendship Observation Checklist

Tony Attwood has studied friendship issues in people with Asperger syndrome. Two observation checklists are available on his Web site, www.tonyattwood.com.au (click on Publications/By Tony Attwood/Archived papers).

Occupational therapists can play a pivotal role in helping all children and youth develop friendships both in and out of school. The first step is to ask children about their friends and friendship issues. Informal interviews and observations of children and youth in natural settings are one way to gather information about friendship skills (Resource 6.1). Attwood (2002) has identified key social behaviors important to making friends, which are highlighted in Box 6.5. Occupational therapy intervention can help teach friendship skills during individual or group interaction. To foster the development of friendships outside of school, it is important to help children identify their interests and join a group or club. The use of coaching strategies, as described in Chapter 2, can assist children who are reluctant or who have limited social skills to successfully enter and participate in a group. Doing enjoyable activities with other children increases the opportunity to develop friendships with those who have similar interests. Participating in a camp program is another strategy for encouraging the development of friendships within a natural context of doing enjoyable activities. Numerous examples of camp programs developed by occupational therapists have been published and are highlighted in Resource 6.2.

Box 6.5. Key Social Behaviors Important for Developing Friendships

- *Entry skills:* Knowing how to join a group of children; welcoming and including children who want to enter and participate in a group activity
- *Assistance:* Recognizing when and how to provide assistance to another child and knowing when to seek assistance from others
- *Compliments:* Providing compliments at appropriate times and knowing how to respond to a friend's compliment
- *Criticism:* Knowing when criticism is appropriate and inappropriate and how to give it and having the ability to accept criticism
- *Accepting suggestions:* Being open to others' ideas and incorporating those ideas
- *Cooperation in groups:* Contributing to common goals; following rules; being aware of personal body space
- *Reciprocity and sharing:* Demonstrating the ability to converse and share materials in an equitable manner
- *Conflict resolution:* Managing disagreements with compromise; recognizing others' opinions; knowing not to respond with aggression or immature behavior; forgiving
- *Monitoring and listening:* Avoiding monologue; speaking at an appropriate volume; and using appropriate humor. Regularly observing other people to monitor their contribution to the activity and what their body language is conveying. Being aware of one's own body language and nonverbal behaviors that indicate interest in another person (e.g., smiling, eye contact, nodding head)
- *Empathy:* Recognizing another person's feelings and responding with appropriate comments and actions
- *Avoiding and ending:* Understanding the appropriate behavior and commenting to maintain a friendship or end the relationship.

Source. Attwood (2002).

Resource 6.2. Examples of Camp Programs for Children and Youth

Banet, J. (2008). Creating participation at a camp for children with autism and Asperger syndrome. *Developmental Disabilities Special Interest Section Quarterly, 31*(4), 1–3.

Cahill, S. M., & Suarez-Balcazar, Y. (2009). Promoting children's nutrition and fitness in the urban context. *American Journal of Occupational Therapy, 63,* 113–116.

Candler, C. (2003). Sensory integration and therapeutic riding at summer camp: Occupational performance outcomes. *Physical and Occupational Therapy in Pediatrics, 23,* 51–64.

Loukas, K. M., & Cote, T. L. (2005). Sports as occupation: A sports camp experience for children who are blind or have visual impairment. *OT Practice, 10*(5), 15–19.

Schmelzer, L. (2006). An occupation-based camp for healthier children. *OT Practice, 11*(16), 18–23.

Obesity

Obesity is a major public health concern in the United States and other Western countries. Approximately 32.7% of U.S. adults age 20 or older are overweight, 34.3% are obese, and 5.9% are extremely obese (Centers for Disease Control and Prevention, 2006). Of significant concern is the accelerating growth in the prevalence of childhood obesity: About 25% of children are overweight, and 11% are obese (Dehghan, Akhtar-Danesh, & Merchant, 2005; Dwyer, Baur, Higgs, & Hardy, 2009).

Causes

The combined effect of overconsumption of calories and reduced physical activity is considered the cause of childhood obesity (Dehghan et al., 2005). Societal influences—such as the overavailability of foods high in sugar and fat, increased food serving sizes, increased time spent in television- and computer-related activities, and decreased physical activity—have contributed to the obesity epidemic (American Occupational Therapy Association, 2007). The decrease in physical activity can be attributed, in part, to less time in physical education class and recess; decreased time spent in outside play; and increased use of automated transportation (Smallfield & Anderson, 2009).

Children at Greater Risk of Obesity

Children living in poverty and those with disabilities are at even greater risk for becoming overweight or obese at young ages, making the problem a social justice issue as well as a public health epidemic. Youth growing up in low-income urban environments in working-class African-American and Latino communities have rates of obesity almost double those of White children (Cahill & Suarez-Balcazar, 2009). Such environments generally provide fewer opportunities for physical activity (e.g., fewer safe public play areas) and less access to nutritional foods (prevalence of fast food outlets and convenience stores vs. grocery stores).

Recent research has also indicated that the prevalence of overweight and obesity is higher among children with developmental disabilities (40%) than among the general population, leading to a greater number of obesity-related secondary conditions (e.g., fatigue, pain, deconditioning, social isolation, difficulty performing activities of daily living; De, Small, & Baur, 2008; Rimmer, Rowland, & Yamaki, 2007). Children with developmental disabilities often have one or more predisposing factors for obesity, including the coexistence of certain genetic syndromes known to be associated with obesity (e.g., Prader-Willi syndrome), reduced levels of physical activity, and the use of medications that can cause weight gain (De et al., 2008). Factors within the physical and social environments may also contribute to a lack of physical activity, such as a lack of access to recreation facilities and limited knowledge among staff on how to adapt programs for youth with disabilities (Rimmer et al., 2007). Finally, studies have shown that by age 3, children with developmental delay are significantly more likely to be obese than their typically developing peers (Emerson, 2009). Such findings make a case for the investment in interventions during the early years of life to prevent the emergence of obesity among children with developmental delay. Occupational therapists must be aware of conditions that put children at greater risk of obesity and embed strategies to prevent obesity and promote health into their interventions.

Resource 6.3. Yale Rudd Center for Food Policy and Obesity

- Key aims: to prevent obesity, reduce weight stigma, and promote positive change in the world's diet by promoting the convergence of academic institutions, food and agricultural industries, governments, nongovernment organizations, and for-profit organizations
- Resources for schools, families, and communities to promote healthy food environment
- Information on weight bias, including research papers, assessment tools, and PowerPoint presentations.

Visit www.yaleruddcenter.org.

Consequences

Obesity in childhood is known to have a significant impact on physical and psychological health and on social interaction (Smallfield & Anderson, 2009). Physical consequences include an increased risk for diabetes, heart disease, high cholesterol, high blood pressure, sleep apnea, and orthopedic problems. Children who are obese may experience negative effects associated with weight bias. *Weight bias* refers to weight-related attitudes and beliefs expressed as stereotypes, rejection, and prejudice because of being overweight or obese (Puhl & Later, 2007). Children may face weight bias from multiple sources, including peers, teachers, health care providers, and even parents. Children who are overweight might encounter verbal teasing (name calling, derogatory remarks), social exclusion (being ignored), and physical bullying (pushed, shoved). About one-third of overweight girls and one-fourth of overweight boys report being teased by peers at school. Obese children who are victimized because of their weight are more vulnerable to depression, anxiety, lower self-esteem, and poor body image (Puhl & Later, 2007). With this awareness, childhood obesity prevention programs in schools and community settings to promote health in overweight and obese children must simultaneously protect them in the face of social stigmatization and its consequences. The Yale Rudd Center for Food Policy and Obesity (Resource 6.3) offers comprehensive resources on obesity prevention.

Occupational Therapy Intervention

Traditional approaches to obesity have emphasized diet and exercise at the individual level; however, these strategies have had little impact on the growing obesity epidemic (Dehghan et al., 2005). Recent efforts have called for broader attention to all of the physical, psychological, social, and spiritual dimensions of children's health in obesity prevention (O'Dea, 2005). Additionally, because it is difficult to reduce excessive weight once it becomes established, prevention strategies need to begin while children are young and continue throughout the growing years. Strategies for intervention with children and youth can be embedded in a number of settings, including preschools and schools, after-school care, and community programs. Without specialized education and training in bariatric medicine, occupational therapy interventions can emphasize the prevention of obesity and the promotion of overall health at the individual, school, and community levels.

Framing Obesity Prevention Efforts

According to O'Dea (2005), it is important to consider the possibility that some well-meaning prevention efforts may be more harmful than beneficial to children who are overweight. Child obesity prevention programs and untested health education messages have the potential to further stigmatize children who are overweight. Most children who are overweight are well aware of their body size and are at risk of developing a poor body image. Negatively focused health messages (e.g., those that emphasize the undesirability of being overweight) may lead students to feel worse about themselves. Professionals must carefully consider how prevention messages are framed to avoid the potential psychosocial (e.g., poor self-esteem) and physical health (e.g., binge dieting) consequences that can result (Puhl & Later, 2007).

Promoting Health Behaviors for All Children

Prevention efforts that focus on health as both the primary motivator for and the desired outcome of positive lifestyle behaviors in all children may be more effective than those focusing on weight reduction in an isolated group (O'Dea, 2005). The "health at any size" movement has been successful in helping health professionals and people who are overweight focus on health improvement rather than weight status. Children of all weights should receive support from peers, adults, teachers, and parents to make healthy food choices and be physically active. Moreover, to foster enjoyment in health behaviors, educators and health care providers need to remove blame from children who are overweight, provide education about weight bias to all adults and students, and implement policies that prohibit weight-based victimization (Puhl & Later, 2007).

Nutrition

A healthy diet has many benefits in addition to obesity prevention, including positive growth, physical development, brain development and cognition, and disease prevention (O'Dea, 2005). Occupational therapists can assess the availability of nutritious foods in children's schools and neighborhoods (Cahill & Suarez-Balcazar, 2009). Attention to family habits and routines related to nutrition and mealtimes may be also be beneficial. Working with school administration and staff to reduce vending machines with high-calorie foods and offer nutritious lunches and snacks is a strategy that supports healthy eating habits for all children.

Physical Activity

Pressuring overweight children who are generally self-conscious of their bodies to participate in sports or physical activity may inadvertently reduce interest in ongoing participation (O'Dea, 2005). In contrast, engaging children in physical activities that they are interested in and enjoy is likely to foster positive feelings about being physically active and can have the added benefit of promoting social interaction and friendships. Exploring a range of physical activity options in addition to traditional exercise can be done individually or with groups of children and include walking clubs, hiking, biking, or swimming, to name a few. If after-school clubs do not offer options for physical activity, occupational therapists might consider developing a program (Smallfield & Anderson, 2009). Supporting school and community programs that offer noncompetitive sports teams can increase the likelihood that all children have opportunities to participate in and enjoy organized sports. In addition, children need to be taught about the mental health benefits of exercise.

A growing body of research has suggested that moderate regular exercise should be considered as a viable means of treating depression and anxiety and improving mental well-being in the general public (Fox, 1999).

Modifying Environments

A socioecological, environmental model for increasing physical activity suggests that focusing on changing the physical environment, urban planning, and modes of transportation is likely to provide significant benefits in obesity prevention (O'Dea, 2005). Such a model emphasizes helping neighborhoods and communities to develop safe, enjoyable, and inexpensive opportunities for physical activity, such as (1) walking networks (designated safe walking paths and hiking trails), (2) cycling networks (designated cycling routes and paths), (3) public open spaces (safe parks and playgrounds), and (4) recreation facilities (safe and inexpensive; Dehghan et al., 2005).

Preventing Weight Bias and Promoting Weight Tolerance

Researchers increasingly agree that obesity prevention programs need to include strategies to prevent weight-based stigmatization in youth and promote weight tolerance (Puhl & Later, 2007). The adoption of school policies that prohibit weight-based teasing and victimization and periodic assessment of bias to prevent unintentional stigmatization are also recommended. Occupational therapists need to become aware of their own biases related to overweight or obese children and youth and help foster school and community environments that promote tolerance (Box 6.6).

Box 6.6. Strategies for Reducing Weight Bias

1. *Increase awareness of personal attitudes about weight.* As a health care provider, you should become aware of your own weight-based assumptions, which are often unintentionally communicated to children. Questions to consider are
   - What are my views about the causes of obesity? Does this affect my attitudes toward obese people?
   - Do I make assumptions about people's character, intelligence, or lifestyle on the basis of their weight?
2. *Use sensitive and appropriate language about weight.* Children are perceptive of people's attitudes, so avoid making negative comments about one's own or other people's weight in front of them. Avoid making negative associations regarding being overweight (e.g., that overweight people are lazy), and avoid making critical statements about body weight. Talk with children about what terms they prefer to use when talking about weight.
3. *Intervene to reduce weight-based teasing.* Health care providers need to look for signs of peer harassment, teasing, or victimization in children who are overweight. It is important to offer support to children in these situations and bring the behavior to the attention of relevant school personnel.
4. *Increase awareness of weight bias at school.* Talk to teachers and school administrators to promote awareness of weight bias. Identify whole-school strategies for addressing bias and promoting weight tolerance.
5. *Find role models to build confidence and self-esteem.* Help children see examples of positive role models who are not thin. Emphasize that overweight people can be successful, accomplish important goals, and feel good about themselves.
6. *Emphasize health rather than thinness.* Although most health care providers encourage children who are overweight to lose weight, make sure to focus on the promotion of physical and emotional health.

Source. Puhl (2007).

Coping With Loss and Grieving

For children experiencing stress as a result of loss, occupational therapists can help promote healthy grieving. *Grief* is defined as conflicting feelings caused by a change in or an end to a familiar pattern of behavior (James, Friedman, & Landon Matthews, 2001). This broad definition encompasses a wide variety of losses that might result in grieving, including death of a loved one (parent, friend), a major move, parental divorce, death of a pet, military deployment of a parent, and loss of function as a result of illness or injury. It is estimated that 1 in 20 children will lose a parent to death before age 18; 1 in 5 families will move each year; and 1 in 3 children under age 18 will have divorced parents. When considering all the possible situations that bring about loss for children and youth, it is likely that occupational therapists will routinely interact with children who are grieving. In fact, a recent survey of occupational therapists working in schools found that the most frequently identified losses included a major move, debilitating injuries to self, and parental divorce (Milliken, Goodman, Bazyk, & Flynn, 2007). Information important to help therapists understand children's grieving, contribute to schoolwide approaches, and provide support on an individual basis follows. Although children may grieve after a variety of losses, information specific to the death of a loved one, along with information on issues specific to military families, follows.

Grieving After the Death of a Loved One

"The death of a loved one can be one of the most severe traumas one may encounter and the sense of loss and grief which follows is a natural and important part of life" (Ayyash-Abdo, 2001, p. 417). The grief process in children differs from that in adults for several reasons (Willis, 2002). First, children often do not have the communication skills to express how they feel, especially young children. Second, grieving tends to be more cyclical, with children revisiting previous feelings and behaviors and processing death in a different way because of developmental changes. The stress associated with grieving may result in a range of behavioral changes, including emotional withdrawal, altered eating and sleeping patterns, behavioral outbursts, regressive behaviors (e.g., bedwetting, clinging to parent), physical symptoms (e.g., headaches, stomachaches), anxiety, difficulty concentrating on schoolwork, and even aggressive behaviors (Ayyash-Abdo, 2001).

When children receive support from parents and other adults around them, that support helps the child and the entire family cope (Schonfeld & Quackenbush, 2009). All school personnel and adults involved in youth activities should learn about grieving as a normal response to significant loss and learn appropriate strategies for supporting healthy grieving and minimizing further stress (Holland, 2004). A child's return to school after the death of a loved one is a key event. Schools are encouraged to have procedures in place to address this return and ongoing interaction. Schoolwide, Tier 1 grief awareness training could be provided to teachers, school nurses, related service personnel, parents, and volunteers to promote interactions that support the grieving process. Tier 2 services could provide targeted small-group programs led by staff with expertise in mental health such as school nurses, occupational therapists, school psychologists, and social workers. Tier 3 services target children and youth who are grief impaired and need individual bereavement counseling (Black, 2005).

The following schoolwide strategies promote a grief-friendly school:

1. Create a grief support team that meets 4 times per year to review bereavement literature on supporting children at various ages.
2. Educate all school staff about grief as a normal response to death, behaviors associated with grieving, the importance of emotional support, and how to talk with children about their feelings.
3. Consider each child's individual response to grieving, taking into account the child's age and home situation.
4. Help staff recognize symptoms that may indicate the need for individual counseling and procedures for making a referral.
5. Help support students to resume their regular school and extracurricular activities with modifications as needed (McGlauflin, 2003).

School staff also need to be educated on what not to do, such as acting as though nothing happened, making comments that minimize the loss (e.g., "You'll be stronger for this."), or telling the student that it is time to move on (McGlauflin, 2003). Finally, teaching the entire student body about what to say to peers who have experienced loss is something that can be embedded in health education or language arts (Box 6.7).

Military Families

According to the U.S. Department of Defense (2008), approximately 44% of active duty forces have children (Swank & Robinson, 2009). These children experience many challenges in their family lives, including deployment of parents and the potential death of a parent while on active duty. When addressing grief issues, several factors are unique to children and adolescents in military families. First,

Box 6.7. Teaching Children to Provide Support to Friends Who Are Grieving

One of the most important things children can do for friends who are grieving is to show they care, using the following strategies:

- *Offer to spend time with the person.* Listen if the person wants to talk; sit quietly if the person just wants company; or do something the person likes to do.
- *Listen more, talk less.* It's fine to share your feelings and express your caring and concern, but keep the focus on the person grieving. Listen to the person's feelings without telling the person how he or she ought to feel.
- *Don't try to take away the grief.* Feelings are often powerful and painful and will last some time. Comments or efforts meant to cheer people up are usually not helpful.
- *Accept strong expressions of feeling.* These expressions are a part of grieving. It is not helpful to encourage people to "be strong" or cover up their feelings.
- *Make routine contact.* Let your friend know that you are thinking of him or her. Call him or her. Send a card.
- *Be available over the long haul.* Grieving takes a long time. Offer ongoing support. Pay special attention to holidays, anniversaries, and other special occasions.

Source. Schonfeld and Quackenbush (2009).

Resource 6.4. Working With Military Children

- *Military Child Initiative at Johns Hopkins University* (www.jhsph.edu/mci)
- *Military Child Education Coalition* (www.militarychild.org)
- *Educator's Guide to the Military Child During Deployment* (www2.ed.gov/about/offices/list/os/homefront/homefront.pdf)
- *Working With Military Children: A Primer for School Personnel* (http://nmfa.convio.net/site/DocServer?docID=642; a primer for school personnel and guidance counselors prepared by the Virginia Military Family Services Board)

deployment is an experience unique to military families that may cause feelings of ambiguous loss for children as a result of parents being physically separated but psychologically present (Betz & Thorngren, 2006). Families may have only a short period of time to prepare emotionally and physically for the change. Experiences associated with the death of a parent in the military also differ in ways that extend the number of changes that occur following the funeral. If families live in military housing, for example, they generally have a limited time to move, reducing the time that children have to say goodbye to friends. Children may attend a new school that is not a Department of Defense school, resulting in the loss of support from other military children. Professionals in the new school may lack an awareness of issues specific to military families. Because these issues are unique to military families, all school personnel need education about how to support grief and loss particular to this group of children (Swank & Robinson, 2009). See Resource 6.4 for sources of information on working with children in military families.

Occupational Therapy's Role in Promoting Healthy Grieving

Occupational therapists can help children recognize that "grieving can last a lifetime, but should not consume a life" (Schonfeld & Quackenbush, 2009, p. 19). As children develop over time, they will gain new ways of thinking about their loss. Occupational therapists can help support children in their grieving process through the use of meaningful occupations and the therapeutic use of self.

Occupation-Based Approaches

After the death of a loved one, getting back to regular routines and activities can have an organizing effect on children's feelings of well-being. In schools, occupational therapists can consult with teachers to help recognize behavioral changes that might cause problems with completing homework or attending in class and suggest strategies for modifying assignments or the learning environment to foster success. Encouraging participation in enjoyable but low-stress activities with close friends can also minimize feelings of isolation once a child returns to school after the funeral.

The benefits of using creative arts in helping children express feelings of loss is well supported in the literature (Milliken et al., 2007; Schonfeld & Quackenbush, 2009; Willis, 2002). Creative arts can be embedded in individual or group work using a variety of methods, including drawing, painting, craftwork, storytelling, music, play, puppetry, and dancing, to name a few. Suggested tasks such as journaling, scrap booking, making memory boards with photographs, and collages lend themselves naturally to meeting the needs of the grieving child while incorporating a fine motor focus (Milliken et al., 2007).

Therapeutic Use of Self

Occupational therapists, who have knowledge and skills in the therapeutic use of self and facilitating therapeutic groups, can help support children's grieving process over time. Everyday interactions can help or hinder this process. Occupational therapists need to be aware that children sometimes worry that they will forget the person who died (Schonfeld & Quackenbush, 2009). Helping the child remember what was valuable in the relationship and preserve such memories through stories, pictures, and mentioning the person in everyday conversation may be beneficial. It is also important to anticipate *grief triggers,* such as anniversaries of important events, the first birthday, and favorite family meals. Such triggers can bring about strong emotions. Reassuring children that these experiences are natural can help normalize the experience (Schonfeld & Quackenbush, 2009). Specific suggestions for talking to children about death are summarized in Box 6.8.

Preventing Participation in Risky Teen Behaviors

> Adolescents and college-age individuals take more risks than children or adults do, as indicated by statistics on automobile crashes, binge drinking, contraceptive use, and crime; but trying to understand why risk taking is more common during adolescence than during other periods of development has challenged psychologists for decades. (Steinberg, 2007, p. 55)

More than 90% of all American high school students have been educated in school about risks associated with teen sex, drug and substance abuse, and reckless driving, yet large proportions of them still have unsafe sex, binge drink, smoke cigarettes, and drive recklessly (Steinberg, 2004). According to developmental neuroscience, a teen's inclination to engage in risky behavior is not the result of a lack of information or logical reasoning abilities (Steinberg, 2007). Instead, a lag in the development of psychosocial capacities (e.g., impulse control, delayed gratification, emotional regulation, resistance to peer influence) that regulate impulses contributes to adolescents' vulnerability for participation in risky behaviors. These findings suggest that changing the contexts in which risky behavior occurs may be more successful than changing the way adolescents think about risk. For example, it is important for adults in home, school, and community settings to have a strong

Box 6.8. Talking With Children About Death

Talking with a child provides an opportunity to share feelings; when feelings are understood, it is easier to cope with them.

Suggestions:

- Let the child know that it's OK to show his or her feelings. Let the child know it's OK to cry and that crying may help him or her feel better.
- Pause the conversation when the child is crying if that seems best. Provide support and comfort. Plan to continue the talk another time soon.
- Acknowledge that these conversations can be difficult. Let the child know that talking about feelings helps to process them.
- Maintain an emotional and physical presence with the child.
- Allow children to express their anger. Recognize that anger is a normal and natural response. Help children identify appropriate ways to express their anger (e.g., doing something physical or expressing anger through creative arts activities).

Source. Schonfeld and Quackenbush (2009).

presence in teens' lives, to be vigilant about teen activities and behavior, and to be knowledgeable about a range of risky behaviors and associated symptoms.

Contextual factors have been linked to the reduction of substance abuse and smoking. VanderWaal, Powell, Terry-McElrath, Bao, and Flay (2005), for example, recommended that communities wishing to reduce smoking and drinking rates among adolescents should continue to provide supervised after-school activities for their youth. They found that adult-supervised after-school activities were significantly related to lower rates of cigarette smoking, alcohol use, and binge drinking. Encouraging all teens to participate in meaningful structured leisure activities during the after-school hours may, in fact, help reduce participation in risky behaviors (VanderWaal et al., 2005). In a related way, the reduction of alcohol use may reduce the risk of suicide. Schilling, Aseltine, Glanovsky, James, and Jacobs (2009) identified the use of alcohol while sad or depressed as being associated with suicidal behavior in adolescents who may not engage in planning before an attempt.

In addition to fostering participation in meaningful activities and maintaining an adult presence in teens' lives, it is important for parents, teachers, and health professionals to be aware of signs associated with various risky behaviors. A risky behavior that many parents and health care professionals are unaware of is the "choking game," which involves self-strangulation or strangulation by another person with the hands or a noose to achieve a brief euphoric state caused by cerebral hypoxia. Although youth have played asphyxiation games for generations, limited information about this activity has been reported in the medical literature (Andrew, Macnab, & Russell, 2009). The use of ligatures to induce asphyxia and solo play has made today's version of this phenomenon more dangerous, resulting in serious neurological injury or death (Toblin, Paulozzi, Gilchrist, & Russell, 2008).

Children who participate in this behavior clearly differ from those who commit suicide or engage in autoerotic activity. Those whose deaths have been reported in the media have tended to be high-achieving and athletic youth who were not engaged in other risk-taking activities. Occupational therapists, along with parents, educators, coaches, and other health care providers, need to promote awareness of the dangers of this activity and of associated symptoms. Warning signs that youth are participating in self-strangulation include frequent severe headaches; seizures; sudden vision loss; behavior change; bloodshot eyes; marks on the neck; disorientation after spending time alone; and ropes, scarves, and belts tied to bedroom furniture or doorknobs (Andrew et al., 2009; Toblin et al., 2008).

Summary

All children face challenges at some point throughout their developing years that require coping skills and additional supports to maintain mental health and function successfully in school, home, and community activities. Some stressors may pose significant challenges, such as poverty, bullying, obesity, death of a loved one, and participation in risky behavior. Occupational therapists need to be aware of these and other situational factors that place children and youth at risk of developing mental or physical health problems and occupational performance challenges. Although it is impossible to address all situational stressors, this chapter presented examples of how occupational therapists can reduce risks and promote competencies in children at both the schoolwide and the individual levels.

References

American Occupational Therapy Association. (2007). Obesity and occupational therapy (position paper). *American Journal of Occupational Therapy, 61,* 701–703.

Andrew, T. A., Macnab, A., & Russell, P. (2009). Update on "the choking game." *Journal of Pediatrics, 155,* 777–779.

Attwood, T. (2002). *The profile of friendship skills in Asperger's syndrome.* Retrieved January 11, 2010, from www.tonyattwood.com.au/pdfs/attwood2.pdf

Ayyash-Abdo, H. (2001). Childhood bereavement: What school psychologists need to know. *School Psychology International, 22,* 417–433.

Batsche, G. M., & Porter, L. J. (2006). Bullying. In G. G. Bear & K. M. Minke (Eds.), *Children's needs III: Development, prevention, and intervention* (pp. 135–148). Bethesda, MD: National Association of School Psychologists.

Bazyk, S., & Bazyk, J. (2009). Meaning of occupation-based groups for low-income urban youth attending after-school care. *American Journal of Occupational Therapy, 63,* 69–83.

Betz, G., & Thorngren, J. M. (2006). Ambiguous loss and the family grieving process. *Family Journal: Counseling and Therapy for Couples and Families, 14*(4), 359–365.

Black, S. (2005). Research: How teachers and counselors can reach out to bereaved students. *American School Board Journal, 192*(8), 28–30.

Bruno, J. (1996). Time perceptions and time allocation preferences among adolescent boys and girls. *Adolescence, 31,* 109–126.

Cahill, S. M., & Suarez-Balcazar, Y. (2009). Promoting children's nutrition and fitness in the urban context. *American Journal of Occupational Therapy, 63,* 113–116.

Catalano, R. F., Hawkins, J. D., Berglund, M. L., Pollard, J. A., & Arthur, M. W. (2002). Prevention science and positive youth development: Competitive or cooperative frameworks? *Journal of Adolescent Health, 31,* 230–239.

Center for the Study and Prevention of School Violence. (2008). *An overview of bullying: Fact sheet.* Retrieved January 15, 2010, from www.colorado.edu/cspv/publications/factsheets/safeschools/FS-SC07.pdf

Centers for Disease Control and Prevention. (2006). *Prevalence of overweight, obesity and extreme obesity among adults: United States, trends 1960–62 through 2005–2006.* Retrieved January 12, 2010, from www.cdc.gov/nchs/data/hestat/overweight/overweight_adult.htm

Collaborative for Academic, Social, and Emotional Learning. (2009). *Social and emotional learning and bullying prevention.* Prepared by K. Ragozzino & M. Utne O'Brien for the National Center for Mental Health Promotion and Youth Violence Prevention. Retrieved February 1, 2010, from http://casel.org/downloads/2009_bullyingbrief.pdf

Crockett, D. (2003). Critical issues children face in the 2000s. *School Psychology Quarterly, 18,* 446–453.

Csikszentmihalyi, M. (1993). Activity and happiness: Towards a science of occupation. *Occupational Science: Australia, 1,* 38–42.

De, S., Small, J., & Baur, L. A. (2008). Overweight and obesity among children with developmental disabilities. *Journal of Intellectual and Developmental Disability, 33,* 43–47.

Dehghan, M., Akhtar-Danesh, N., & Merchant, A. T. (2005). Childhood obesity, prevalence, and prevention. *Nutrition Journal, 4,* 1–8.

Demir, M., & Weitekamp, L. A. (2007). I am so happy cause today I found my friend: Friendship and personality as predictors of happiness. *Journal of Happiness Studies, 8,* 181–211.

Demir, M., Zdemir, M., & Weitekamp, L. A. (2007). Looking to happy tomorrows with friends: Best and close friendships as they predict happiness. *Journal of Happiness Studies, 8,* 243–271.

Dwyer, G., Baur, L., Higgs, J., & Hardy, L. (2009). Promoting children's health and well-being: Broadening the therapy perspective. *Physical and Occupational Therapy in Pediatrics, 29,* 27–43.

Emerson, E. (2009). Overweight and obesity in 3- and 5-year-old children with and without developmental delay. *Public Health, 123,* 130–133.

Espelage, D. L., & Swearer, S. M. (2003). Research on school bullying and victimization: What have we learned and where do we go from here? *School Psychology Review, 32*(3), 365–383.

Fox, K. R. (1999). The influence of physical activity on mental well-being. *Public Health Nutrition, 2,* 411–418.

Garey, A. I. (2002). Social domains and concepts of care: Protection, instruction, and containment in after-school programs. *Journal of Family Issues, 23,* 768–790.

Goleman, D. (1995). *Emotional intelligence: Why it can matter more than IQ.* New York: Bantam.

Grant, K. E., Katz, B. N., Kina, T. K., O'Koon, J. H., Meza, C. M., DiPaquale, A.-M., et al. (2004). Psychological symptoms affecting low-income urban youth. *Journal of Adolescent Research, 19,* 613–634.

Hall, G., Israel, L., & Shortt, J. (2004). *It's about time: A look at out-of-school time for urban teens.* Retrieved August 8, 2010, from www.wcwonline.org/component/page,shop.getfile/file_id,17/product_id,827/option,com_virtuemart/Itemid,175/www.niost.org/AOLTW.pdf

Heinrich, R. H. (2003). A whole-school approach to bullying: Special considerations for children with exceptionalities. *Intervention in School and Clinic, 38,* 195–204.

Holland, J. (2004, December). "Lost for Words" in Hull. *Pastoral Care,* pp. 22–26.

James, J. W., Friedman, R., & Landon Matthews, L. (2001). *When children grieve.* New York: HarperCollins.

Jarrett, R. (1998). African American children, families, and neighborhoods: Qualitative contributions to understanding developmental pathways. *Applied Developmental Science, 2,* 2–16.

Jenson, J. M., & Dieterich, W. A. (2007). Effects of a skills-based prevention program on bullying and bully victimization among elementary school children. *Prevention Science, 8,* 285–296.

Kusche, C. A., & Greenberg, M. T. (1994) *The PATHS curriculum.* Seattle: Developmental Research & Programs.

Mason, M. J., & Chuang, S. (2001). Culturally based after-school arts programming for low-income urban children: Adaptive and preventive effects. *Journal of Primary Prevention, 22,* 45–54.

McCown, K. S., Jensen, A. L., Freedman, J. M., & Rideout, M. C. (1998). *Self-science: The emotional intelligence curriculum.* San Mateo, CA: Six Seconds.

McGlauflin, H. (2003). *Encouraging your school to be grief friendly.* Retrieved August 8, 2010, from www.cgcmaine.org/article1.html

McLoyd, V. C. (1990). The impact of economic hardship on Black families and children: Psychological distress, parenting, and socioemotional development. *Child Development, 61,* 311–346.

Milliken, B., Goodman, G., Bazyk, S., & Flynn, S. (2007). Establishing a case for occupational therapy in meeting the needs of children with grief issues in school-based settings. *Occupational Therapy in Mental Health, 23,* 75–100.

Nabors, L., Proescher, E., & DeSilva, M. (2001). School-based mental health prevention activities for homeless and at-risk youth. *Child and Youth Care Forum, 30,* 3–18.

Nansel, T. R., Overpeck, M., Pilla, R. S., Ruan, W. J., Simons-Morton, B., & Scheidt, P. (2001). Bullying behaviors among U.S. youth: Prevalence and associations with psychosocial adjustment. *JAMA, 285*(16), 2094–2100.

National Institute on Out-of-School Time. (2004). *Making the case: A fact sheet on children and youth in out-of-school time.* Retrieved January 8, 2005, from http://niost.org/publications/Factsheet_2004.pdf

O'Dea, J. A. (2005). Prevention of child obesity: "First, do no harm." *Health Education Research, 20,* 259–265.

Passmore, A. (1998). Does leisure have an association with creating cultural patterns of work? *Journal of Occupational Science, 5,* 161–165.

Puhl, R. M. (2007). Child obesity and stigma. *Your Weight Matters Magazine, 2*(3), 1–3. Retrieved August 8, 2010, from www.obesityaction.org/magazine/oacnews7/Childhood%20Obesity%20and%20Stigma.pdf

Puhl, R. M., & Later, J. D. (2007). Stigma, obesity, and health of the nation's children. *Psychological Bulletin, 133,* 557–580.

Rimmer, J. H., Rowland, J. L., & Yamaki, K. (2007). Obesity and secondary conditions in adolescents with disabilities: Addressing the needs of an underserved population. *Journal of Adolescent Health, 41,* 224–229.

Schilling, E. A., Aseltine, R. H., Glanovsky, J. L., James, A., & Jacobs, D. (2009). Adolescent alcohol use, suicidal ideation, and suicide attempts. *Journal of Adolescent Health, 44,* 335–341.

Schonfeld, D., & Quackenbush, M. (2009). *After a loved one dies—How children grieve and how parents and other adults can support them.* New York: New York Life Foundation. Retrieved January 14, 2010, from www.nylgriefguide.com/Artworks/333866_Preview.pdf

Smallfield, S., & Anderson, A. J. (2009). Using after-school programming to support health and wellness: A physical activity engagement program description. *Early Intervention Special Interest Section Quarterly, 16*(3), 1–4.

Snyder, C., Clark, F., Masunaka-Noriega, M., & Young, B. (1998). Los Angeles street kids: New occupations for life program. *Journal of Occupational Science, 5,* 133–139.

Steinberg, L. (2004). Risk-taking in adolescence: What changes, and why? *Annals of the New York Academy of Sciences, 1021,* 51–58.

Steinberg, L. (2007). Risk taking in adolescence: New perspectives from brain and behavioral science. *Current Directions in Psychological Science, 16,* 55–59.

Stiller, B., Ross, S., & Horner, R. (n.d.-a). *Bully prevention manual—Elementary school level.* Retrieved January 10, 2010, from www.pbis.org/common/pbisresources/publications/bullyprevention_ES.pdf

Stiller, B., Ross, S., & Horner, R. (n.d.-b). *Bully prevention manual—Middle school level.* Retrieved January 10, 2010, from www.pbis.org/common/pbisresources/publications/BullyPrevention_PBS_MS.pdf

Storey, K., Slaby, R., Adler, R., Minotti, J., & Katz, R. (2008). *Eyes on bullying: What you can do.* Retrieved August 8, 2010, from www.eyesonbullying.org/pdfs/toolkit.pdf

Swank, J. M., & Robinson, E. H. M. (2009, March). *Addressing grief and loss issues with children and adolescents of military families.* Paper based on a program presented at the American Counseling Association Annual Conference and Exposition, Charlotte, NC.

Swearer, S. M., Espelage, D. L., Love, K. B., & Kingsbury, W. (2008). School-wide approaches to intervention for school aggression and bullying. In B. Doll & J. A. Cummings (Eds.), *Transforming school mental health services* (pp. 187–212). Thousand Oaks, CA: Corwin Press.

Toblin, R. L., Paulozzi, L. J., Gilchrist, J., & Russell, P. J. (2008). Unintentional strangulation deaths from the "Choking Game" among youths aged 6–19 years—United States, 1995–2007. *Journal of Safety Research, 39,* 445–448.

Townsend, E. (1999). Enabling occupation in the 21st century: Making good intentions a reality. *Australian Occupational Therapy Journal, 46,* 147–159.

Ttofi, M. M., & Farrington, D. P. (2009). What works in preventing bullying: Effective elements of anti-bullying programs. *Journal of Aggression, Conflict, and Peace Research, 1*(1), 13–24.

U.S. Department of Defense. (2008). *Casualty report.* Retrieved September 20, 2008, from www.defenselink.mil/news/casualty.pdf

U.S. Department of Education, Office of Special Education Programs Technical Assistance Center on Positive Behavioral Interventions and Supports. (2010). *Bully prevention.* Retrieved June 15, 2010, from www.pbis.org/pbis_resource_detail_page.aspx?PBIS_ResourceID=785

VanderWaal, C. J., Powell, L. M., Terry-McElrath, Y. M., Bao, Y., & Flay, B. R. (2005). Community and school drug prevention strategy prevalence: Differential effects by setting and substance. *Journal of Primary Prevention, 26,* 299–320.

Vreeman, R. C., & Carroll, A. E. (2007). A systematic review of school-based interventions to prevent bullying. *Archives of Pediatric Adolescent Medicine, 161*(1), 78–88.

Wentzel, K., Baker, S., & Russell, S. (2009). Peer relationships and positive adjustment in school. In R. Gilman, E. S. Huebner, & M. J. Furlong (Eds.), *Handbook of positive psychology in schools* (pp. 229–244). New York: Routledge.

Whitehouse, E., & Pudney, W. (1996). *Volcano in my tummy: Helping children to handle anger.* Gabriola Island, British Columbia: New Society.

Wilcock, A. A. (1993). A theory of the human need for occupation. *Journal of Occupational Science: Australia, 1,* 17–24.

Wilcock, A. A. (1998). *An occupational perspective of health.* Thorofare, NJ: Slack.

Willis, C. A. (2002). The grieving process in children: Strategies for understanding, educating, and reconciling children's perceptions of death. *Early Childhood Education Journal, 29,* 221–226.

Wilson, W. J. (1999). *Successful youth in high-risk environments* (Urban Seminar Series on Children's Health and Safety). Retrieved August 8, 2010, from www.hks.harvard.edu/urbanpoverty/urbsem_december1999.html

CHAPTER 7

Occupational Therapy for Youth at Risk of Psychosis and Those With Identified Mental Illness

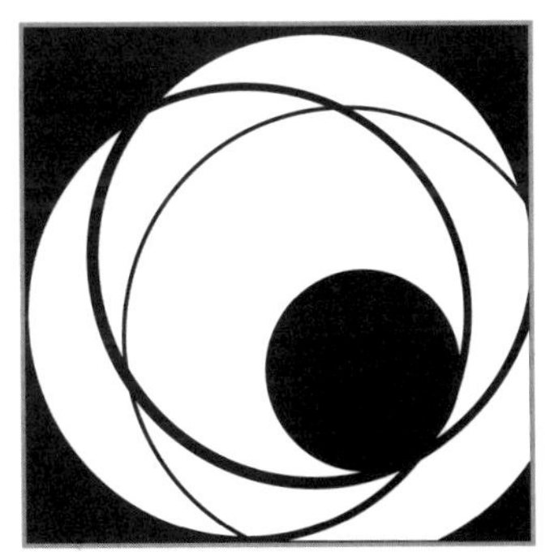

Donna Downing, MS, OTR/L

Learning Objectives

After reading this material and completing the examination, readers will be able to

- Identify specific early symptoms of the prepsychotic phase of a serious mental illness to become an "early identifier";
- Recognize specific early cognitive and sensory changes that occur in the prepsychotic phase and how they affect functioning;
- Recognize the role of substance use in the prepsychotic phase;
- Determine how early detection of and intervention with psychosis can lead to more rapid recovery and improved functioning in all performance areas;
- Identify the emerging role for occupational therapists in working with prepsychotic youth, their families, and school professionals;
- Recognize current international research for early detection of and intervention with psychosis; and
- Distinguish emerging psychosis from typical adolescent behaviors.

One of the tasks of adolescence is participation in school, whether public or private. It is not simply the act of learning that is important at this stage of life; the process of engaging with peers and community activities is equally important (Simpson, 2001). Mental health consists of positive emotions and psychosocial function (Keyes, 2007), which together allow a person to fully participate in school and benefit from that experience. Positive mental health, also known as *flourishing* (Keyes, 2007), allows a person to progress through the necessary developmental tasks of adolescence toward healthy adulthood (Simpson, 2001).

According to Keyes (2007), less than 20% of today's adult population has positive mental health, and only approximately 50% of youth between the ages of 12 and 14 have positive mental health. The decline in flourishing seen in adults places a burden on health systems and should be a call to action for all health care professionals to promote positive mental health in all areas of society and at all age levels (Keyes, 2007).

Growing evidence has supported that mood disorders and psychotic illnesses emerge in early to mid-adolescence, when the brain is still in development (Aamodt & Wang, 2008). Adolescence is the time when a person assumes more responsibility, develops a personal identity, becomes more independent from parents, builds interpersonal relationships, establishes a sexual identity, regulates emotions, sharpens opinions about morality and religion, and so forth (Simpson, 2001). An emerging mental illness can interrupt those developmental tasks, which can be a confusing situation for the person and family members (Downing, 2006).

This chapter addresses the occupational performance needs of adolescents and young adults who are experiencing new difficulties as a result of emergent mental illnesses that affect learning and general functioning. The main focus is on people who appear to be at a clinically high risk of developing psychosis, although it also addresses other mental illnesses that interfere with everyday performance issues. The early signs of psychosis are discussed along with related cognitive, social, sensory, and behavioral changes that can occur during the phases leading to a full psychotic episode.

Role of the School Environment

School is the predominant environment in which multiple components of adolescent development are shaped and in which a student's mental health is affected by social and academic stresses (Marin & Brown, 2008). Therefore, it is important that school personnel address the mental well-being of all students. Two federal acts have reinforced the need for assisting students with mental health issues: (1) the No Child Left Behind Act of 2001, which focuses on the emotional health of all children by creating specific school programs that target safety issues (e.g., bullying, violence) and healthy development in multiple performance areas, and (2) the Individuals With Disabilities Education Improvement Act of 2004 (IDEA), which mandates that schools address the mental health needs of students with emotional disabilities that interfere with academic achievement (Bazyk, 2007).

Occupational therapists have the necessary skills to address mental health issues in youth because of their medical training, knowledge of occupational performance areas, understanding of developmental tasks of adolescence, and ability to detect changes in cognition and functioning. School occupational therapists are in a position to assist with the early detection of and intervention with psychotic illnesses and the emergence of other mental health issues because they have frequent contact with students and participate in school team meetings. They can help shape school environments that promote positive mental health and can provide education to colleagues and parents about preventing or averting mental health issues. For example, some school occupational therapists collaborate with teachers to develop classroom environments and activities that promote socialization and acceptance while reducing stress (Bazyk, 2007).

Occupational therapists, whether outside consultants or school-based providers, can assist with the early detection of mental illnesses and collaborate with colleagues to make recommendations for accommodations. If school occupational therapists are knowledgeable about the early warning signs of mental illnesses, then early detection and intervention can be implemented. For example, even without direct interaction with a student who is experiencing early symptoms, classroom observations of the student's behavior and teacher reports of behavioral, social, and cognitive changes can serve as important screening data to alert the team to the need for further evaluation and early intervention. Occupational therapists who function as outside consultants can offer recommendations for enhancing school performance based on specific assessments (Downing, 2006).

Understanding Psychosis

Psychosis is defined as a medical condition of the brain that creates loss of touch with reality. It is characterized by a specific set of symptoms that occur either individually or in combination (Mueser & Gingerich, 2006). The three main symptom categories of psychosis are (1) hallucinations, (2) delusions, and (3) disorganized thinking and speech (Mueser & Gingerich, 2006). These symptoms are often referred to as *positive symptoms,* not because they are good or helpful but because they "are viewed as an excess or distortion of the individual's normal functioning" (Vancouver/Richmond Early Psychosis Intervention Program, n.d.).

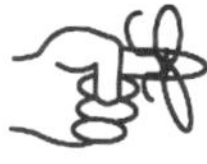

Remember this. . . .

- ***Positive symptoms of psychosis:*** hallucinations, delusions, disorganized thinking and speech
- ***Negative symptoms of psychosis:*** "absence of normal thoughts, behaviors, or feelings" (Mueser & Gingerich, 2006, p. 24).

Psychosis is considered the hallmark of schizophrenia, but it also occurs in some cases of bipolar disorder, major depression, posttraumatic stress disorder, borderline personality disorder, and substance abuse. It is also present in some medical conditions, such as malignant lung neoplasm and Alzheimer's disease (American Psychiatric Association, 2000). Although psychosis affects a small percentage of the population, it can lead to disability that disrupts the person's life in every way for a long time or a lifetime, depending on the severity of its course and whether the person gets help early (Mueser & Gingerich, 2006).

As with most medical illnesses, psychosis seems to exist on a continuum. It may begin with subtle changes that are not bothersome to the person or noticeable to someone close to him or her (Bota, Sagduyu, & Munro, 2005). As it progresses, psychosis can lead to declines in cognition and everyday functioning. It is not the positive symptoms so much as the negative symptoms that precede or accompany psychosis that seem to have the most impact on functioning, cognition, and participation in activities (Lucas, Redoblado-Hodge, Shores, Brennan, & Harris, 2009). Negative symptoms are "characterized by the *absence* of normal thoughts, behaviors, or feelings" (Mueser & Gingerich, 2006, p. 24) and are evidenced by a lack of interest in activities and people, loss of motivation, lack of facial expression, difficulty experiencing pleasure, and difficulty expressing thoughts (Mueser & Gingerich, 2006). The presence of such symptoms signals the lack of positive mental health (Keyes, 2007).

Some young people, especially those who have moved away from home to attend school, take a new job, or join the military, are able to conceal emerging symptoms from their families and close friends for long periods, even when the symptoms reach psychotic levels. This period when illness is not detected or treated is known as the *duration of untreated psychosis* (DUP; Fusar-Poli et al., 2009). Some young people experience a long DUP before their illness is detected and treatment is sought. A long DUP is now associated with a poor prognosis for recovery to a previous level of functioning (Fusar-Poli et al., 2009; Valmaggia et al., 2009).

Neuroimaging studies, such as functional magnetic resonance imaging, are providing better understanding of the psychotic process, but they have not yet revealed what distinguishes the brains of healthy participants from those who develop psychosis (Wood et al., 2008). New evidence has suggested that multiple factors, such as intense environmental stress and genetic predisposition, may trigger neurological changes (Wood et al., 2008). An international, multisite study is finding that specific features identified in the early phase before psychosis fully emerges can predict a conversion to psychosis (Cannon et al., 2008).

Recent findings have also suggested that the best protection against developing psychosis and disability is to detect symptoms of psychosis early and intervene quickly with clinical services (Auther, Gillett, & Cornblatt, 2008; Hardy, Dickson, & Morrison, 2009). The early attenuated symptoms are now believed to be a risk factor for more severe disorders. Therefore, rapid intervention to help the person preserve role function is critical, even though social functioning may not be altered with treatment (Cornblatt et al., 2007; McGorry, 2006). Intervention might involve a variety of evidence-based psychosocial treatments instead of the traditional wait-and-see approach (Edwards & McGorry, 2002). At present, no solid data exist regarding specific psychosocial interventions and their effectiveness during the early phase of emerging illness. However, Auther et al. (2008) found that families and people with attenuated positive symptoms seem to accept and engage more readily in psychosocial treatments than they do medications.

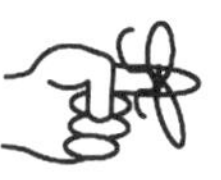

Remember this. . . .
The best protection against developing psychosis and disability is to detect symptoms of psychosis early and intervene quickly with clinical services.

Understanding Early Psychosis

During the past 2 decades, advances have been made in detecting the early signs of a developing psychosis, referred to as the *prepsychotic prodrome* (Edwards & McGorry, 2002), or *prodromal phase*. The term *prodrome* is commonly used in medicine to describe a group of symptoms indicating the onset of an illness process (Anderson, 1998). Although varied, the prodromal symptoms of psychosis are becoming better defined and can lead to improved identification of the condition (Cannon et al., 2008; Phillips, Yung, & McGorry, 2000). Note that the prepsychotic prodrome can be thought about in two ways: (1) the onset of a psychotic illness process or (2) a syndrome indicating increased vulnerability to or risk of a psychotic illness (Edwards & McGorry, 2002).

Being "at risk" does not necessarily mean that psychosis will follow (Auther et al., 2008), but it is becoming clearer that during the prodromal phase, a person's social and role functioning begin to deteriorate because of changes in the brain that affect cognition (Cornblatt et al., 2007; Woodberry et al., 2010) and, consequently, daily function. For example, a student may find he or she cannot stay focused on studies because of external or internal distractions or that he or she cannot retain verbal information during class lectures while trying to take notes. As a result, the student slowly falls behind in academics.

Studies have shown that mental illnesses accompanied by a psychotic process, such as schizophrenia, bipolar disorder, and major depression, tend to share early symptoms that may not lead to a specific diagnosis unless the person can be followed over time (Auther et al., 2008). More recent studies that have targeted early bipolar I disorder symptoms are identifying specific symptoms that are more likely to appear as part of the mania prodrome, which differ from those seen during the prodrome of schizophrenia spectrum disorders (Correll et al., 2007). Regardless of the diagnostic course of illness, people who are prodromal experience challenges in their cognitive and functional abilities. See Table 7.1 for psychiatric illnesses accompanied by psychosis and their identifying symptoms.

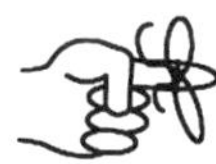

Remember this. . . . **Recognizing prodromal symptoms of psychosis can lead to early intervention for and prevention of psychosis. Early symptoms are characterized by deteriorating social and role function and appear out of character for the person (e.g., isolation from typical activities, academic decline).**

Experiential Phase of the Prepsychotic Prodrome

The continuum of psychotic symptoms begins with subtle, experiential symptoms that ebb and flow in frequency, intensity, and duration, sometimes lasting as long as 4 years before the manifestation of an illness (Bota et al., 2005). When a person who has had good mental health begins to experience the world differently because of the early symptoms of psychosis, challenges to participate in any performance area may occur because of difficulties with concentration, staying focused on tasks or conversations, and difficulties in organizing thoughts. Initially, the symptoms seem to be fleeting experiences for the person and therefore may not be considered bothersome, because they are easily ignored or normalized, even though the person may feel "This is strange" or ask "Why is this so difficult?" Over time, an increase in the frequency, intensity, and duration of the experiences leads to a decreased tolerance of daily stress and to behavior changes (Bota et al., 2005). According to Bota et al., only a small subset of people at risk of psychosis has a rapid trajectory to illness.

The experiential symptoms are frequently at a cognitive level (such as poor concentration and difficulty remembering information; Edwards & McGorry, 2002) and at a sensory level. Early sensory experiences are referred to as *perceptual distortions* (Edwards & McGorry, 2002; McGlashan et al., 2003). Examples of perceptual distortions are seeing shadows or quick-moving objects out of the corner of one's eyes while recognizing that nothing is there; hearing one's name called, but on investigation, learning that no one has been calling; or having the sensation that there is a presence standing beside oneself, but no one is there. Suddenly, sounds can seem too loud or lights too bright. These experiences can occur for a few seconds once a month and then, over an indeterminate period of time, may increase to several times a month for a few more seconds or minutes (McGlashan et al., 2003). Eventually, they become the basis for developing delusional systems (Bota et al., 2005).

As positive symptoms intensify and occur more frequently, they may become bothersome and interfere with daily functioning, but the person may not know how to describe them and may fear ridicule or rejection if he or she shares the experiences. According to Edwards and McGorry (2002), once families understand their loved one is experiencing prodromal symptoms, they may not seek help because (1) religious or cultural beliefs prevent them from seeking help; (2) they have prior negative experiences with mental health services; (3) there is a tendency to deny that a problem exists; or (4) there is a lack of knowledge of available resources.

Table 7.1. Mental Illnesses, Symptoms, Performance Effects for School or Work, and Accommodations and Supports

Diagnosis	Common Symptoms	Performance Effects	Suggested Accommodations and Supports for Occupational Therapists
Thought disorders (peak age of onset is between ages 16 and 25)			
Schizophrenia and schizoaffective disorder	• Hallucinations—visual, auditory, olfactory, and tactile sensory distortions • Delusions—beliefs that are fixed and false • Paranoia or suspiciousness • Low registration • Reduced sense of smell • Poor insight about symptoms • Reduced ability to process information • Slowed visual scanning abilities • Mood fluctuations • Reduced facial expressions (blunting)	• Distracted by internal stimulation, making it difficult to orient to tasks and stay focused and adding to the appearance of being "odd" • Difficulty organizing thoughts and articulating well, which affects school or work performance and social relationships • Isolation and difficulties making and keeping friends because of moodiness, sensory sensitivities, suspiciousness, delayed responses, and odd behaviors • Tendency to miss key information because of poor awareness of visual cues and surroundings and slowed information processing • Difficulty reading facial expressions, which can lead to inappropriate emotional responses and poor understanding of social situations • Difficulty multitasking and understanding complex directions • May need to start at the beginning when an activity is interrupted • Suicidal thoughts and acts can be persistent, often leading to suicide completion	*Note.* Medication and other therapies may be prescribed to treat these disorders; suggestions made here are to help guide occupational therapy intervention. • Use activities to help organize thoughts and behaviors, such as deep proprioceptive tasks (e.g., calisthenics, pulling a wagon filled with soil or rocks, pushing a broom, playing tug-of-war, swinging from a rope). • Use environments with few distractions in which to perform school or work tasks, for example, quiet spaces, few interruptions, predictable changes, and not crowded. • Use clear, simple instructions that are repeated, written down, or both to ensure success; use a calm tone, but not a patronizing one. • Demonstrate a new task or step first, and then allow the person to practice several times while being observed. Offer extra demonstrations and practice sessions as necessary. • Provide individualized assistance when organizing tasks, asking the person to help develop the strategies; this approach aids with recall. • Create and support opportunities for socialization with peers and coworkers, especially when social situations are not overwhelming, for example, small gatherings. Introduce client to one person who shares a common interest and assist with small talk. • Respond to signs of depression and talk of suicide. Help the person seek professional assistance when necessary.
Mood disorders (These disorders have multiple diagnostic variations, and not everyone experiences all the listed symptoms.) Bipolar I disorder and bipolar II disorder	Shifts in mood from sadness (depression) to elation (hypomania or mania) *Mania:* • Irritable • Decreased need for sleep • More talkative than usual • Too many ideas at once—thoughts race • Easily distracted • Poor judgment • Impulsive • Increase in goal-directed activities that may seem risky or reckless • Inflated self-esteem and ideas of special abilities • Psychomotor agitation • Delusions, hallucinations, or both (i.e., psychotic features)	*Mania:* • May react to frustration with lengthy explosive outbursts, which can lead to destruction, assault, or both • May react defiantly to authority • Can appear disorganized and scattered, leaping from one task to another with enthusiasm and sharing grand ideas, but never completing anything • People associating with someone with hypomania or mania feel worn out (as though they cannot keep up) • Engage in risky behaviors, such as sexual promiscuity, overspending, reckless driving	*Mania:* • Do not engage in arguments, and call for help if the person becomes explosive, dangerous, or both. • Ignore comments about superior skills and gently encourage the person to engage in a task he or she finds meaningful. • Allow autonomy when possible. • Redirect energies to perform physical activities, either alone or with one other person (to minimize opportunities for arguments and outbursts and to help with organization of thoughts and actions). • Offer simple, structured tasks that the person finds enjoyable as a way to improve attention and focus.
Major depression	• Sadness that lingers • Irritability • Low energy • Loss of interest in activities • Difficulty initiating tasks	• Affect appears sad, and person may not respond to or understand humor • Can appear argumentative or short tempered, which affects social relationships	• Eliminate decision making to increase activity engagement and reduce stress. • Offer simple, structured, familiar tasks to promote self-efficacy and productivity, one at a time.

Table 7.1. (*cont.*)

Diagnosis	Common Symptoms	Performance Effects	Suggested Accommodations and Supports for Occupational Therapists
Major depression (*cont.*)	• Sleep and appetite disturbances • Withdrawal from friends and social activities • Children and adolescents may refuse school attendance • Decreased mental functioning • Thoughts of death and suicide	• Falls asleep easily, in class, at work, in social situations • May not be able to get out of bed all day • Overeats or refuses to eat, both of which are worrisome to family and friends • Difficulty starting tasks, so may fall behind at school or work • Difficulty sustaining attention with any task or activity and difficulty processing information • Difficulty making decisions • May complete suicide attempt after suicide talk or gestures	• Encourage the development of daily routines that include good nutrition and some physical activity. • Advocate for shorter school and work days, with reduced tasks and expectations, even if only temporarily. • Offer to consult with employers, school personnel, and service providers to help with accommodations. • Invite participation, but do not push. • Keep conversations short and simple. • Set reasonable goals that are within the person's reach (e.g., "try doing this in the next 10 minutes"). • Be alert to signs and talk of suicide, then get help quickly.
Anxiety disorders (There are multiple diagnostic variations for these disorders, and not everyone experiences all the symptoms listed.) Posttraumatic stress disorder (PTSD)	• Avoiding places, people, or situations • Reexperiencing the event through images ("flashbacks"), thoughts, or perceptions • Experiencing high states of arousal, such as difficulty falling or staying asleep, irritability or outbursts of anger, difficulty concentrating, hypervigilance, exaggerated startle response • Feeling depressed or numb • Fatigue • Restlessness • Sleep disturbance because of distressing dreams of the event	• Tendency to isolate from others and withdraw from activities—may refuse school or work or drop out of extracurricular activities • Difficulty completing tasks because of fatigue, distractibility, poor concentration, restlessness, and hypervigilance • Lack of enjoyment from socializing and participating in activities • May appear fearful when asked to do something in an unfamiliar setting or with multiple people • Tends to startle easily, especially when there are loud or unexpected noises; person may have difficulty reengaging in the activity	• Explore enjoyable, calming activities, especially deep breathing, meditation, and physical exercise. • Help establish a bedtime routine that prepares for restful sleep, for example, no caffeine 5–6 hours before sleep (includes soda and chocolate), no TV 1 hour before bed, consistent bedtime. • Explore enjoyable physical activities that can be done with one other person (as a means of increasing socialization, as well). • Identify tasks the person needs to complete, then break them into easy, manageable steps with a realistic time frame (i.e., extra time allowed, but within a finite period). • People may need advocacy for environmental adaptations at school or work that reduce hypervigilance.
Generalized anxiety disorder	• Excessive anxiety and worry that is difficult to control and causes disability in social, work, school, or other important areas of functioning • Feeling keyed up or on edge • Easily fatigued • Difficulty concentrating or mind going blank • Irritability • Muscle tension • Difficulty falling or staying asleep or restless, unsatisfying sleep	• Tendency to isolate from others and withdraw from activities as a way to reduce anxiety; may refuse school or work or drop out of extracurricular activities • Difficulty completing tasks because of fatigue, distractibility, poor concentration, or low frustration tolerance • May forget thoughts when talking, which increases distress • May fall asleep in school or at work • May appear restless or have difficulty engaging in tasks • May be avoided by peers because of his or her irritability • May complain of soreness in different body areas or may appear stiff during physical activities (even when walking or sitting)	• Explore enjoyable, calming activities, especially deep breathing, meditation, and physical exercise. • Identify tasks the person needs to complete, then break them into easy, manageable steps with a realistic time frame (i.e., extra time allowed, but within a finite period). Posting a daily schedule can help reduce anxiety because expectations and tasks are clear. • Discuss ways to decrease muscle tension, for example, warm baths, yoga, stretching, heating pads on muscles. • Encourage writing thoughts on paper before speaking so there is a reference and to increase confidence. • Help establish a bedtime routine that prepares for restful sleep, for example, no caffeine 5–6 hours before sleep (includes soda and chocolate), no TV 1 hour before bed, consistent bedtime. • Explore options for dealing with restlessness in socially acceptable ways at school and work, for example, asking to take a 10-minute walk break, doing gross motor stretching. • Identify socially acceptable methods to increase arousal when sleepy in school or at work.

Sources. American Psychiatric Association (2000); Minnesota Association for Children's Mental Health (2009).

Brain Changes and Their Impact on Occupational Performance Areas

During adolescence, some regions of the brain are more active than others, and some areas, such as the prefrontal cortex, which helps regulate and select behaviors needed to meet goals, continue their development until early adulthood (Aamodt & Wang, 2008). The areas of the brain that seem to be the most active during the teen years are those areas that regulate emotional responses and seek novelty. The healthy adolescent brain is completely mature in terms of reflexes and its ability to acquire new information (Aamodt & Wang, 2008).

During the prepsychotic prodrome, a person may demonstrate behavioral changes, such as isolation or withdrawal from typical activities, and academic decline. As the psychotic process progresses, weak positive symptoms may intensify so that the person is consistently bothered by sunlight or bright lights, thinks that friends are talking about him or her, feels afraid for no clear reason, or all of these. Subsequently, the symptoms progress at varying paces to a severe level just below psychotic proportions (Cornblatt et al., 2003).

Brain Changes and Their Impact on Relationships

Most youth in the prepsychotic prodromal phase suspect that something is wrong with their brains, but they do not understand what is happening. Parents may see their teen or young adult start to fail academically and drop out of extracurricular activities while becoming more withdrawn and irritable. They may wonder whether the changes are the influence of new friends or drugs or are simply normal adolescent behavior. Peers may wonder why their friend seems irritable, withdrawn, and unapproachable, but they may not know what to say or how to help. Teachers may notice that the student is less engaged with classroom discussions, has poor concentration, is turning in homework late or not at all, and is failing academically. Employers may consider firing the employee because of behaviors, such as frequently arriving late to work, appearing distracted on the job, and being short tempered with other employees and customers. Teachers and employers may wonder what is wrong with the young person and may feel uncertain about how to help, especially when conversations have yielded little information or insight (Downing, 2006).

It is important to understand how the biological changes that occur in the prepsychotic prodromal phase can affect relationships in addition to other performance areas. Cornblatt et al. (2003) found a connection between the underlying biological vulnerability for schizophrenia and impaired social relationships. Another study suggested that once schizophrenia emerges as an illness, social skills development is arrested (Hafner, Loffler, Maurer, Hambrecht, & an der Heiden, 1999). That same study found that depression is not a reaction to emerging symptoms or a response to medications but a definite symptom of the illness (Hafner et al., 1999). Lack of motivation, social withdrawal, and lack of interest (all negative symptoms) are characteristic symptoms of depression that affect functioning and relationships.

Cornblatt et al. (2003) suggested that during the prepsychotic prodrome, as the person begins to experience cognitive decline along with increased difficulty filtering environmental sensations, anxiety increases, leading to social isolation and subsequent school failure. With increased stress or triggers, psychosis can develop (Cornblatt et al., 2003). That this progression of events increases not only the youth's anxiety but also the parents' level of apprehension and confusion about what is happening is understandable (Cornblatt et al., 2003). Although parents may appear anxious and overly concerned during the prodromal phase, they remain emotionally connected and invested in their child's welfare, especially when therapists offer support and hope (McFarlane & Cook, 2007). This finding differs from studies of people who have developed schizophrenia, in which parents and family members tend to be detached emotionally and highly critical of their ill relative (McFarlane & Cook, 2007).

Resource 7.1. Early Detection and Intervention Programs

- Portland Identification and Early Referral (PIER) Program: www.preventmentalillness.org
- Early Detection and Intervention for the Prevention of Psychosis Program (EDIPPP): www.changemymind.org

Associated Risks: Early Psychosis and Substance Use

During the prodromal phase, the young person may engage in substance use (especially marijuana and alcohol) as a way to cope with negative emotions, enhance a sense of well-being, socialize with peers, or avoid negative social consequences (Hides et al., 2008). Establishing strong connections with peers and relying on them for emotional support and a sense of connectedness is within the realm of normal teen behavior (Simpson, 2001). The limbic system, which is highly active during adolescence, can lead a young person to choose risky activities, such as experimentation with substances (Aamodt & Wang, 2008). This experimentation may not be related to symptoms, as has been previously believed, but rather may be a way to maintain social relationships and deal with the challenges of adolescence (Rey, 2007). Unfortunately, new research is showing that marijuana use in particular may trigger psychosis in someone who is biologically vulnerable (Rey, 2007).

As the illness process progresses, the young person may use substances to self-medicate symptoms, causing further decline in social functioning, cognition, and school performance (Pencer & Addington, 2008). In their study sample, Pencer and Addington (2008) also found that negative affect was predictive of substance use. Therefore, during the prepsychotic prodromal phase when negative symptoms are apparent, it seems especially important for the family, service providers, and educators to be vigilant about substance use and its effects on symptoms, learning, and general functioning.

Early Detection of and Intervention With Psychosis

The past 2 decades have seen an international effort to study the effects of identifying youth in the early stages of psychosis or in the prepsychotic prodromal phase of illness and the benefits of intervening quickly with a variety of psychosocial interventions (Auther et al., 2008; Canon et al., 2008; Hardy et al., 2009). One such program in the United States is the Portland Identification and Early Referral (PIER) Program in Portland, Maine (Resource 7.1).*

*Donna Downing, the author of this chapter, is clinical team leader of the PIER Program and is the former director of clinical training for the Early Detection and Intervention for the Prevention of Psychosis Program, which is replicating PIER in five sites across the United States.

Portland Identification and Early Referral Program

The PIER Program can be considered a public health effort (Davis, 2002) because of its focus on communitywide education about early detection of and intervention for severe mental illness, evaluation and monitoring of interventions, access to services, and epidemiological data and analyses. This family-focused research treatment program is imbedded in the Center for Psychiatric Research at Maine Medical Center but sits in a nondescript building in the community, next to a minor league baseball park. The placement of this program is purposeful: Many families experiencing the onset of illness have had no previous contact with the mental health system and tend to avoid seeking help because of the stigma of mental illness (Edwards & McGorry, 2002). Moreover, many families with a strong history of mental illness have had negative experiences associated with the mental health system and are reluctant to seek help early (Edwards & McGorry, 2002). PIER's location, which is a distance from the main hospital and outpatient mental health center, tends to eliminate such barriers.

The PIER Program began in late 2000 with minimal grant funding from local supporters and a part-time staff, which included me as the team leader and program occupational therapist. During the next few years, more substantial funding was secured through the National Institute of Mental Health, the Center for Mental Health Services, and the Robert Wood Johnson Foundation Local Funding Partnerships.

Today, the PIER Program continues as a family-focused research treatment program with grant funding. Services are subsidized, thereby eliminating another barrier to seeking help: inability to pay for services. Because the PIER Program is a research project, it has parameters, such as a contained service area for accepting referrals and a limited client age range of 12 to 25. The PIER team is multidisciplinary, consisting of a child psychiatrist, nurse practitioner, nurse, social worker, occupational therapist, employment specialist, and research interviewers. A research team and administrative staff also provide ancillary support. To date, the PIER team has provided services to approximately 150 families in the community and is working to become sustainable in some format in the future. PIER's continuation would not just promote a public health initiative by offsetting a serious illness process early: According to one British study, intervening early can have significant financial benefits over a 2-year period (Valmaggia et al., 2009).

Since 2007, the PIER Program has served as the model for a larger replication project funded by the Robert Wood Johnson Foundation, the Early Detection and Intervention for the Prevention of Psychosis Program (EDIPPP). After an application process, four EDIPPP sites were chosen: California, Oregon, Michigan, and New York, with the PIER Program serving as the National Program Office and fifth site (Downing & Spring, 2007). In 2008, the University of New Mexico joined the study with major funding from private donors and some assistance from EDIPPP. The Robert Wood Johnson Foundation considers EDIPPP the basis for a paradigm shift in the prevention and treatment of mental illness, which according to Davis (2002) is lacking in the United States even though such national agendas exist in Australia, New Zealand, and Canada (Davis, 2002). EDIPPP is building the evidence to change the way mental health services are delivered in the future.

Engaging the Community

The PIER Program's original mission was to reduce the incidence of psychosis in the greater Portland area by identifying young people at risk of psychosis and then offering treatment before its onset. That mission has evolved to include offsetting an illness process at the earliest possible point to preserve functioning. To promote PIER's original mission, an extensive outreach campaign was implemented in 2000 to educate community stakeholders about the importance of early detection of and intervention for psychosis while training them to become early identifiers and referrers. This education involved learning the early warning signs of the prepsychotic phase (Box 7.1). During the past 9 years, most PIER staff have participated in outreach activities, regardless of their professional discipline.

A list of community members who were considered potential early identifiers and referrers was developed, such as school, mental health, and medical professionals. School professionals included teachers, occupational therapists, guidance counselors, psychologists, social workers, nurses, and administrators. Later, the list expanded to include parents, youth workers, students, employers, and clergy. All audiences were taught the specific early symptoms of the prepsychotic prodromal phase and the benefits of identifying and intervening early in the illness process. The message to trainees was that they were perfectly positioned to be early identifiers because of their frequent interactions with youth. Thus, they were considered by PIER staff to be gatekeepers (Downing & Spring, 2007).

The outreach efforts paid off within a few months when referrals to PIER began to occur with frequency. Today, referrals continue to be made to PIER on a regular basis because of enduring outreach. An evaluation process conducted by a local, independent research team is showing that those referrals can be traced directly to outreach activities (Joly, Pukstas, Williamson, Mittal, & Pratt, 2009). Additionally, over time the referrers have become more accurate in their identification of the early

Box 7.1. Early Warning Signs in the Prepsychosis Phase

People experiencing a combination of at least two of the following (new experiences) may be in the prepsychosis phase; concern is warranted:

- Jumbled speech or writing
- Trouble speaking clearly, not understanding others
- Feeling "something's not quite right"
- Declining interest in people, activities, and self-care
- Being fearful for no good reason
- Hearing sounds or voices that no one else hears
- Declining mental acuity, memory, or attention
- Seeing things that no one else sees
- Suicidal thoughts
- Belief that he or she has special powers
- Dramatic changes in sleep or appetite
- Unwarranted suspiciousness of others
- Extreme and unreasonable resentments or grudges
- Jumbled thoughts or confusion.

warning signs of psychosis (McFarlane et al., 2010). Referrers report that they are seeking services for students earlier than in the past because of increased awareness of the benefits of early detection and intervention. Consequently, even if a young person does not appear to be appropriate for PIER services, he or she is referred to services (e.g., counseling, medication evaluation, personal care physician) in the community earlier than in the past.

PIER Program Services

The PIER staff initiate a partnership with the family from the first contact to promote an environment conducive to recovery and improved functioning. According to the systems-of-care paradigm, family involvement and partnerships are critical to improving outcomes by minimizing the effects of stress on psychological well-being, creating supportive environments, and advocating for services (Fette & Estes, 2009). *Systems of care* refers to community resources that are child and family centered and deliver coordinated care to meet children's mental health needs (Fette & Estes, 2009).

PIER is considered to be a family program because it includes parents, siblings, and secondary relatives in all phases of treatment, beginning with the first phone contact (either the referral call or call to family if they have been referred by someone else in the community), and continuing through the research evaluation process and treatment phase. See Box 7.2 for examples of how families and youth are included in the PIER model.

PIER's research assessments are important because they offer information about family relationships and levels of stress experienced by all family members in the prodromal phase, as well as insight into what families need during this phase. Some research assessments provide insight into the course of illness and the effectiveness of specific interventions over time. Although analysis of study results is not yet complete, preliminary results have shown that families are invested in their loved ones'

Box 7.2. Areas of Portland Identification and Early Referral Program Family Inclusion

- *Baseline research appointments:* These sessions consist of answering questions (either verbally or through written self-reports) about the referred person's developmental history, family history of mental illness, recent symptoms, person's social and role functioning, and family relationships.
- *Educational sessions:* All family members are asked to participate to share with and receive information from the treatment team, such as symptoms, occupational performance issues, strengths, challenges, social networks, support systems, and the like. During these sessions, the treatment team offers information about what is happening on a biological level, answers questions about the treatment, provides information about the program services, and, most important, starts partnering with family members.
- *Psychoeducational multifamily groups:* These 1.5-hour structured, problem-solving sessions are held every other week with five to six other families. One problem is worked on each session by the entire group, and the family with the problem leaves with an action plan to work on for the next 2 weeks. The family then reports their results back to the group.
- *One-day educational workshop:* This classroom-style, 4- to 5-hour workshop helps prepare family members for the psychoeducational multifamily group by gathering more information about the illness process and psychosocial interventions while meeting other families who will be in their group. Parents, grandparents, siblings, and clients are encouraged to attend.
- *Regularly scheduled or as-needed meetings.* These meetings are held with the clinical team, psychiatrist, or both.
- *Key research appointments:* Research evaluations, questionnaires, and surveys are repeated at 6, 12, and 24 months by family members and the client.

lives, clients' functional levels are improving (e.g., working, graduating from high school, regularly attending school), and progression to a first episode of psychosis is infrequent and low compared with that found in other international studies (Canon et al., 2008; McFarlane et al., 2010).

The PIER Program uses a combination of psychosocial interventions considered to be evidence-based practices for people with chronic and persistent mental illness but offers them to youth and young adults in the prodromal phase. Treatments offered are family psychoeducation, medication management, substance use counseling, assertive community treatment, supported employment, supported education, and supportive counseling (Box 7.3).

Toolkits for the first five interventions are available on the Center for Mental Health Services' Web site (see http://mentalhealth.samhsa.gov/cmhs/CommunitySupport/toolkits/illness). These interventions are being researched with the prodromal population to determine whether they help preserve functioning and social relationships while reducing stresses that influence illness symptoms.

Occupational Therapy Services

Once a young person meets criteria for PIER services, the team occupational therapist completes an assessment to determine baseline functioning in areas of occupational performance (i.e., play and leisure, activities of daily living [ADLs], instrumental activities of daily living [IADLs], social participation, education, work, sleep, rest) and sensory, motor, and cognitive abilities. The occupational therapist first meets with the client and family to gather information, explore goals, and discuss assessment options and the rationale for the evaluation process. Structured observations and selected standardized assessment tools are part of the evaluation process (Table 7.2). Once the evaluation is completed, a report is written in a user-friendly format that is shared with the client, family, and treatment team. This report should focus on the client's strengths and provide recommendations for addressing any occupational performance challenges. If the family gives permission, the report is shared with the client's service providers (e.g., family doctor, counselor) and school team.

The PIER occupational therapist contributes to the client's treatment plan by sharing strengths, challenges, and goals identified during the evaluation process. The therapist also participates in regular case reviews to better understand each client's level of symptoms, family involvement, family issues, general functioning, and symptom acuity. The occupational therapist then collaborates with the team employment specialist regarding supported education and employment interventions. Although the PIER employment specialist generally attends a client's individualized education program (IEP) or 504 plan meeting at school, the PIER occupational therapist attends the meetings when the evaluation report contains information to share.

On the basis of the evaluation findings, the occupational therapist makes recommendations to support the client's functional goals. For example, the therapist may recommend strategies to enhance school performance on the basis of a client's learning style and sensory preferences, such as sitting in a particular seat in the classroom to decrease environmental distractions, recording lectures to compensate for delayed information-processing abilities, or taking additional time in a quiet setting to complete an exam because of distractibility. Similarly, the therapist

Box 7.3. Psychosocial Treatments Offered to Portland Identification and Early Referral (PIER) Families

- *Family psychoeducation:* This term refers to individual and group educational opportunities for all family members. From the first point of contact, youth and young adults and their families are given information about their experiences in a hopeful manner and in a form they can understand at that moment (e.g., people in crisis have difficulty processing and remembering information). The sessions provide opportunity for discussions, questions, and reinforcing messages while learning about the psychotic prodromal phase or first episode phase of illness. Once the family is engaged in the program, they are encouraged to participate in one of the multifamily groups (see Box 7.2).
- *Medication management:* Program participants who receive medication to help with symptoms (i.e., positive, negative, generalized anxiety) are seen regularly by a psychiatrist or family nurse practitioner to monitor effects and side effects of medications. PIER and the other Early Detection and Intervention for the Prevention of Psychosis Program (EDIPPP) sites offer low-dose medications to participants who can benefit from them, then medical staff track weight gain (in relation to normal growth) and extrapyramidal signs that may be caused by medications. The youth or young adult and his or her families are encouraged to be forthcoming about side effects and to openly discuss medications with the treatment team rather than stop them independently.
- *Substance use counseling:* The EDIPPP treatment teams provide substance use counseling to program participants and their families as part of their treatment. On occasion, a participant needs residential treatment to help combat addictions, but such interventions tend to be rare.
- *Assertive community treatment:* This term refers to the entire team's (clinical and research) ability to be mobile; they can meet the youth or young adult and family in their home, at school, in the physician's office, at the private counselor's office, and so forth. The team becomes an assertive community treatment team when it has this capability and consequently is able to decrease barriers to services and advance early engagement.
- *Supported employment:* This intervention refers to assistance with work in any manner that may be helpful to the youth or young adult and, on occasion, to another family member. The team's employment specialist meets with the person to discuss work history, present functional difficulties, work interests, and goals. The occupational therapist offers information to the person, employment specialist, family, and team about the person's strengths and challenges, based on cognitive and functional assessments. Sometimes the program participant simply needs encouragement to look for work or help with developing a resume. Other times, the person needs assistance with keeping the job, such as analysis of the job tasks and the work environment so that accommodations can be recommended.
- *Supported education:* This is not an evidence-based practice as yet, but the EDIPPP study hopes to contribute to the data regarding the usefulness of this intervention with youth at risk or ultra-high risk of a psychotic illness. Evidence is being collected with young people who have developed a major mental illness and who are receiving support with their educations. Most young people in EDIPPP receive some form of support with their educations from the occupational therapist and employment specialist in their program. The treatment team, person, family, and school personnel work together to discuss needed supports and possible accommodations to promote improved school performance.
- *Supportive counseling:* As the name implies, these sessions are supportive in nature and are not psychotherapy. The EDIPPP young person meets with the clinician to work on issues of everyday functioning. Many times, family members are invited into the sessions, particularly when the person is young (12–14) and has difficulties with occupational performance areas such as social relationships, school, sleep, and nutrition.

Note. The first five psychosocial interventions are considered evidence-based practices for severe, persistent mental illness and are being trialed with prepsychotic and high-risk youth in the EDIPPP study. Toolkits for these evidence-based practices are available on the Center for Mental Health Services Web site (see http://mentalhealth.samhsa.gov/cmhs/CommunitySupport/toolkits/illness).

may recommend ways to enhance success in the work setting by restructuring tasks, modifying environments, or increasing or decreasing the amount and type of supervision needed. When appropriate and with the family's or client's permission, the occupational therapist provides education about the early phase of illness to increase educators' or employers' level of understanding about the illness process and how it affects the person's functioning in all areas.

Table 7.2. Portland Identification and Early Referral Occupational Therapy Assessments

Assessment Tool	Areas Assessed
Allen Cognitive Level Screen (Allen et al., 2007): Leather lacing task with progressive complexity	Executive functioning
Adolescent/Adult Sensory Profile (Brown & Dunn, 2002): Self-report questionnaire about sensory preferences	Sensory preferences
Assessment of Motor and Process Skills (Fisher, 2003): Two familiar daily activities of client's choosing are performed	Cognitive and motor skills
Canadian Occupational Performance Measure–4th edition (Law et al., 2005): Individual interview to better understand the client's satisfaction and motivation with all performance areas	Daily functioning; role performance and satisfaction
Contextual Memory Test (Toglia, 1993): Uses pictures with or without a theme to measure recall and strategy use	Short-term visual memory; executive skills
Motor-Free Visual Perceptual Test–3rd Edition (Colarusso & Hammill, 2003): Uses shapes in a visual multiple-choice format	Visual perception in five areas
Rivermead Behavioural Memory Test–II (Wilson, Cockburn, & Baddeley, 1986): Varied tasks to assess multiple areas of recall	Gross memory
Test of Everyday Attention–Child and Adult versions (Robertson, Ward, Ridgeway, & Nimmo-Smith, 1994): interactive, broad measure of the most important clinical aspects of attention	Selective attention, sustained attention, attentional switching, divided attention, and working memory

Note. Tools are selected on the basis of the client's needs.

A case example illustrating the PIER occupational therapist's interventions with an adolescent experiencing attenuated positive symptoms and a decline in functioning is presented in Box 7.4. This example can guide a school-based occupational therapist's interventions as well.

School Occupational Therapy Involvement With the PIER Program

When a PIER client requires educational support, it is important that the school team, the family, and the PIER Program team collaborate. The school occupational therapist can bridge the gaps between the outside mental health services, the home, and the school setting (Downing, 2006). Marin and Brown (2008) noted that peer and teacher support can increase motivation to achieve academically while helping psychologically. The school occupational therapist has the necessary skills to carry out the PIER occupational therapist's recommendations while introducing her or his own suggestions for enhanced learning and social opportunities at school.

Three-Tiered Model of Mental Health Promotion and Supports

In most school districts, unless students with prodromal symptoms or mental illness are eligible for special education, the occupational therapist may not have an opportunity to include them in her or his caseload. With increasing opportunities to integrate services in the classroom setting and provide early intervention services, occupational therapists need to be watchful for students who may be demonstrating signs of early psychosis and advocate for early accommodations and supports. When adopting a three-tiered public health model of mental health promotion and

Box 7.4. Case Example: Allison

Allison, a 13-year-old seventh grader, is referred to the Portland Identification and Early Referral (PIER) Program by the school social worker and meets criteria for the program on the basis of attenuated positive symptoms, a steady decline in school performance, and withdrawal from peers. She is living with her mother, stepfather, and 6-year-old half-brother. Her biological father, who carries a diagnosis of bipolar I disorder with psychosis, is not involved with her life, but her stepfather seems to be caring and involved. The school social worker is aware of the early signs of psychosis because of recent PIER outreach training. She is also aware of Allison's biological father's history of psychosis, which places her at high risk of psychosis.

After the research intake assessment process, the PIER occupational therapist meets with Allison and her mother for a first session. They report that Allison is having increasing trouble processing auditory information but does not have a learning disability. She also demonstrates a heightened response to environmental stimuli, resulting in sensory avoidance. During assessment with the Canadian Occupational Performance Measure (Law et al., 2005), Allison reports that she no longer likes school and is dissatisfied with her academic performance and socialization. She still enjoys some hobbies, such as writing poetry, which she does in her bedroom. Writing is an area of satisfaction for her. She tends to avoid school and is at risk of having too many absences, which could result in the need to take summer classes. Allison is not completing or handing in assignments, which is a performance change. In the past, she has been a conscientious student, handing in assignments on time.

Allison and her mother agree on two major goals: (1) attend school each day and (2) complete class assignments on time. They want to know what they can do to reduce stimuli so that she will be less distracted in class, feel more motivated to be social, and feel less stressed. The occupational therapist discusses the occupational therapy evaluation process and which assessment tools will provide information about her cognitive and functional abilities and her sensory preferences. She schedules a second assessment session for later in the week and discusses what she and Allison will do during that meeting: Complete (1) the Adolescent/Adult Sensory Profile (Brown & Dunn, 2002) to better understand Allison's sensory preferences and (2) the Test of Everyday Attention–Child Version (Robertson et al., 1994), to better understand Allison's difficulties with attention. The occupational therapist schedules a third session for Allison to participate in two activities of daily living (ADLs) that she chooses as part of the Assessment of Motor and Process Skills (Fisher, 2003). Allison decides to make a sandwich and sweep the floor, which are two familiar activities.

Before ending the first session, the occupational therapist asks Allison and her mother to help make a plan for Allison get to school the next day. Together, they develop a detailed action plan that includes specifics about (1) how Allison will wake up (i.e., she will set her clock radio that night for earlier than usual to allow more time to get ready); (2) what will help her feel less anxious so that she will more easily leave the house (i.e., have her mother drive her to school with her best friend); and (3) whom she can contact at school if she starts to feel anxious (i.e., the school nurse or a favorite teacher). They identify specific tasks for each of them to carry out to make the plan successful. Allison and her mom create a reward system that consists of spending time together the next evening if Allison attends school on time and stays there for the day. The end result is that Allison and her mother feel more positive, hopeful, and less stressed because they have a clear plan. Mother and daughter agree to tackle the homework issue at home later that day, using some of the techniques they learned in the session with the occupational therapist.

Results of the Adolescent/Adult Sensory Profile reveal that Allison rates "much more than most people" in the areas of sensory sensitivity and sensory avoidance. This finding matches reports of Allison's recent experiences and behaviors. When she makes a sandwich and sweeps the floor for the Assessment of Motor and Process Skills activities, she demonstrates significant difficulties with executive functioning skills (especially with planning and sequencing), crossing the midline, and trunk stability. During the Test of Everyday Attention, it is clear that Allison has difficulty with divided attention, visual scanning, and verbal working memory. All of these difficulties have an impact on multiple occupational performance areas at school and home, including her desire to be social. The assessments also reveal Allison's strengths (e.g., motivation, good social skills, pleasant manner, ability to sustain attention when distractions are minimal, insight about deficits), which the occupational therapist includes in her report.

The PIER occupational therapist develops a short report that is easy for parents and school staff to understand, that is, jargon is eliminated. The report includes Allison's strengths and challenges and recommendations for addressing her sensitivities, specific learning style, extracurricular activities, and social opportunities. All of the recommendations are easy to implement and nonstigmatizing, especially for the classroom setting, which is an important issue at Allison's age. The PIER occupational therapist asks the family whether she can share her assessment results during the pending individualized education program meeting and whether she can enlist the aid of the school occupational therapist to help implement some of the recommendations. The family agrees to both requests.

supports, efforts to function outside a caseload model will be essential. Because of increased demands for their services, decreased time to see students, and limited school district funds, the school occupational therapist may not have time to work directly with a student with prodromal symptoms or with the student's classroom teacher to develop accommodations (A. Lachance, personal communication, June 20, 2009). However, a range of services reflecting promotion, prevention, and intervention may be provided within a tiered model. Occupational therapy's role within each tier is discussed in the following sections.

Tier 1: Universal Interventions

As an example of a primary prevention–level service, occupational therapists can offer in-service professional development training sessions to teachers and professional staff about sensory preferences and ways to alter environments to decrease stress and promote learning and socialization. In addition, the educational staff can benefit from information about designing classroom environments for enhanced learning while minimizing problem behaviors and decreasing sensory overload for students like the young woman described in the case example in Box 7.4 (Bazyk, 2007). The school staff can learn that specific school areas, such as the cafeteria, library, and playground, can be designed to reduce environmental stress, thereby reducing the number of behavioral issues at school while promoting positive social participation (Bazyk, 2007). These three areas are venues in which approximately half of all behavior problems occur (Bazyk, 2007).

Tier 2: Targeted Interventions

An example of the school occupational therapist's participation at the secondary prevention level is for the therapist to consult with or assist the school social worker with developing a small social skills group for youth displaying difficulties interacting with peers because of behavioral issues (e.g., aggressiveness, bullying) or emotional difficulties (e.g., anxiety, depression, trauma, early psychosis). Many schools already offer groups co-led by occupational therapists and social workers, but these groups tend to address sensory, motor, or eating issues. In a group for youth displaying behavioral or emotional difficulties, the occupational therapist guides the intervention by recommending age-appropriate, enjoyable activities that reduce stress and promote socialization, organization of thoughts, self-confidence, and self-efficacy. The therapist may recommend a small group size (approximately four to six youth) to help students feel more comfortable, which in turn fosters social participation and successful activity engagement.

For example, the coleaders may ask the fifth and sixth graders in the small group to pair up to trace the outline of their partners' bodies and then decorate their own outlines. The interactions are not forced, and opportunity to work alone after a brief interaction with one peer is provided. The therapist and social worker guide and assist throughout. If there is time during the same session, the students talk about their body drawings and contribute one positive comment about their peers' drawings. Otherwise, they wait until the next session to complete their body drawings and then discuss them. Another activity could be a joint project to help other people in the community, such as baking cookies for the neighborhood nursing home and then delivering them or making one large holiday decoration to display in the school lobby. When a group activity has a common goal, one person is not responsible for the outcome.

Tier 3: Intensive, Individualized Interventions

For intensive individualized interventions, which are considered to be at the tertiary prevention level, the school occupational therapist offers direct service to the student with behavioral or mental health issues. At this level, the practitioner works directly with the student and teachers to identify useful accommodations that decrease sensory stimuli, reduce stress, and enhance learning (Table 7.3).

For a high school student who has symptoms of prodromal psychosis and has difficulty getting to school on time, an intervention may be to review bedtime rituals and develop a step-by-step plan for getting to school on time (see Box 7.4). Accommodations can be simple and easy to implement, such as waiting to leave each class until just before the next bell rings because fewer people are passing in the hallways at that time; changing seats to decrease visual and auditory stimulation; organizing homework assignments and breaking them into small steps to complete them on time; and finding a friend to assist with note taking. At this level, the occupational therapist should discuss interests outside of school and ways in which the student can reengage with them over time, such as reconnecting with a friend with whom the student has enjoyed playing tennis or riding mountain bikes. The student may need assistance to develop a plan for reconnecting with friends, just as he or she does for improving academics or work performance (Downing, 2006).

Summary

Occupational therapists' work with adolescents and young adults in the early phases of psychosis is an emerging area of practice that is dependent on advances in mental health. International research has found that when a psychotic illness is detected and treated early, there is a greater chance of preserving cognition and functioning while preventing severe disability. Social skills, which affect a person's life in every conceivable way, are at particular risk of declining as psychosis advances.

Occupational therapists have the necessary training and skills to identify young people at risk of psychosis and then offer appropriate interventions to improve functioning in all performance areas. They are trained to view a person holistically while collaborating with him or her and other service providers to develop the best possible treatment plan. School-based occupational therapists are well situated to identify young people at risk of developing a serious mental illness and to then intervene early with appropriate treatments.

References

Aamodt, S., & Wang, S. (2008). *Welcome to your brain.* New York: Bloomsbury.

Allen, C. K., Austin, S. A., David, S. K., Earhart, C. A., McCraith, D. B., & Riska-Williams, L. (2007). *Manual for the Allen Cognitive Level Screen–5 (ACLS–5).* Camarillo, CA: ACLS & LACLS Committee.

American Psychiatric Association. (2000). *Diagnostic and statistical manual of mental disorders* (4th ed., text rev.). Washington, DC: Author.

Anderson, K. N. (Ed.). (1998). *Mosby's medical, nursing, and allied health dictionary.* St. Louis, MO: Mosby.

Table 7.3. Prodromal Symptoms and Their Effects on Performance Areas

Areas of Occupational Performance	Symptoms (Intensity Varies)	Occupational Performance Limitations (Vary According to Symptom Intensity)	Occupational Therapy Strategies
Education	Poor concentration, low registration, sensory sensitivity and bombardment, low motivation, avolition, slow information processing, declining verbal memory, disorganized thoughts and speech, difficulty understanding social situations, difficulty articulating problems and symptoms, mild to moderate perceptual distortions	Difficulty understanding verbal and written information, difficulty absorbing new information, slow or unable to complete tasks, difficulty engaging in tasks, withdrawal or isolation from social situations	Reduce environmental stimulation to enhance learning, encourage physical activity to increase alertness and energy, assist with organization of assignments to accommodate cognitive and sensory challenges, advocate for academic modifications.
Play and leisure	Low energy, avolition, difficulty sustaining attention and interest, perceptual distortions, difficulty organizing thoughts, difficulty with sequencing	Strong tendency to withdraw or isolate because of sensory overload and increased difficulty understanding social rules; low energy and low interest make engagement difficult, even with previously enjoyable and familiar activities.	Decrease activity demands, assist with organization, encourage brief participation (e.g., 10-minute blocks), encourage participation with a familiar person to increase socialization and help with motivation, encourage physical activity to increase alertness and energy.
Activities of daily living and instrumental activities of daily living	Poor concentration, low registration, sensory sensitivity or overload, low motivation, avolition, slow information processing, declining verbal memory, disorganized thoughts and speech, difficulty understanding social situations, difficulty with sequencing	Decreased participation, less thorough completion of tasks, refusal to engage in tasks, disorganized approach; cannot recall task sequences; may try to cover disability by delaying tasks or refusing to do them; may appear argumentative to avoid engagement	Offer strategies to assist with organization; break tasks into small, manageable steps; assist with prioritizing tasks; help develop routines that include medication management, exercise, good sleep hygiene, and healthy nutrition.
Social participation	Difficulty understanding complex social situations, desire to withdraw or isolate, low energy, difficulty sustaining attention and interest, difficulty with sequencing	Strong tendency to withdraw or isolate because of sensory overload and increased difficulty understanding social rules; low energy and low interest make engagement difficult, even with previously enjoyable and familiar activities, such as family gatherings; may not understand conversations or may lose track of what is being said	Encourage participation in social situations in which there is reduced sensory overload and numbers of people; discourage settings in which there is sensory overload (e.g., large parties, the mall); assist with planning ahead for social situations through role playing, developing strategies to keep track of conversations and people's names, when to take breaks, and so forth.
Sleep and rest	Disrupted sleep patterns because of perceptual distortions when falling asleep, nightmares, or bad dreams; difficulty settling down to sleep; appears tired with low energy	May appear tired all the time, with low energy; reduced quality of sleep interferes with all other performance areas.	Assist with sleep hygiene (preparation for sleep) and bedtime routine; identify ways to rest during the day to increase productivity.
Work	Poor concentration, low registration, sensory sensitivity and bombardment, low motivation, avolition, slow information processing, declining verbal memory, disorganized thoughts and speech, difficulty understanding social situations, difficulty articulating problems and symptoms, mild to moderate perceptual distortions	Difficulty understanding verbal and written information, difficulty absorbing new information, slow or unable to complete tasks, difficulty engaging in tasks, withdrawal or isolation from social situations	Help the person identify accommodations (based on learning style, sensory preferences, and strengths) that would improve work performance; offer support that is acceptable to the client (e.g., task analysis, coaching regarding talking with the employer, help with résumé writing)

Auther, A. M., Gillett, D. A., & Cornblatt, B. A. (2008). Expanding the boundaries of early intervention for psychosis: Intervening during the prodrome. *Psychiatric Annals, 38*(8), 528–537.

Bazyk, S. (2007). Addressing the mental health needs of children in schools. In L. Jackson (Ed.), *Occupational therapy services for children and youth under IDEA* (3rd ed.). Bethesda, MD: AOTA Press.

Bota, R. G., Sagduyu, K., & Munro, J. S. (2005). Factors associated with the prodromal progression of schizophrenia that influence the course of the illness. *CNS Spectrums, 10*(12), 937–942.

Brown, C., & Dunn, W. (2002). *Adolescent/Adult Sensory Profile.* San Antonio, TX: Therapy Skill Builders.

Cannon, T. D., Cadenhead, K., Cornblatt, B. A., Woods, S. W., Addington, J., Walker, E., et al. (2008). Prediction of psychosis in youth at high clinical risk: A multisite longitudinal study in North America. *Archives of General Psychiatry, 65*(1), 28–37.

Colarusso, R. P., & Hammill, D. D. (2003). *Motor-Free Visual Perception Test: Third edition.* Novato, CA: Academic Therapy.

Cornblatt, B. A., Auther, A. M., Niendam, T., Smith, C. W., Zinberg, J., Bearden, C. E., et al. (2007). Preliminary findings for two new measures of social and role functioning in the prodromal phase of schizophrenia. *Schizophrenia Bulletin, 33*(3), 688–702.

Cornblatt, B., Lencz, T., Smith, C. W., Correll, C. U., Auther, A., & Nakayama, E. (2003). The schizophrenia prodrome revisited: A neurodevelopmental perspective. *Schizophrenia Bulletin, 29*(4), 633–651.

Correll, C. U., Penzner, J. B., Frederickson, A. M., Richter, J. J., Auther, A. M., Smith, C. W., et al. (2007). Differentiation in the preonset phases of schizophrenia and mood disorders: Evidence in support of a bipolar mania prodrome. *Schizophrenia Bulletin, 33*(3), 703–714.

Davis, N. J. (2002). The promotion of mental health and the prevention of mental and behavioral disorders: Surely the time is right. *International Journal of Emergency Mental Health, 4*(1), 3–29.

Downing, D. T. (2006). The impact of early psychosis on learning: Supported education for teens and young adults. *OT Practice, 11*(12), 7–10.

Downing, D., & Spring, E. (2007). Community collaboration helps to target early detection and intervention for psychosis. *National Council Magazine, 3,* 32–33.

Edwards, J., & McGorry, P. D. (2002). *Implementing early intervention in psychosis: A guide to establishing early psychosis services.* London: Cromwell.

Fette, C., & Estes, R. (2009). Community participation needs of families with children with behavioral disorders: A systems of care approach. *Occupational Therapy in Mental Health, 25,* 44–61.

Fisher, A. G. (2003). *Assessment of Motor and Process Skills: Volume 1—Development, standardization, and administration manual* (5th ed.). Fort Collins, CO: Three Star Press.

Fusar-Poli, P., Meneghelli, A., Valmaggia, L., Allen, P., Galvan, F., McGuire, P., et al. (2009). Duration of untreated prodromal symptoms and 12-month functional outcome of individuals at risk of psychosis. *British Journal of Psychiatry, 194,* 181–182.

Hafner, H., Loffler, W., Maurer, K., Hambrecht, M., & an der Heiden, W. (1999). Depression, negative symptoms, social stagnation and social decline in the early course of schizophrenia. *Acta Psychiatrica Scandinavica, 100,* 105–118.

Hardy, K., Dickson, J., & Morrison, A. (2009). Journey into and through an early detection of psychosis service: The subjective experience of persons at risk of developing psychosis. *Early Intervention in Psychiatry, 3*(1), 52–57.

Hides, L., Lubman, D. I., Cosgrave, E. M., Buckby, J. A., Killackey, E., & Yung, A. (2008). Motives for substance use among young people seeking mental health treatment. *Early Intervention in Psychiatry, 2*(3), 188–194.

Individuals With Disabilities Education Improvement Act of 2004, Pub. L. 108–446, 20 U.S.C. § 1400 *et seq.*

Joly, B. M., Pukstas, K., Williamson, M. E., Mittal, P., & Pratt, J. (2009). *Early detection and intervention for the prevention of psychosis: Outreach evaluation report—Year 2.* Portland: University of Southern Maine, Muskie School of Public Service.

Keyes, C. L. (2007). Promoting and protecting mental health as flourishing: A complementary strategy for improving national mental health. *American Psychologist, 62,* 95–108.

Law, M., Baptiste, S., Carswell, A., McColl, M. A., Polatajko, H., & Pollock, N. (2005). *Canadian Occupational Performance Measure* (4th ed.). Ottawa: CAOT Publications.

Lucas, S., Redoblado-Hodge, A., Shores, A., Brennan, J., & Harris, A. (2009). Factors associated with functional psychosocial status in first-episode psychosis. *Early Intervention in Psychiatry, 3*(1), 35–43.

Marin, P., & Brown, B. (2008, November). The school environment and adolescent well-being: Beyond academics. *Child Trends, 26,* 1–11.

McFarlane, W. R., & Cook, W. (2007). Family expressed emotion prior to onset of psychosis. *Family Process, 46*(2), 185–197.

McFarlane, W. R., Cook, W. L., Downing, D., Verdi, M., Woodberry, K., & Ruff, A. (2010). Portland Identification and Early Referral: A community-based system for identifying and treating youths at high risk of psychosis. *Psychiatric Services, 61*(5), 512–515.

McGlashan, T., Miller, T., Woods, S., Rosen, J. L., Hoffman, R., & Davidson, L. (2003). *Structured Interview for Prodromal Syndromes* (Version 4.0). New Haven, CT: Yale School of Medicine, Prime Clinic.

McGorry, P. D. (2006). The recognition and optimal management of early psychosis: Applying the concept of staging in the treatment of psychosis. In J. O. Johannessen, B. V. Martindale, & J. Cullberg (Eds.). *Evolving psychosis* (pp. 19–34). London: Routledge.

Minnesota Association for Children's Mental Health. (2009). *Mental health fact sheets for the classroom.* Retrieved October 8, 2009, from www.schoolmentalhealth.org/Resources/Educ/MACMH/MACMH.html

Mueser, K., & Gingerich, S. (2006). *The complete family guide to schizophrenia.* New York: Guilford Press.

No Child Left Behind Act of 2001, Pub. L. 107–110, 115 Stat. 1425 (2002).

Pencer, A., & Addington, J. (2008). Models of substance use in adolescents with and without psychosis. *Journal of the Canadian Academy of Child and Adolescent Psychiatry, 17*(4), 202–209.

Phillips, L. J., Yung, A. R., & McGorry, P. D. (2000). Identification of young people at risk of psychosis: Validation of Personal Assessment and Crisis Evaluation Clinic intake criteria. *Australian/New Zealand Journal of Psychiatry, 34*(Suppl.), S164–S169.

Rey, J. M. (2007). Does marijuana contribute to psychotic illness? *Current Psychiatry, 6*(2), 36–47.

Robertson, I., Ward, T., Ridgeway, V., & Nimmo-Smith, I. (1994). *The Test of Everyday Attention.* London: Harcourt Assessment.

Simpson, A. R. (2001). *Raising teens: A synthesis of research and a foundation for action.* Boston: Harvard School of Public Health, Center for Health Communication.

Toglia, J. (1993). *Contextual Memory Test.* San Antonio, TX: Therapy Skill Builders.

Valmaggia, L. R., McCrone, P., Knapp, M., Woolley, J. B., Broome, M. R., Tabraham, P., et al. (2009). Economic impact of early intervention in people at high risk of psychosis. *Psychological Medicine, 39,* 1617–1626.

Vancouver/Richmond Early Psychosis Intervention Program. (n.d.). *Positive and negative symptoms of psychosis.* Retrieved May 17, 2009, from www.hopevancouver.com/Symptoms_of_Psychosis.html

Wilson, B., Cockburn, J., & Baddeley, A. (1986). *The Rivermead Behavioural Memory Test: Second supplement.* London: Thames Valley Test Company.

Wood, S. J., Pantelis, C., Velakoulis, D., Yucel, M., Fornito, A., & McGorry, P. D. (2008). Progressive changes in the development toward schizophrenia: Studies in subjects at increased symptomatic risk. *Schizophrenia Bulletin, 34*(2), 322–329.

Woodberry, K. A., McFarlane, W. R., Giuliano, A. J., Verdi, M. B., Cook, W. L., & Seidman, L. J. (2010, April). *Neuropsychological changes over one year for youth at clinical high risk for psychosis.* Poster session presented at the annual conference of the Schizophrenia International Research Society, Florence, Italy.

CHAPTER 8

Autism: Promoting Social Participation and Mental Health

Lisa Crabtree, PhD, OTR/L, and
Janet V. DeLany, DEd, OTR/L, FAOTA

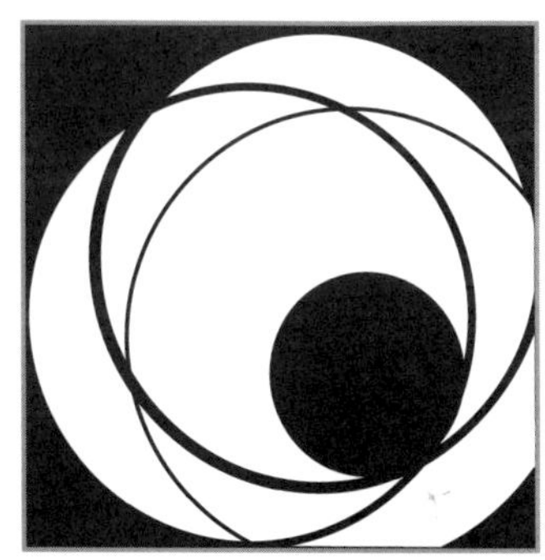

Learning Objectives

After reading this material and completing the examination, readers will be able to

- Identify characteristics of autism that hinder children's and youth's development of social participation and occupational engagement;
- Identify occupational therapists' role in promoting social opportunities that support positive mental health of children and youth on the autism spectrum;
- Identify secondary mental health challenges and co-occurrence of other mental health diagnoses of children and youth on the autism spectrum;
- Identify occupation-based intervention strategies that occupational therapists can use to support positive mental health and social participation of children and youth on the autism spectrum in collaboration with the interdisciplinary team; and
- Recognize the use of a three-tiered approach in the application of current intervention models to promote positive life experiences for children and youth on the autism spectrum.

> People on the autism spectrum are integral members of their families and communities, and have the right to fully participate in the educational, social, cultural, political, and economic life of society.
>
> —Towson University (2009)

In 2009, the Centers for Disease Control and Prevention (CDC; 2010) identified the prevalence of autism as approximately 1% of the population, a significant increase from previous estimates made in the past 10 years. This growth has made it increasingly essential for occupational therapists to promote positive mental health and social participation for this group of children and youth so that they may lead productive and fulfilling lives as integrated members of their communities. This chapter describes strategies that occupational therapists can use for the development of skills and supportive environments for children and youth on the autism spectrum.

Defining Autism

The autism spectrum is described as "a group of developmental disabilities that can cause significant social, communication and behavioral challenges" (CDC, 2010). The disorders within the autism spectrum are described in the *Diagnostic and Statistical Manual of Mental Disorders* (4th ed., text rev.; *DSM–IV–TR;* American Psychiatric Association [APA], 2000) as pervasive developmental disorders and include autistic disorder, Asperger disorder, childhood disintegrative disorder, and pervasive developmental disorder–not otherwise specified. In the planned fifth edition of the *DSM* (APA, 2010), the proposed single diagnostic category within which these individual diagnoses will be subsumed is autism spectrum disorder (ASD). Individual specifiers, such as severity of behavioral symptoms, will be used to describe a person's clinical presentation.

These lifelong developmental disabilities, which have an onset before age 3, are associated with a range of abilities across the lifespan. Although all people on the autism spectrum demonstrate challenges with social interaction and communication and display restricted, repetitive, and stereotyped patterns of behavior, many also demonstrate strengths and abilities beyond those of typically developing children and youth. It is particularly imperative, therefore, that families and occupational therapists collaborate to promote the mental health and social participation of these children and youth through early identification of their individual learning styles and the development of environments that promote meaningful participation in the home, school, and community.

Characteristics of Children and Youth on the Autism Spectrum

Children and youth on the autism spectrum have social–cognitive challenges and interpret language in a literal way, having to "think about every social interaction" (Grandin, 1995, p. 133). They may have difficulty with nonverbal behaviors such as maintaining eye contact, recognizing gestures, and interpreting others' facial expressions. Also, they may struggle with establishing and maintaining peer relationships, engaging in social and emotional reciprocity, and spontaneously participating in social activities (Macintosh & Dissanayake, 2006). As a result, they have fewer opportunities to interact with peers; this limitation can further diminish their social experiences and lead to isolation and loneliness unless they receive appropriate interventions and support.

For example, Church, Alisanski, and Amanullah (2000) described the social behaviors of 40 children and youth on the autism spectrum ranging in age from preschool to high school. The children and youth had difficulty reading others' social cues; they frequently violated social boundaries and blurted out socially inappropriate comments. The children and youth who did participate socially with others focused on common and circumscribed interests but interacted only minimally. Their difficulty with peers was a "constant source of frustration, anxiety, and confusion" for them (p. 19).

Although not a key indicator of autism according to *DSM* diagnostic criteria, 92% of children with autism demonstrate sensory processing challenges such as sensory over- or underresponsiveness and restricted food and tactile preferences (Ben-Sasson et al., 2009; Hilton, Graver, & LaVesser, 2007) that negatively influence their social participation and mental health. Retrospective studies of infants later diagnosed with autism have concluded that their unusual posturing and touch aversion, restricted gestures and expressive postures, hypoactivity, and difficulty orienting to social and nonsocial sensory stimuli affect interactions with their parents and siblings (Watson et al., 2007). Other researchers have found positive correlations between sensory modulation difficulties and communication and social difficulties (Liss, Saulnier, Fein, & Kinsbourne, 2006); between tactile, movement, and auditory sensitivities and oppositional behavior and academic underachievement (McIntosh, Miller, Shyu, & Dunn, 1999); and between sensory processing difficulties and anxiety, antisocial behavior, and communication and social challenges (Baker, Lane, Angley, & Young, 2008).

As children and youth on the autism spectrum transition to adulthood, most of them report that they face significant obstacles to employment, independence, meaningful social support, and positive mental health. In a large-scale survey of 405 children and adults on the autism spectrum in the United States, Seltzer et al. (2003) found that 73% of respondents older than age 21 reported living with their parents; only 4% lived independently, and 13% lived semi independently. In addition, 95% of respondents reported difficulty making and keeping friends, and 90% of those old enough to work could not gain or maintain competitive employment. To change these outcomes for future generations of children and youth on the autism spectrum, it is increasingly important to change the approach to intervention. Promoting positive mental health and opportunities for social participation and occupational engagement, rather than primarily focusing on remediation and skill development, is critical. The Ohio Center for Autism and Low Incidence (see www.ocali.org) is one resource for accessing current information related to best practices with children and youth on the autism spectrum (Resource 8.1).

Impact of Autism on Social Participation

The American Occupational Therapy Association (AOTA) maintains that occupational therapy intervention for children and youth on the autism spectrum should be "individualized to foster occupational engagement and social participation" (AOTA, 2005, p. 681). The social and communication challenges of these children and youth affect their social participation, which in turn influences their health and well-being (Klin, Volkmar, & Sparrow, 2000; Myles & Simpson, 2002). For instance, Macintosh and Dissanayake (2006) completed a study of the social interactions of boys with and without autism, ages 4 through 10, who were

Resource 8.1. Autism Internet Modules

Written by autism spectrum disorder experts from across the United States, the Autism Internet Modules available from the Ohio Center for Autism and Low Incidence provide information on assessment, recognizing and understanding behaviors and characteristics, transition to adulthood, employment, and numerous evidence-based practices and interventions. The modules are available at www.autisminternetmodules.org.

attending mainstream schools. Both groups of boys displayed similar diversity in the types of playground activities in which they engaged. However, compared with their neurotypical peers, the boys on the autism spectrum interacted with fewer peers, less often and for a shorter duration. Although the neurotypical boys spent most of their time in simple social play with three or more peers, the boys on the autism spectrum spent more time either unoccupied or engaged with only one peer. Factors of skill level, opportunities, and relationship development influence participation.

Social Skills

Social skills training curricula that address the particular social challenges of children and youth on the autism spectrum have been developed during the past decade. The intent of these programs is for children to learn skills for interacting and participating in social activities with others, such as playing on the playground or in the neighborhood. However, children on the autism spectrum often do not generalize skills beyond the social skills groups and do not sustain them over time (Elder, Caterino, Chao, Shacknai, & De Simone, 2006; Hillier, Fish, Cloppert, & Beversdorf, 2007). In contrast, programs that incorporate peers and provide opportunities to generalize skills to settings outside the intervention group have been shown to help children increase their social competence (Barry et al., 2003; Quinn, Kavale, Mathur, Rutherford, & Forness, 1999).

Promotion of social participation, therefore, includes integration of strategies for practicing explicitly taught social skills in natural environments with typically developing peers. For youth on the autism spectrum, the development of social skills is critical for the successful transition to adulthood. In a qualitative study of 6 adults with Asperger syndrome, Hurlbutt and Chalmers (2004) identified that one of the most critical challenges with employment was difficulty with social interaction. Struggles with getting along with employers and coworkers in the workplace had "a devastating effect on mood, mental health and self-esteem" (p. 220).

Social Isolation

Often, children on the autism spectrum do not master or are slower in learning the social competency skills necessary for experience-sharing relationships with siblings and peers—skills that most other children acquire in a developmental hierarchy starting in infancy. Although some children on the autism spectrum with limited to no verbal skills use simple gestures or augmentative communication systems to communicate basic needs and feelings, the intentionality of their actions may not be apparent to their families and caregivers. Other children on the autism spectrum develop expansive vocabularies but struggle with the pragmatics and nuances of social exchanges. Preadolescents often become more aware of their limitations in communication and social skills in comparison to their neurotypical peers and, as a result, may deliberately avoid interacting with others at home, at school, and in the community. Hilton, Crouch, and Israel (2008) found that children on the autism spectrum participated in fewer physical and social activities with fewer participants and in places closer to home than do typically developing children. Their limited engagement contributed to feelings of loneliness, isolation, and depression, which may have further restricted opportunities to develop communication and social skills for successful engagement in play, educational, and social activities with peers.

By adolescence, many youth on the autism spectrum struggle with social anxiety and social stress. They are more likely to experience poor-quality friendships and greater feelings of loneliness than their peers (Bauminger & Kasari, 2000). In a study of 235 adolescents and adults on the autism spectrum, nearly half (46.4%) reported that they did not have peer relationships (Orsmond, Krauss, & Seltzer, 2004). Instead, they reported primary engagement in solitary recreational activities, such as exercising and hobbies. Youth who were more socially adept were more likely to have peer relationships. Having the social skills and the opportunity to practice them in social and recreational contexts during childhood increased social participation and maintenance of friendships in later years (Orsmond et al., 2004).

Friendship

Bauminger and Kasari (2000) studied the prevalence and quality of friendships in children with high-functioning autism. Each child in the study perceived him- or herself as having at least one friend. A later study completed by Bauminger et al. (2008) examined the characteristics of friendships by observing interactions of dyads of typical children and children on the autism spectrum. Although the children on the autism spectrum described their friendships as less close, helpful, intimate, and fun than did typically developing children, both groups demonstrated similar patterns of leader and follower roles. The researchers suggested that although children on the autism spectrum struggle with forming friendships, they do have the capacity to form meaningful relationships and benefit from interventions that foster friendship formation and sustainment.

Co-Occurrence of Autism and Other Mental Health Diagnoses

In addition to challenges with social participation and friendship, many children and youth on the autism spectrum also cope with secondary mental health challenges. Understanding the co-occurrence of mental health challenges is important for designing effective prevention, early intervening, and individualized intensive intervention programs. Understanding the positive mental health attributes of these children and youth is equally important because doing so shifts the perspective on autism from a focus on disability to a focus on neurological diversity, consistent with some autism advocacy initiatives (Paradiz, 2005). AOTA has developed many autism-related resources, which are available on its Web site (see www.aota.org/Practitioners/Autism.aspx). The resources, which include frequently asked questions and research articles related to autism, provide practitioners with current information and strategies.

People on the autism spectrum are diagnosed with affective disorders, anxiety disorders, bipolar disorders, and attention deficit hyperactivity disorder (ADHD) at a rate similar to or higher than that in the general population. Ghaziuddin (2002) reported that as many as 40% of people referred for an evaluation of Asperger syndrome manifest additional psychiatric symptoms, including ADHD and depression.

The reasons for these high incidences are not clear, but they may be related to genetic predisposition, additional daily living stressors associated with autism, and difficulty coping with change.

Depression

Kim, Szatmari, Bryson, Streiner, and Wilson (2000) found that 20% of their sample of 49 children demonstrated clinical levels of depression 6 years after being diagnosed with high-functioning autism or Asperger syndrome. Some studies have suggested that people on the autism spectrum who (1) have higher cognitive and communication capacities; (2) have higher rates of obsessions, compulsion, and anxiety; and (3) experience peer victimization are more likely to have lower levels of self-perceived social competence and increased incidence of depression (Shtayermman, 2007; Vickerstaff, Heriot, Wong, Lopes, & Dossetor, 2007). The increased rates of depression in youth with higher cognitive and communication abilities may more accurately reflect their ability to verbalize their feelings than actual differences in the rates of depression compared with peers who have lower cognitive and communication abilities. Other authors have recognized that in diagnosing depression, it is important to attend to changes in nonverbal behaviors, such as loss of interest in preferred activities; flattened facial expressions; and increased episodes of crying, irritability, aggressiveness, self-abuse, social withdrawal, and appetite or sleep disturbance (Cooper & Hanstock, 2009; Stewart, Barnard, Pearson, Hasan, & O'Brien, 2006). Although some of those behaviors are associated with autism, the change in their intensity or frequency may provide clues to the dual diagnosis of depression in the absence of standardized tools to support such a conclusion.

Anxiety Disorders

Anxiety disorders follow depression as the most prevalent mental health conditions co-occurring with autism. Sukhodolsky et al. (2008) found that 43% of a sample of 171 children on the autism spectrum exhibited one or more anxiety disorders—a rate twice that in the general population. Although the level of social anxiety tends to increase as children on the autism spectrum age, it tends to decrease as children in the general population age (Kuusikko et al., 2008). Farrugia and Hudson (2006) found that adolescents on the autism spectrum experience anxiety at a rate similar to that of adolescents with diagnoses of anxiety disorders, but those on the autism spectrum had significantly higher rates of automatic negative thoughts, behavioral problems, obsessive–compulsiveness, and social phobias, with social phobias being the greatest source of anxiety. In a study by Shtayermman (2007), 30% of the participants with autism met the diagnostic criteria for an anxiety disorder; however, they also reported high levels of peer victimization, suggesting that environmental influences may affect clinically significant levels of anxiety.

Bipolar Disorders

The co-occurrence of autism and bipolar disorders is under investigation, and reported rates vary from 2% to 75% (Bradley, Summer, Wood, & Bryson, 2004; Munesue et al., 2008). Part of this variance stems from criteria for participant inclusion. As with trying to assess the incidence of depression, standardized assessment tools do not exist for measuring bipolar disorders for those on the autism spectrum. Thus, an astute analysis of changes in behavior is necessary to make an accurate diagnosis.

Obsessive–Compulsive Disorder

Little is known about the incidence of obsessive–compulsive disorder in children and youth with autism. One study found that 37% of 109 children on the autism spectrum also had a diagnosis of obsessive–compulsive disorder (Leyfer et al., 2006). Other authors have suggested that ritualistic behaviors exhibited during childhood can be diagnosed as obsessive–compulsive disorder in adulthood. Part of the focus on the ritualistic behaviors is associated with an intense interest as to how objects work and for a desire for predictable routines. In contrast, subjective feelings of stress and concern for how people work differentiate obsessive compulsions from ritualistic behaviors of youth on the autism spectrum (Gillott & Standen, 2007).

Attention Deficit Hyperactivity Disorder

Controversy exists as to whether ADHD occurs concurrently with autism. According to the *DSM–IV–TR,* ADHD occurs independently of pervasive developmental disorder (APA, 2000). Yet, studies have indicated that behaviors associated with both conditions occur simultaneously. Leyfer et al. (2006) and Sinzig, Bruning, Morsch, and Lehmkuhl (2008) concluded that 50% and 31% of their respective samples of children on the autism spectrum exhibited behaviors consistent with a diagnosis of ADHD. Additional studies have suggested that the quality of attention and hyperactivity symptoms may differ in youth with and without autism. For example, Corbett and Constantine (2006) found that children on the autism spectrum and those with ADHD demonstrated similar difficulties with visual and auditory attention as typically developing peers, but those on the autism spectrum exhibited greater difficulty with behavioral inhibition and sustained effort. Sinzig et al. (2008) suggested that the children with a dual diagnosis have more difficulty with divided attention, whereas those with only ADHD have more difficulty with sustained attention.

Impact of Autism on the Mental Health of the Family

Autism also affects the mental health and social participation of family members. The life of families of children on the autism spectrum who have severe behavioral challenges often centers on meeting the daily demands associated with the condition. These families indicate having only fleeting moments when they are able to engage in shared occupations that promote their sense of connectedness. Dreaming about the future and a sense of peace is not part of their experience (DeGrace, 2004). Parents also report greater levels of stress, less involvement with community and social activities, and diminished quality of life. Because of the child care demands, some parents need to quit their jobs, adding to financial burden. Chronic concerns persist about learning difficulty, bullying, social isolation, physical safety, strained marital relationships, and compromised attention to siblings (Lee, Harrington, Louie, & Newschaffer, 2008). The level of parental stress, in turn, negatively influences the mental health of children on the autism spectrum.

Promotion of Mental Health

In her influential book *Elijah's Cup,* Valerie Paradiz (2005) reframed the emphasis on the limitations of people on the autism spectrum to their strengths. On the basis of her journey with her son who has Asperger syndrome, she states in the preface, "I hope that what I have learned from Elijah—to think of autism not as a mental illness that absolutely needs a cure, but rather as a way of life that possesses a deep history and a rich culture—makes its way across [in this book]" (p. 13). Paradiz struggled for several years to find appropriate medical, child care, and educational support for her son, and she wrote of the physical and emotional exhaustion and social isolation she experienced as a single parent trying to address the complexity of his needs. Yet, as part of the journey, she also discovered an empathically sensitive son who displays deep, sustained interests; intellectual curiosity; and a sense of humor. She unearthed her own diagnosis of Asperger syndrome and the importance of modulating environments; tempering the pace and structure of daily life routines; and designing a social network to promote one's physical, mental, cognitive, and social health. By shifting her lens for interpreting how her son engages in occupations, she came to appreciate his view and the meaning he held for such occupations. For example, rather than judge his rocking and moaning behaviors as self-stimulatory, she learned to read them as signals of stress and strategies for self-calming. Rather than criticize her son's repetitive drawing of the same cartoon characters, she began to see the subtle variations in them that reflect an exploration of the visual relationship of objects to one another from various angles. Rather than become frustrated with Elijah's daily insistence about purchasing helium balloons only to release them into the air on exiting the store, she learned that it is not the possession of the balloons but rather the study of the change in their size and light composition as they ascend that is important to him. Central to Elijah's mental health and social participation is a sustained connection to a community of advocates who help the family value their own self-worth and the power of communal efficacy.

On the basis of an ethnographic study of young, nonverbal children on the autism spectrum, Spitzer (2003, 2004) also concluded that different meaning and importance may be assigned to occupations. Thus, to promote health and participation in daily life, it is important to examine how and why children on the autism spectrum engage in occupations. Emphasizing that meaning and importance are subjectively determined, Spitzer recommended attending to the children's physical movement and use of time, space, and objects to understand the sensory, emotional, symbolic, and social meaning of the occupations for them. What looks like nonresponsiveness or overfixation on minute details may reflect difficulty with or an alternative way of filtering and processing information. What appears to be self-isolating or aggressive behaviors may be self-defense or communication strategies in the absence of adequate language (DeLany & Pendzick, 2009; Notbohm, 2005). Notbohm (2005) offered thoughtful reflections from the perspective of the child, which are useful to remember when providing programs and can contribute to the mental health and social acceptance of children and youth on the autism spectrum (Box 8.1).

Box 8.1. Ten Things Every Child With Autism Wishes You Knew

1. "I am first and foremost a child. I have autism. I am not primarily 'autistic.' My autism is only one aspect of my total character. It does not define me as a person" (p. xx).
2. "My sensory perceptions are disordered. . . . I may appear withdrawn or belligerent to you but I am really just trying to defend myself" (p. xxi).
3. "Please remember to distinguish between won't (I choose not to) and can't (I am not able to). It isn't that I don't listen to instructions. It's that I can't understand you" (p. xxiii).
4. "I am a concrete thinker. This means I interpret language very literally . . . Idioms, puns, nuances, double entendres, inference, metaphors, allusions and sarcasm are lost on me" (p. xxiv).
5. "Please be patient with my limited vocabulary. It's hard for me to tell you what I need when I don't know the words to describe my feelings. I may be hungry, frustrated, frightened or confused but right now those words are beyond my ability to express. Be alert for body language, withdrawal, agitation or other signs that something is difficult for me" (p. xxv).
6. "Because language is so difficult for me, I am very visually oriented. Please show me how to do something rather than just telling me. And please be prepared to show me many times. Lots of consistent repetition helps me learn" (p. xxvi).
7. "Please focus and build on what I can do rather than what I can't do. Like any other human, I can't learn in an environment where I'm constantly made to feel that I'm not good enough and that I need 'fixing' . . . Look for my strengths and you will find them" (p. xxvii).
8. "Please help me with social interactions. It may look like I don't want to play with the other kids on the playground, but sometimes it's just that I simply do not know how to start a conversation or enter a play situation" (p. xxviii).
9. "Try to identify what triggers my meltdowns. Meltdowns, blow-ups, tantrums or whatever you want to call them are even more horrid for me than they are for you. They occur because one or more of my senses has gone into overload. If you can figure out why my meltdowns occur, they can be prevented" (p. xxix).
10. "If you are a family member, please love me unconditionally. Banish thoughts like, "If he would just . . ." and "Why can't she. . . ." I did not choose to have autism. But remember it is happening to me, not you" (p. xxx).

Source. From *Ten Things Every Child With Autism Wishes You Knew,* by E. Notbohm, 2005, Arlington, TX: Future Horizons. Copyright © 2005 by Ellen Notbohm, www.ellennotbohm.com. Reprinted with permission of author.

Interventions to Support Children and Youth on the Autism Spectrum

Because each child and youth on the autism spectrum possesses a unique constellation of strengths and limitations, interventions to support mental health and social participation must be individualized. Interventions depend on the chronological and developmental age of the child or youth and the strength and limitations of his or her occupations, performance skills, performance patterns, environments and contexts, and body functions (AOTA, 2008). Integral to intervention is consideration of the child or youth as a member of a family and a community.

Research to build evidence that documents the effectiveness of the wide range of interventions implemented with children and youth on the autism spectrum is expanding. The most documented interventions in the literature are related to applied behavior analysis (ABA) and include methods such as pivotal response treatment (PRT) and modeling (National Autism Center, 2009). *PRT* focuses on pivotal areas rather than specific behaviors, such as the child's development, motivation, self-management, and responsivity to multiple cues, and it incorporates opportunities for making choices and reinforcement of approximations of the desired behavior using natural reinforcers (Koegel Autism Center, 2010). *Modeling* includes demonstrations of appropriate behaviors by an adult and can incorporate video modeling methods (National Autism Center, 2009).

Evidence related to the efficacy of other interventions, however, will require greater systematic documentation (Baranek, 2002; Case-Smith & Arbesman, 2008). It is imperative for occupational therapists to document effective intervention strategies that support goals related to positive outcomes for children and youth on the autism spectrum. The next section describes several interventions that occupational therapists can integrate into practice to support positive mental health and social participation at each stage of development, either directly or through the role of supportive team member.

Occupational therapy interventions for infants and toddlers frequently focus on engagement in social co-occupations with parents and siblings; sensory and motor development; foundational feeding, child care, and sleeping needs; and environmental safety. Interventions developed for preschoolers may address emerging communication and social interactions, behavioral and emotional regulation, sensory modulation, and the development of cognitive and play skills. Interventions for school-age children may emphasize learning how to negotiate peer relationships; understanding social rules and social behaviors for home, school, and community; and developing social participation opportunities. In addition to a continued focus on peer relationships, occupational therapy interventions for adolescents often address hormonal influences and body changes, identity and self-determination, and transition planning.

Intervention for Infants and Young Children

Policymakers, clinicians, and caregivers are increasingly appreciating that early intervention programs help ameliorate secondary mental health and social participation challenges; as a result, additional services, such as those available from the *Learn the Signs: Act Early* campaign of the CDC (Resource 8.2), are becoming available for infants and young children on the autism spectrum. In collaboration with the interdisciplinary team, occupational therapists use a variety of approaches, including sensorimotor and sensory integration approaches; Developmental, Individual Difference, Relationship-Based (DIR)/Floortime®; early intensive behavioral intervention; and positive behavioral strategies. The integration of these approaches with occupation-based models to promote "health and participation in life through engagement in occupations" (AOTA, 2008, p. 624) distinguishes occupational therapy services from those provided by other disciplines.

Sensorimotor and Sensory Integration Approaches

Sensorimotor and sensory integration challenges, possibly the earliest at-risk indicators for autism (Flanagan, LaVesser, & Landa, 2008), negatively affect young children's ability to explore the environment, play, regulate emotion, and engage in social interactions. As children enter school, the multiple-sensory

Resource 8.2. Learn the Signs

The Centers for Disease Control and Prevention has initiated a campaign titled "Learn the Signs: Act Early" to promote early identification and intervention for children on the autism spectrum. Resource materials can be obtained from www.cdc.gov/ncbddd/actearly/index.html.

environment of the typical classroom can be a source of stress. Thus, interventions that address these challenges within the context of the family and school dynamics hold promise. "Occupational therapy using sensory integration theory and methods is designed to improve a person's ability to interact adaptively in the environment, learn, behave, and to prevent future adaptive difficulties and thus improve quality of life" (AOTA, 2009, p. 826).

Several studies have found that sensory integration approaches help to improve speech, play, attention, social interactions, and behavioral control of young children on the autism spectrum (Linderman & Stewart, 1999; Roberts, King-Thomas, & Boccia, 2007). Sensory integration approaches have also helped reduce stereotypical mannerisms and increase goal attainment (Pfeiffer, Kinnealy, & Koenig, 2008). Group-based sensorimotor play programs that encourage language and social participation have resulted in increased child-initiated sharing and turn taking. Reducing extraneous sensory stimuli and providing structured activities and predictable routines have helped reduce stress-induced disruptive behaviors and improve classroom success (Ashburner, Ziviani, & Rodger, 2008). In addition, deep proprioceptive input from nightly therapeutic massages given by parents may help improve attention, relational behaviors, and sleep patterns of young children on the autism spectrum (Escalona, Field, Singer-Strunk, Cullen, & Hartshorn, 2001). Because of the challenges to home life, families value sensory integration interventions that are connected to functional performance of daily occupations rather than those focused solely on sensory processing capacities (Cohn, Miller, & Tickle-Degnen, 2000).

DIR/Floortime

Greenspan and Wieder pioneered an approach called DIR/Floortime, which uses playful situations and appropriately matched environments to foster positive social interaction for infants and young children (Case-Smith & Arbesman, 2008; Greenspan, 1992a, 1992b; Greenspan & Wieder, 1998; Interdisciplinary Council for Developmental and Learning Disorders [ICDL], 2009a). As noted earlier, DIR stands for "developmental, individual difference, relationship-based" and is structured around six developmental milestones that Greenspan and Wieder believed are essential for healthy social, emotional, and intellectual growth. This framework allows practitioners and families to "construct a program tailored to the child's unique challenges and strengths" (ICDL, 2009b). The adult uses humanistic and developmental approaches to build on the child's limited repertoire of skills by interacting with the child on activities or actions the child finds interesting and engaging, which can include repetitive body actions or sustained focus on a particular object or toy.

The goal is to slowly and deliberately build two-way communications by guiding the child through the six stages of interaction: (1) shared attention, (2) engagement, (3) two-way purposeful interactions, (4) two-way purposeful problem-solving interactions, (5) elaborating ideas, and (6) connecting ideas for thinking (ICDL, 2000). Greenspan and Wieder (1997) proposed that 8 to 10 sessions for 20 to 30 minutes every day is optimal for promoting emotional and cognitive development and appreciated that additional support systems, such as siblings and family friends, may be needed to provide such programming. When feasible, the sessions are

Table 8.1. DIR/Floortime Stages

Stage	Goal	Intervention Examples
Stage 1: Shared attention	Encourage the child to briefly attend to the same object or action as the adult.	Direct the child's attention to the object. Strategies include • Tapping into the child's preferred sensory system by making noises or light patterns with the toy • Using playful obstruction to momentarily block access to the desired object.
Stage 2: Engagement	Establish a warm, trusting, and personal relationship.	Follow the child's lead, rather than direct the child's behavior. Strategies include • Setting up a sensory-based play environment, then joining the child in play • Expanding on the child's interests to promote more elaborate and functional play routines.
Stage 3: Two-way purposeful interactions	Build on and expand the child's nonverbal gestures and facial expressions.	Observe the child's emotional expressions and model appropriate strategies for labeling and communicating them.
Stage 4: Two-way purposeful problem solving	Foster preverbal problem solving.	Seek the child's assistance to resolve basic reality-based dilemmas that occur within the daily routine. Strategies include • Subdividing the problem into manageable chunks • Pretending not to be able to accomplish the task • Prompting the child to assist in solving the problem.
Stage 5: Elaborating ideas	Encourage the child to move beyond concrete objects to engage in imaginary play.	Use toy props to model communicating ideas and feelings with others.
Stage 6: Connecting ideas for thinking	Encourage child to functionally interact in his or her natural settings.	Prompt the child to use language during play to connect actions to ideas and to expand the range of emotional expression.

Note. DIR = developmental, individual difference, relationship-based.

Source. Interdisciplinary Council for Developmental and Learning Disorders (2000).

incorporated into the family's daily routine and within the natural setting (ICDL, 2009a). Table 8.1 provides examples of the six stages of the DIR/Floortime model that occupational therapists may incorporate into their intervention strategies.

Early Intensive Behavioral Intervention

Early intensive behavioral intervention incorporates ABA, using positive reinforcement strategies coupled with other methods such as incidental teaching and peer support to shape the behaviors of children on the autism spectrum. A highly researched method because of its systematic approach, early intensive behavioral intervention is based on the initial work of Charles Ferster, Ivar Lovaas, Montrose Wolf, and Todd Risley in the 1960s (Autism Resource Foundation, n.d.). The approach requires careful analysis of the skill to be learned, then subdivision of that skill into smaller, measurable steps that are taught using repeated drilling—a process labeled *discrete trial* teaching. The instructor uses positive reinforcers to reward the child for closer and closer approximations of the targeted behavior (Lovaas, 1987;

Sheinkopf, & Siegel, 1998). The approach also requires the instructor to systematically record the child's responses and the rewards offered. Initially, the behavior may be learned in a contrived environment until the child acquires sufficient competency to apply and generalize it in the natural environment.

Most commonly used to teach self-care, preacademic, or academic skills when working with young children, early intensive behavioral intervention also can be used to shape appropriate behaviors; develop foundational communication skills; and facilitate basic social interactions such as developing motor and verbal imitation skills, following basic directions, making simple requests, and playing with others. Intensive ABA school- and home-based programs typically require one-on-one instruction for 35 to 40 hours per week (Lovaas Institute, 2009). Usually, a behavioral specialist with advanced training in ABA methods is responsible for designing and overseeing the program's implementation. Because of this level of intensity, families and school professionals may opt for a modified ABA approach to teaching selected skills. Occupational therapists may use this approach in collaboration with other professionals to address targeted behaviors.

Positive Strategies for Managing and Preventing Out-of-Control Behaviors

Baker (2008) offered a pragmatic four-step program that emphasizes positive strategies for minimizing and managing out-of-control behaviors and increasing opportunities for social participation and positive self-esteem. His program is not discipline specific, thereby allowing for interdisciplinary and family collaboration.

The program's first step contributes to the family's mental health by acknowledging that the child's out-of-control behavior is not a reflection of their failure to provide adequate caregiving. Rather, Baker clarified that out-of-control behaviors are not abnormal but an intense fight-or-flight response to a situation that the child perceives as overwhelming or threatening. Factors such as the child's temperament, developmental age, amount of sleep, tolerance of environmental sensory inputs, motor capacities to communicate, health status and pain levels, and cognitive capacities to engage in abstract and flexible thinking affect emotional regulation and self-control. Difficulties in these areas increase the likelihood of out-of-control behaviors, and strengths in these areas increase the likelihood of positive emotional regulation and behavioral control. The four steps of the program, with examples of occupational therapy interventions, are described in Table 8.2.

Tiered Interventions for Infants and Young Children

Clinical reasoning, grounded in occupation-based and other theoretical models and shaped by evidence, guides the occupational therapist in determining which approaches to use to provide the most appropriate level of service. As part of an interdisciplinary team, occupational therapists may collaborate with other professionals and family members in the approaches they use to provide consistency of expectations and program goals across disciplines. A case example depicting examples of Tier 1, 2, and 3 approaches that occupational therapists may implement in collaboration with family members and other professionals to support the mental health and social participation of preschoolers is presented in Box 8.2.

Table 8.2. Positive Strategies for Managing and Preventing Out-of-Control Behaviors

Step	Purpose	Intervention Examples
Step 1: Caregiver's acceptance and appreciation of the child	Identify and gain control over frustrated feelings about the child's behaviors, accept that the out-of control behaviors are only temporary, and acknowledge that behaviors do not reflect caregiver incompetence.	Create an atmosphere of safety and success that promotes the child's sense of confidence. • Allow the child to succeed at simpler tasks before expecting the child to complete more challenging ones. • Help the child to understand that frustration is part of the learning. • Avoid power struggles over situations in which the child does not yet possess the skills to cope successfully.
Step 2: Deescalation of the meltdown or out-of-control behavior	Help child gain self-control to successfully complete task.	Use distractions and calming strategies such as humor and secret signals, validation of child's feelings, favorite toys, safety zones, deep breathing, and walking without talking.
Step 3: Identification of ABC sequence	Clearly identify the trigger or antecedent (A), the behavior the child manifests (B), and the consequence of the behavior (C).	Use concrete terms to describe triggers and consequences. • Triggers include sensory stimulation that is too intense, a lack of clear structure and understanding about the expected activity, internal or biological triggers, demands and performance requirements of others, the expectation to wait for or stop a desired activity, threats to self-image, and unmet desires for attention. • Consequences of the out-of-control behavior include avoiding the situation or task, receiving attention, obtaining the desired object or activity, venting frustration, soothing self, or getting pleasure.
Step 4: Intervention plan to reduce the frequency of repetitive meltdowns and out-of-control behaviors	Create an intervention plan that alters or eliminates the triggers, teaches coping skills for dealing with the triggers, implements a reward or loss system, and considers biological and physical strategies.	• Change triggers by alternating the activity's sensory, time, and task demands and providing visual supports. • Teach coping strategies such as learning to ask for help, first observing others perform the task, negotiating about the task demands, learning perspective taking, recognizing one's strengths, and practicing self-calming techniques. • Subdivide the task or activity into small enough units so that the child will be successful. • Incorporate reward systems such as hugs, points earned, or time with favorite activity or object. • Incorporate biological strategies such as getting appropriate nutrition and sleep and engaging in vigorous exercise. • Use loss systems such as time-outs, lost privileges, and loss of attention only after child has learned about and received prompting to use a positive coping strategy to deal with the situation but continues with the disruptive behavior.

Source. Baker (2008).

Interventions for School-Age Children and Adolescents

Expectations for understanding social rules and demonstrating appropriate social behaviors increase as children enter elementary school and expand their participation in extracurricular activities. This time is important for children to develop meaningful friendships and explore personal interests. During adolescence, social participation becomes more critical; it contributes to the formation of self-concept and self-esteem and leads to an awareness of personal attributes.

As mentioned earlier, children and youth on the autism spectrum often struggle with social isolation and restricted social participation patterns. Those who are able to verbalize their feelings express frustration with social challenges along with a desire for social relationships and community contributions. Transitioning into adolescence may result in a confusing and emotionally charged period of life for people on the autism spectrum and their families as the hormonal, emotional, and social issues associated with puberty exacerbate these feelings of frustration and isolation (Bolman, 2008; Wehman, Smith, & Schall, 2009).

Box 8.2. Case Example: Kahil

Occupational Profile

Kahil, age 4, lives with his parents and three siblings. He is able to identify some photos of common objects and activities and uses picture schedules with adult assistance. He has started to use a few short phrases by repeating adult speech and video clips. With one-to-one guidance, he follows basic routines. He can attend to objects and watch his siblings and peers engage in activities for several minutes. When he plays, he prefers to line up objects on the floor and open and close containers. Occasionally, he will hand a toy to or take a toy from his siblings and peers. He also prefers to watch the same video repeatedly and becomes angry if his parents try to turn it off before the story is over. They calm him by hugging him firmly and rubbing his back.

Kahil enjoys touching and feeling objects, but he struggles with prewriting and manipulative tasks. Although he climbs easily, he has difficulty figuring out how to move his body to get down from high places or play on the playground equipment. He is hypersensitive to auditory stimuli. When he hears loud sounds he often cries, covers his ears, and tries to escape the noisy activity. Bright lights also are difficult for him to tolerate; he sometimes responds by biting his hand. He prefers a firm touch and activities that involve deep pressure such as rolling with bolsters.

In public spaces, Kahil wanders. To make sure he is safe, one parent needs to continually supervise him while the other parent plays with Kahil's siblings. They are able to take him to the local playground where he can roam, but they do not take him to restaurants or community events that require him to sit. They avoid going to shopping centers or amusement parks because he becomes overwhelmed by the noises and begins to bite his hand and to scream. Kahil's meltdowns in these public places negatively affect his siblings, who then begin to have behavioral and emotional meltdowns.

The occupational therapist meets with Kahil's parents and the educational team to develop intervention strategies. Together, they decide to first provide interventions at the Tier 1 level. If more intense services are needed, they will then implement those at Tier 2 and then Tier 3, if necessary, to support Kahil's occupational performance and social participation.

Tier 1 Interventions

The occupational therapist provides in-services to the educational staff and family groups at Kahil's school regarding the effects of the sensory environment on children's emotional regulation and social behaviors. The therapist recommends strategies for

- Gradually modulating the amount of sensory stimuli during transitions, creating quiet zones within the classroom, home, or community where children can calm themselves;
- Providing equipment and activities that provide deep, proprioceptive input in collaboration with the local autism society, the occupational therapist, and the occupational therapy assistant;
- Negotiating with local store and restaurant owners to set aside selected off-hours in which families with children with autism can shop and eat in a stimulus-reduced environment;
- Providing workshops for family friends and potential babysitters regarding child care strategies so that they can offer the families respite; and
- Providing workshops for staff at local community setting regarding inclusion strategies for recreational program for families with children with autism.

Tier 2 Interventions

The occupational therapist educates the school staff and family in how to use Social Stories to help Kahil identify and follow social rules for specific contexts and to help his siblings and peers respond positively to Kahil.

Using strategies suggested in the Developmental, Individual Difference, Relationship-Based/Floortime model, the occupational therapist systematically interacts with Kahil in shared activities to expand his ability to engage in play and facilitate his ability to participate socially. As Kahil gains skills, the therapist routinely includes Kahil's siblings and peers in these shared interactions.

Tier 3 Interventions

Using Baker's (2008) four-step program, the occupational therapist analyzes triggers that generate Kahil's out-of-control behaviors and develops a plan that his parents and school staff can use to deescalate the behaviors when they occur and reduce or prevent reoccurrences.

In collaboration with Kahil's parents and teachers, the occupational therapist designs and implements a program using discrete trial teaching from applied behavior analysis to teach Kahil how to follow directions, complete routine tasks, remain seated for selected activities, and verbalize basic requests and feelings.

Using sensory integrative approaches, the occupational therapist helps Kahil to increase his tolerance of auditory, tactile, and visual stimuli and strengthen his praxis skills to control his body movements so that he can participate in community activities with his family.

Inclusionary interventions found to promote social participation incorporate (1) peer support to decrease barriers and increase acceptance and (2) opportunities to learn and apply social skills. Children and youth who become more adept at social, reciprocal relationships are more likely to participate in social and recreational activities as adults (Orsmond et al., 2004) and have greater opportunities for success in becoming productive members of society.

Occupational therapists use a variety of strategies in collaboration with families and other team members to promote social participation and mental health in children and youth on the autism spectrum. Those strategies include cognitive–behavioral therapy (CBT), Social Stories, relationship development intervention (RDI), and peer support programs. The Ziggurat model (Aspy & Grossman, 2008) is an evidence-based framework that incorporates these strategies into a comprehensive intervention approach used in collaboration with families and other team members.

Cognitive–Behavioral Therapy

A cognitive–behavioral approach to social development developed by Attwood (Sofronoff, Attwood, & Hinton, 2005) is highly structured and targets specific emotions and behaviors of children and youth on the autism spectrum. This approach is focused on explicit exploration of cognitive control of emotions and recognizing emotions in others. Role playing and practice with strategies to deal with feelings of frustration and anger can be effective in assisting children and youth in understanding the component steps to addressing confusing feelings. The success of a cognitive–behavioral approach is contingent on practicing skills in a supportive, naturalistic environment (Attwood, 2007). Refer to Chapter 3 for further information on CBT.

Social Stories™

Social stories™ are short scenarios written in clear, concise terms designed to teach children and youth on the autism spectrum appropriate social behaviors for a particular situation (Gray & White, 2002). Social stories can be developed by the adult or in collaboration with the child or youth to describe a skill or situation, its relevant social cues, and possible appropriate behavioral responses. Often, the story is a few sentences in length and written in short, declarative statements. The story includes a description of the situation, examples of visual or auditory cues to anticipate, and the steps to take to complete the task or handle the social dilemma. The stories can also depict other people's emotions or behaviors. Single stories can be collated into a set of stories around a common topic. The occupational therapist can use the story as part of Tier 1, 2, or 3 interventions to inform, teach, praise, or redirect a single child or a group of children about how to respond in social situations. How frequently the child uses the same story depends on his or her interest in it and mastery of the concepts. The occupational therapist can adjust the details and complexity of the story to meet the child's needs and capacities and can incorporate role playing to rehearse real-life scenarios.

Relationship Development Intervention

Developed by Gutstein and Sheely (2002), RDI is an intervention that addresses the social relationship challenges of people on the autism spectrum, such as developing friendships, understanding and displaying empathy, and sharing personal experiences with others. The developers of this approach differentiate social skills into *instrumental skills* (behaviors such as eye contact and smiling) and *relationship skills* (such as creating emotional connections). Instrumental skills, taught through direct instruction and behavior shaping, assist people in behaving appropriately. Alternatively, relationship skills, taught through systematic, layered strategies of referencing social partners, assist them with developing friendships and empathy for others.

The RDI curriculum consists of six levels with four stages at each level (Table 8.3). A Relationship Development Questionnaire (Gutstein & Sheely, 2002) identifies a starting point for the program, which is geared for children through adulthood. A certified consultant can be used to guide family members or professionals through the program. Although not specifically designed for use by any one profession, occupational therapists can apply RDI strategies to promote social relationships that are critical for successful engagement in work, school, play, and leisure occupations and instrumental activities of daily living.

Table 8.3. Relationship Development Intervention

Level	Description	Intervention Example
Level 1: Novice	Develop core relationship with a coach. Activities should be exciting, and the child should be encouraged to share enjoyment through face-to-face emotion.	The occupational therapist instructs family members in how to establish a relationship with the novice through a series of interactive games using exaggerated facial expressions that encourage the child to attend to the adult and imitate actions.
Level 2: Apprentice	Introduce peer partners to teach people to take responsibility for coordinating actions with social partners.	The occupational therapist works with classmates to create opportunities for playful exploration of novelty in favorite games and activities. Humor is introduced by incorporating silly movements or making up new rules.
Level 3: Challenger	Add variation while maintaining coordination with a peer partner.	The occupational therapist supports two children working as a team to follow a treasure map and locate the treasure within an obstacle course. Each child is given a role to play: One is the map reader, and the other retrieves each new clue, experiencing excitement in acting as partners in a creative process.
Level 4: Voyager	Individuals share inner perceptions and reactions with others	The occupational therapist facilitates an after-school club designed to develop experience sharing through photography. Students take photographs of their favorite people and places, and the adult facilitates group discussions about personal meaning.
Level 5: Explorer	Coordinate unique perceptions, emotional reactions, and imaginative embellishments into shared experiences.	The occupational therapist coordinates a weekly social group for teenage girls on the autism spectrum. Included in the activities are role-plays that put each girl into another's shoes, story writing, and problem-solving discussions.
Level 6: Partner	Explore innermost beliefs, dreams, and fears in an atmosphere of trust and confidentiality.	The occupational therapist facilitates a social group for transitional youth who have been working on the Relationship Development Intervention curriculum together for several years. Discussions of topics related to transition to work environments center around assertiveness, peer pressure, and working effectively to balance task demands and emotional needs of coworkers.

Source. Gutstein and Sheely (2002).

Peer Support Programs

As youth develop increased awareness of peers, they become more amenable to accepting support from peers than from adults (Connor, 2000). Peer support systems such as Circle of Friends (Pallis, 2008), lunchtime clubs, and Best Buddies (Best Buddies International, 2010) have been useful in preventing isolation and bullying while promoting greater peer understanding of adolescents with disabilities. Various approaches can be used to implement a peer support program that incorporates service learning at the classroom, school, or district level. For example, an occupational therapist can recruit students in the inclusion classroom to work cooperatively with a student on the autism spectrum for a particular project. In collaboration with the athletic department, the occupational therapist could recruit school athletes to work on exercise machines and in the swimming pool with youth on the autism spectrum who struggle to succeed in typical physical education classes. The occupational therapist could also serve on the schoolwide or systemwide curriculum committee to provide training programs for students who serve as peer buddies as part of a service-learning course. Peer-based supports for students on the autism spectrum are less intrusive than teacher- or paraprofessional-based supports.

Ziggurat Model

The Ziggurat Model, developed by Aspy and Grossman (2008), is a structured framework for addressing the complex needs of people on the autism spectrum. It uses a focused, step-by-step approach to assess the underlying characteristics of autism and the student's strengths and skills to craft targeted, comprehensive, positive interventions. This model incorporates five critical levels to consider when planning interventions that can include the intervention strategies previously described (Figure 8.1).

Occupational therapists' knowledge about and skills for assessing task demands, performance skills, environmental factors, underlying sensory and other body functions, and physical and social supports position them well to use the Ziggurat Model. This model is consistent with research-based trends in the field of autism intervention and addresses four critical areas of behavior intervention: (1) prevention of challenging behaviors, (2) functional assessment based on a functional behavior analysis, (3) comprehensive interventions that address underlying characteristics of autism and the students' strengths and skills, and (4) systems change that allows for maintenance of learned skills.

Tiered Interventions for School-Age Children and Adolescents

Similar to the process for developing programs for preschoolers, occupational therapists use occupation-based models and other theoretical frameworks to select Tier 1, 2, and 3 intervention approaches that best promote the ability of children and youth on the autism spectrum to fully participate in the daily life of their home, school, and community. To do so requires occupational therapists to attend to the fit among the youth's personal capacities, their environmental supports and barriers, and the occupations they need and want to accomplish. In school-based settings,

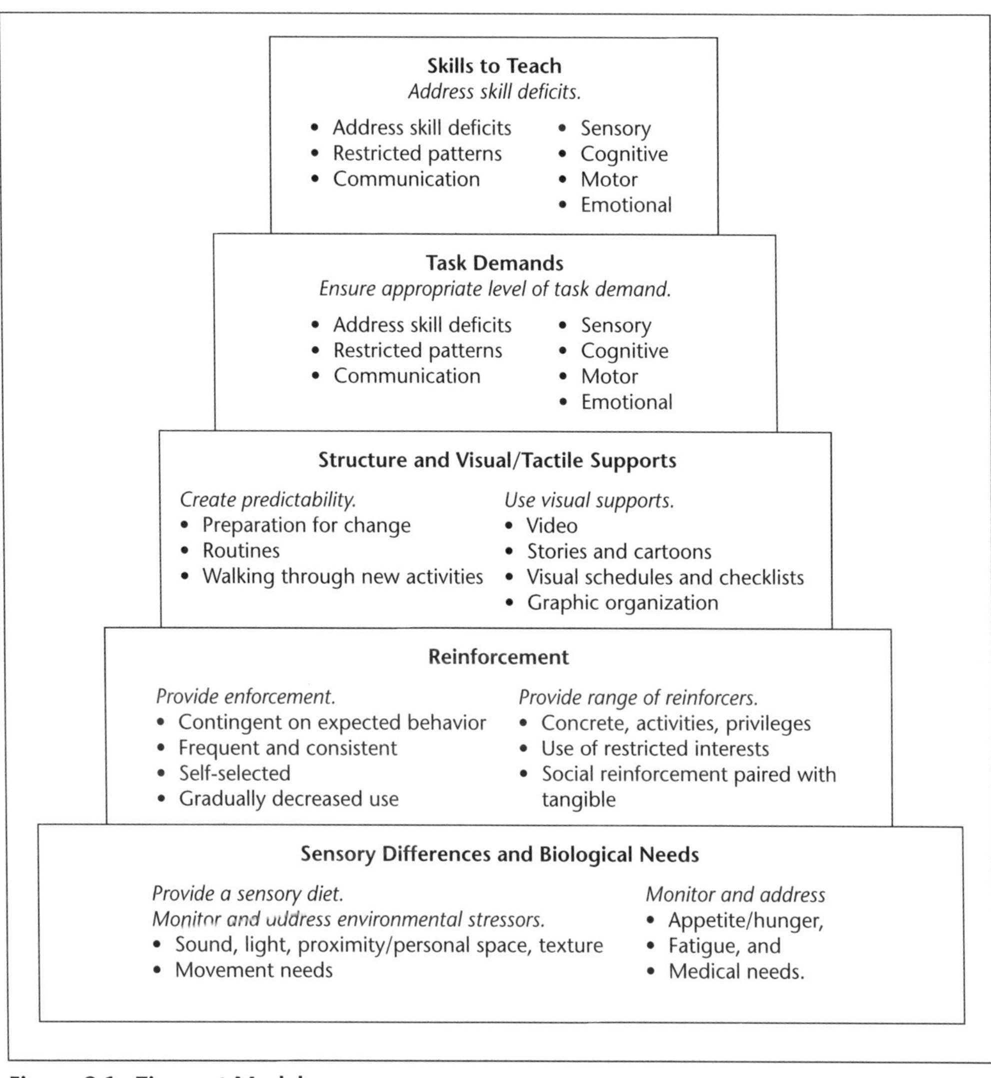

Figure 8.1. Ziggurat Model.

Source. From *Designing Comprehensive Interventions for Individuals With High-Functioning Autism and Asperger Syndrome: The Ziggurat Model* (p. 332), by R. Aspy and B. Grossman, 2008, Shawnee Mission, KS: Autism Asperger Publishing Co. Copyright © 2008 by Autism Asperger Publishing Co. Used with permission.

occupational therapists collaborate with the interdisciplinary team to design and determine which tier level of interventions is needed to support the mental health of the children and youth with autism. Sometimes, only Tier 1–level interventions are needed. Tier 2– or Tier 3–level interventions are introduced only when more intense services are needed. At other times, all three levels of interventions are provided concurrently to support the occupational performance of the person on the autism spectrum and improve the social context for that performance. The case example of Hester in Box 8.3 provides examples of how an occupational therapist might provide Tier 1, 2, and 3 interventions concurrently in collaboration with the family and other school personnel to promote her mental health and social participation.

Box 8.3. Case Example: Hester

Occupational Profile

Hester, age 13, lives with her mother and her 9-year-old twin brothers. She was colicky as a baby, was hypersensitive to changes in her food and to noises and lights, and developed language skills slowly. She often recites dialogue from movies, particularly *Beauty and the Beast,* when she feels anxious or stressed. Usually, she is content to play by herself with the same few games for several hours, but she abandons playing when her brothers try to join her or gets upset if the game pieces are rearranged. Her mother enjoys her humor and is proud of how gentle and courageous she is.

She functions at a fifth-grade level at school, receiving all of her core instruction in a resource room. Hester participates in the general education setting for physical education, library, art, and computer instruction. Her teacher has reported instances of teasing and bullying in the hallways. When she becomes anxious or upset, she starts to moan and throws objects. This behavior has caused her peers to avoid interacting with her. She enjoys participating in ballet and tap dance class once weekly, although she does not know the names of the other girls in the dance classes.

The occupational therapist meets with Hester, her mother, and the educational team. Together, they decide that providing interventions at Tiers 1, 2, and 3 concurrently will best educate the community about autism and support Hester's successful participation at home and in school.

Tier 1 Interventions

The occupational therapist

- Serves on a committee to develop a schoolwide antibullying initiative and to promote a positive supportive environment for all children and
- Offers a 1-hour informational program about promoting social participation and positive mental health to Hester's dance instructors and is available for consultation as needed.

Tier 2 Interventions

The occupational therapist and the classroom teacher facilitate a "Circle of Friends" for Hester that includes

- An initial orientation session about autism and the importance of friendship and
- Monthly pizza parties with Hester and four girls from her class to support their efforts to encourage Hester to join them as they walk between classes and work on class projects.

The occupational therapist and speech–language pathologist

- Organize a weekly "lunch-bunch" group that includes three typical peers and two other children from Hester's resource room class to develop friendship skills and
- Share with Hester's mother strategies that can be incorporated into the home to facilitate play interactions between Hester and her brothers.

Tier 3 Interventions

The occupational therapist

- Administers two assessment tools (Underlying Characteristics Checklist and the Individual Strengths and Skills Inventory) to target specific areas to address Hester's individualized social participation and mental health needs;
- Uses the Ziggurat Model to develop individualized interventions to address Hester's anxiety and stress and resultant behavioral outbursts; and
- Recommends strategies that Hester's mother can incorporate at home to help Hester manage her stress and contribute to peace in the household.

Summary

This chapter has addressed the social participation and mental health of children and youth on the autism spectrum; additional general resources on autism are listed in Resource 8.3. The complexity of the autism spectrum requires an interdisciplinary team approach and a variety of strategies to ensure that people can lead productive and fulfilling lives as integrated members in their communities. Strategies that foster meaningful social participation and support positive mental

Resource 8.3. Web Resources

- *Autism Society of America:* Current information and resources related to the autism spectrum. www.autism-society.org/site/PageServer
- *Corbett, B.* (2009, December). Understanding autism through peers, play, and performance [Video]. Retrieved August 13, 2010, from http://kc.vanderbilt.edu/site/newsandevents/podcastandvideo/page.aspx?id=1820
- *Deudney, D.* (2008). Mental health and Asperger syndrome. London: National Autistic Society. Retrieved November 22, 2010, from www.autism.org.uk/working-with/health/mental-health-and-asperger-syndrome.aspx
- *Interactive Autism Network (IAN):* An online autism research community incorporating the nation's largest online database. www.ianproject.org/
- *Interactive Collaborative Autism Network (ICAN):* Supported by a grant from the U.S. Department of Education, this site has a series of modules used to train individuals about children on the autism spectrum. www.autismnetwork.org/modules/index.html
- *Ohio Center for Autism and Low Incidence (OCALI):* A source for Webinars, Internet modules, and other resources that can be downloaded. www.ocali.org/view.php?nav_id=9
- *Organization for Autism Research:* Focused on applied research, this Web site has resources for individuals on the autism spectrum across the lifespan, their families, and the professionals that work with them. www.researchautism.org/
- *Pennsylvania State University National Autism Conference:* Archived conference presentations on a variety of topics related to autism. www.outreach.psu.edu/programs/Autism/index.htm

health include promoting personal growth, modifying contexts in which they play and work, and providing opportunities to participate with others in a supportive environment. Temple Grandin, an adult on the autism spectrum, identified a key issue when she stated,

> Learning to be part of the social world around me is an ongoing process: I keep learning and doing better all the time. It's going to be that way for most kids on the spectrum; there's not a magic turning point after which things will become natural and effortless—it's a process. . . . To me, "success in life" is defined by my job, my friends, my contribution to society. (Grandin & Barron, 2005, p. 378)

References

American Occupational Therapy Association. (2005). The scope of occupational therapy services for individuals with autism spectrum disorders across the lifespan. *American Journal of Occupational Therapy, 59,* 680–683.

American Occupational Therapy Association. (2008). Occupational therapy practice framework: Domain and process (2nd ed.). *American Journal of Occupational Therapy, 62,* 626–688.

American Occupational Therapy Association. (2009). Providing occupational therapy using sensory integration theory and methods in school-based practice. *American Journal of Occupational Therapy, 63,* 823–842.

American Psychiatric Association. (2000). *Diagnostic and statistical manual of mental disorders* (4th ed., text rev.). Washington, DC: Author.

American Psychiatric Association. (2010). 299.00: Autistic disorder. In *DSM–5 development.* Washington DC: Author. Retrieved August 13, 2010, from www.dsm5.org/ProposedRevisions/Pages/proposedrevision.aspx?rid=94

Ashburner, J., Ziviani, J., & Rodger, S. (2008). Sensory processing and classroom emotional, behavioral, and educational outcomes in children with autism spectrum disorder. *American Journal of Occupational Therapy, 62,* 564–573.

Aspy, R., & Grossman, B. (2008). *Designing comprehensive interventions for individuals with high-functioning autism and Asperger syndrome: The Ziggurat Model.* Shawnee Mission, KS: Autism Asperger.

Attwood, T. (2007). *The complete guide to Asperger's syndrome.* Philadelphia: Jessica Kingsley.

Autism Resource Foundation. (n.d.). *Applied behavioral analysis and autism.* Retrieved August 2, 2010, from www.autismresourcefoundation.org/info/info.ABA.html

Baker, A. E. Z., Lane, A., Angley, M. T., & Young, R. L. (2008). The relationship between sensory processing patterns and behavioural responsiveness in autistic disorder: A pilot study. *Journal of Autism and Developmental Disorders, 38,* 867–875.

Baker, J. (2008). *Positive strategies for managing and preventing out-of control behaviors: No more meltdowns.* Arlington, TX: Future Horizons.

Baranek, G. T. (2002). Efficacy of sensory and motor interventions for children with autism. *Journal of Autism and Developmental Disorders, 32*(5), 397.

Barry, T. D., Klinger, L. G., Lee, J. M., Palardy, N., Gilmore, T., & Bodin, S. D. (2003). Examining the effectiveness of an outpatient clinic–based social skills group for high-functioning children with autism. *Journal of Autism and Developmental Disorders, 33,* 685–701.

Bauminger, N., & Kasari, C. (2000). Loneliness and friendship in high-functioning children with autism. *Child Development, 2,* 447–456.

Bauminger, N., Solomon, M., Aviezer, A., Heung, K., Gazit, L., Brown, J., et al. (2008). Children with autism and their friends: A multidimensional study of friendship in high-functioning autism spectrum disorder. *Journal of Abnormal Child Psychology, 36*(2), 135–150.

Ben-Sasson, A., Hen, L., Fluss, R., Cermak, S. A., Engel-Yeger, B., & Gal, E. (2009). A meta-analysis of sensory modulation symptoms in individuals with autism spectrum disorders. *Journal of Autism and Developmental Disorders, 39,* 1–11.

Best Buddies International. (2010). *Best buddies.* Retrieved August 13, 2010, from www.bestbuddies.org/best-buddies

Bolman, W. M. (2008). Brief report: 25-year follow-up of a high-functioning autistic child. *Journal of Autism and Developmental Disorders, 38,* 181–183.

Bradley, E. A., Summer, J. A., Wood, H. L., & Bryson, S. E. (2004). Comparing rates of psychiatric and behavior disorders in adolescents and young adults with severe intellectual disability with and without autism. *Journal of Autism and Developmental Disorders, 34*(2), 151–161.

Case-Smith, J., & Arbesman, M. (2008). Evidence-based review of interventions for autism used in or of relevance to occupational therapy. *American Journal of Occupational Therapy, 62,* 416–429.

Centers for Disease Control and Prevention. (2010). *Facts about ASDs.* Retrieved August 13, 2010, from www.cdc.gov/ncbddd/autism/facts.html

Church, C., Alisanski, S., & Amanullah, S. (2000). The social, behavioral, and academic experiences of children with Asperger syndrome. *Focus on Autism and Other Developmental Disabilities, 15*(1), 12–20.

Cohn, E., Miller, L. J., & Tickle-Degnen, L. (2000). Parental hopes for therapy outcomes: Children with sensory modulation disorders. *American Journal of Occupational Therapy, 54,* 36–43.

Connor, M. (2000). Asperger syndrome (autistic spectrum disorder) and the self-reports of comprehensive school students. *Educational Psychology in Practice, 16*(3), 285–296.

Cooper, K. L., & Hanstock, T. L. (2009). Confusion between depression and autism in a high functioning child. *Clinical Case Studies, 8*(1), 59–71.

Corbett, B. A., & Constantine, L. J. (2006). Autism and attention deficit hyperactivity disorder: Assessing attention and response control with the integrated visual and auditory continuous performance test. *Child Neuropsychology, 12,* 335–348.

DeGrace, B. W. (2004). The everyday occupations of families with children with autism. *American Journal of Occupational Therapy, 58,* 543–550.

DeLany, J., & Pendzick, M. (2009). *Working with children and adolescents. A guide for the occupational therapy assistant.* Upper Saddle River, NJ: Pearson/Prentice Hall.

Elder, L. M., Caterino, L. C., Chao, J., Shacknai, D., & De Simone, G. (2006). The efficacy of social skills treatment for children with Asperger syndrome. *Education and Treatment of Children, 29*(4), 635–663.

Escalona, A., Field, T., Singer-Strunck, R., Cullen, C., & Hartshorn, K. (2001). Brief report: Improvements in the behavior of children with autism following massage therapy. *Journal of Autism and Developmental Disorders, 31*(5), 513–516.

Farrugia, S., & Hudson, J. (2006). Anxiety in adolescents with Asperger syndrome: Negative thoughts, behavioral problems, and life interference. *Focus on Autism and Other Developmental Disabilities, 21*(1), 25–35.

Flanagan, J., LaVesser, P., & Landa, R. (2008, April). *Implications for early intervention based on indicators of autism in high-risk infants.* Paper presented at the AOTA Annual Conference & Expo, Long Beach, CA.

Ghaziuddin, M. (2002). Asperger syndrome: Associated psychiatric and medical conditions. *Focus on Autism and Other Developmental Disabilities, 17*(3), 138–144.

Gillott, A., & Standen, P. J. (2007). Levels of anxiety and sources of stress in adults with autism. *Journal of Intellectual Disabilities, 11,* 359–370.

Grandin, T. (1995). *Thinking in pictures: And other reports from my life with autism.* New York: Doubleday.

Grandin, T., & Barron, S. (2005). *Unwritten rules of social relationships: Decoding social mysteries through the unique perspectives of autism.* Arlington, TX: Future Horizons.

Gray, C., & White, A. L. (2002). *My social stories book.* Philadelphia: Jessica Kingsley.

Greenspan, S. I. (1992a). *Infancy and early childhood: The practice of clinical assessment and intervention with emotional and developmental challenges.* Madison, CT: International Universities Press.

Greenspan, S. I. (1992b). Reconsidering the diagnosis and treatment of very young children with autistic spectrum of pervasive developmental disorder. *Zero to Three, 13*(2), 1–9.

Greenspan, S. I., & Wieder, S. (1997). Developmental patterns and outcomes in infants and children with disorders in relating and communicating: A chart review of 200 cases of children with autistic spectrum diagnoses. *Journal of Developmental and Learning Disorders, 1,* 87–141.

Greenspan, S. I., & Wieder, S. (1998). *The child with special needs: Intellectual and emotional growth.* Reading, MA: Addison-Wesley/Longman.

Gutstein, S. E., & Sheely, R. K. (2002). *Relationship development intervention with children, adolescents, and adults: Social and emotional development activities for Asperger syndrome, autism, PDD, and NLD.* Philadelphia: Jessica Kingsley.

Hillier, A., Fish, T., Cloppert, P., & Beversdorf, D. Q. (2007). Outcomes of a social and vocational skills support group for adolescents and young adults on the autism spectrum. *Focus on Autism and Other Developmental Disabilities, 22*(2), 107–115.

Hilton, C. L., Crouch, M. C., & Israel, H. (2008). Out-of-school participation patterns in children with high-functioning autism spectrum disorders. *American Journal of Occupational Therapy, 62,* 554–563.

Hilton, C., Graver, K., & LaVesser, P. (2007). Relationship between social competence and sensory processing in children with high functioning autism spectrum disorders. *Research in Autism Spectrum Disorders, 1,* 164–173.

Hurlbutt, K., & Chalmers, L. (2004). Employment and adults with Asperger syndrome. *Focus on Autism and Other Developmental Disabilities, 19*(4), 215–222.

Interdisciplinary Council for Developmental and Learning Disorders. (2000). *Interdisciplinary Council on Developmental and Learning Disorders' clinical practice guidelines: Redefining the standards of care for infants, children, and families with special needs.* Bethesda, MD: Author.

Interdisciplinary Council for Developmental and Learning Disorders. (2009a). *Guidelines for comprehensive approach to DIR/Floortime Program.* Retrieved August 13, 2010, from www.icdl.com/dirFloortime/overview/GuidelinesforComprehensiveApproach.shtml

Interdisciplinary Council for Developmental and Learning Disorders. (2009b). *What's DIR/Floortime?* Retrieved August 13, 2010, from www.icdl.com/dirFloortime/overview/index.shtml

Kim, J. A., Szatmari, P., Bryson, S. E., Streiner, D. L., & Wilson, F. J. (2000). The prevalence of anxiety and mood problems among children with autism and Asperger syndrome. *Autism, 4*(2), 117–132.

Klin, A., Volkmar, F. R., & Sparrow, S. S. (2000). *Asperger syndrome.* New York: Guilford Press.

Koegel Autism Center. (2010). *Welcome to USCB Koegel Autism Center.* Retrieved August 2, 2010, from education.ucsb.edu/autism/index.html

Kuusikko, S., Pollock-Wurman, R., Jussila, K., Carter, A. S., Mattila, M., Ebeling, H., et al. (2008). Social anxiety in high-functioning children and adolescents with autism and Asperger syndrome. *Journal of Autism and Developmental Disorders, 38,* 1697–1709.

Lee, L. C., Harrington, R. A., Louie, B. B., & Newschaffer, C. J. (2008). Children with autism: Quality of life and parental concerns. *Journal of Autism and Developmental Disabilities, 381,* 1147–1160.

Leyfer, O. T., Folstein, S. E., Bacalman, S., Davis, N. O., Dinh, E., Morgan, J., et al. (2006). Comorbid psychiatric disorders in children with autism: Interview development and rates of disorders. *Journal of Autism and Developmental Disorders, 36,* 849–861.

Linderman, T. M., & Stewart, K. B. (1999). Sensory integrative–based occupational therapy and functional outcomes in young children with pervasive developmental disorders: A single-subject study. *American Journal of Occupational Therapy, 53,* 207–213.

Liss, M., Saulnier, C., Fein, D., & Kinsbourne, M. (2006). Sensory and attention abnormalities in autistic spectrum disorders. *Autism, 10,* 155–172.

Lovaas Institute. (2009). *The Lovaas approach.* Retrieved August 13, 2010, from www.lovaas.com/about.php

Lovaas, O. I. (1987). Behavioral treatment and normal educational and intellectual functioning in young autistic children. *Journal of Consulting and Clinical Psychology, 55,* 3–9.

Macintosh, K., & Dissanayake, C. (2006). Social skills and problem behaviors in school aged children with high-functioning autism and Asperger's disorder. *Journal of Autism and Developmental Disorders, 36*(8), 1065–1076.

McIntosh, D. N., Miller, L. J., Shyu, V., & Dunn, W. (1999). Overview of the Short Sensory Profile. In W. Dunn (Ed.), *The Sensory Profile examiner's manual* (pp. 59–73). San Antonio, TX: Psychological Corporation.

Munesue, T., Ono, Y., Mutoh, K., Shimoda, K., Nakatani, H., & Kikuchi, M. (2008). High prevalence of bipolar disorder comorbidity in adolescents and young adults with high-functioning autism spectrum disorder: A preliminary study of 44 outpatients. *Journal of Affective Disorders, 111,* 170–175.

Myles, B. S., & Simpson, R. L. (2002). Asperger syndrome: An overview of characteristics. *Focus on Autism and Other Developmental Disabilities, 17*(3), 132–137.

National Autism Center. (2009). *National autism standards report.* Retrieved August 13, 2010, from www.nationalautismcenter.org/affiliates/reports.php

Notbohm, E. (2005). *Ten things every child with autism wishes you knew.* Arlington, TX: Future Horizons.

Orsmond, G., Krauss, M., & Seltzer, M. (2004). Peer relationships and social and recreational activities among adolescents and adults with autism. *Journal of Autism and Developmental Disorders, 34*(3), 245–256.

Pallis, B. (2008). *Circle of friends: Testimonials.* Retrieved August 13, 2010, from www.circleofriends.org/

Paradiz, V. (2005). *Elijah's cup: A family journey into the community and culture of high-functioning autism and Asperger's syndrome.* Philadelphia: Jessica Kingsley.

Pfeiffer, B., Kinnealey, M., & Koenig, K. (2008, April). *The effectiveness of sensory intervention treatment interventions with children diagnosed with autism spectrum disorders.* Paper presented at the AOTA Annual Conference & Expo, Long Beach, CA.

Quinn, M., Kavale, K., Mathur, S. R., Rutherford, R. B., Jr., & Forness, S. R. (1999). A meta-analysis of social skill interventions for students with emotional or behavioral disorders. *Journal of Emotional and Behavioral Disorders, 7,* 54–67.

Roberts, J. E., King-Thomas, L., & Boccia, M. L. (2007). Behavioral indices of the efficacy of sensory integration. *American Journal of Occupational Therapy, 61,* 555–562.

Seltzer, M. M., Krauss, M. W., Shattuck, P. T., Orsmond, G., Swe, A., & Lord, C. (2003). The symptoms of autism spectrum disorders in adolescence and adulthood. *Journal of Autism and Developmental Disorders, 33*(6), 565–581.

Sheinkopf, S., & Siegel, B. (1998). Home-based behavioral treatment for young autistic children. *Journal of Autism and Developmental Disorders, 28,* 15–23.

Shtayermman, O. (2007). Peer victimization in adolescents and young adults diagnosed with Asperger's syndrome: A link to depressive symptomatology, anxiety symptomatology, and suicidal ideation. *Issues in Comprehensive Pediatric Nursing, 30,* 87–107.

Sinzing, J., Bruning, N., Morsch, G., & Lehmkuhl, D. (2008). Attention profiles in autistic children with and without comorbid hyperactivity and attention problems. *Acta Neuropsychiatrica, 20*(4), 207–215.

Sofronoff, K., Attwood, T., & Hinton, S. (2005). A randomised controlled trial of a CBT intervention for anxiety in children with Asperger syndrome. *Journal of Child Psychology and Psychiatry, 46*(11), 1152–1160.

Spitzer, S. L. (2003). With and without words: Exploring occupation in relation to young children with autism. *Journal of Occupational Science, 10*(2), 67–79.

Spitzer, S. L. (2004). Common and uncommon daily activities in individuals with autism: Challenges and opportunities for supporting occupation. In H. Miller-Kuhaneck (Ed.), *Autism: A comprehensive occupational therapy approach* (pp. 83–106). Bethesda, MD: AOTA Press.

Stewart, M. E., Barnard, L., Pearson, J., Hasan, R., & O'Brien, G. (2006). Presentation of depression in autism and Asperger syndrome. *Autism, 10*(1), 103–116.

Sukhodolsky, D. G., Scahill, L., Gadow, K. D., Arnold, L. E., Aman, M. G., McDougle, C. J., et al. (2008). Parent-rated anxiety symptoms in children with pervasive developmental disorders: Frequency and association with core autism symptoms and cognitive functioning. *Journal of Abnormal Child Psychology, 36,* 117–128.

Towson University. (2009). *Post baccalaureate certificate program in autism studies.* Retrieved August 13, 2010, from http://grad.towson.edu/program/certificate/auts-pbc/

Vickerstaff, S., Heriot, S., Wong, M., Lopes, A., & Dossetor, D. (2007). Intellectual ability, self-perceived social competence, and depressive symptomatology in children with high-functioning autistic spectrum disorders. *Journal of Autism and Developmental Disorders, 37,* 1647–1664.

Watson, L. R., Baranek, G. T., Crais, E. R., Reznick, J. S., Dykstra, J., & Perryman, T. (2007). The first year inventory: Retrospective parent response to a questionnaire designed to identify one-year-olds at risk for autism. *Journal of Autism and Developmental Disabilities, 37,* 49–61.

Wehman, P., Smith, M. D., & Schall, C. (Eds.). (2009). *Autism and the transition to adulthood.* Baltimore: Paul H. Brookes.

CHAPTER 9

Children and Youth With Disabilities: Enhancing Mental Health Through Positive Experiences of Doing and Belonging

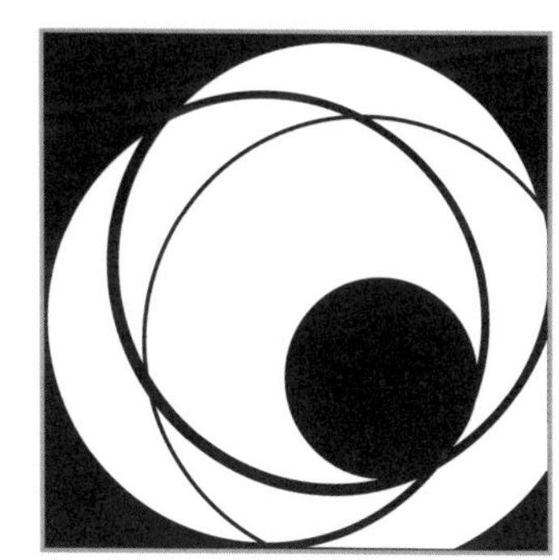

Theresa M. Petrenchik, PhD, OTR/L; Gillian A. King, PhD; and Beata Batorowicz, MSc, OT Reg(Ont)

Learning Objectives

After reading this material and completing the examination, readers will be able to

- Identify positive aspects of child mental health;
- Identify risk and protective factors for children with disabilities;
- Recognize the ways in which participation experiences serve to buffer the negative effects of life adversities and promote positive mental health for children with disabilities; and
- Identify the principles of mental health promotion and prevention in assessment and intervention planning.

> There is no health without mental health.
>
> —World Health Organization (2010)

Children with disabilities are at increased risk for developing mental, emotional, and behavioral (MEB) difficulties. Yet, the promotion of mental health and the prevention of secondary MEB problems for children and youth with disabilities remain neglected topics in the fields of child health and pediatric rehabilitation. Too often the social–emotional and mental health needs of children with disabilities are overshadowed by the attention given to the rehabilitation of obvious physical impairments and functional limitations. As a result, practical concerns for a child's personal happiness, social connectedness, and sense of hope and well-being often languish on the margins of practice. When the worlds of mental health and childhood disability do intersect, the focus is often corrective, fixated primarily on the management and treatment of mental illness, including disruptive or harmful behaviors (Schwartz, Garland, Waddell, & Harrison, 2006).

An integrated, more balanced view of health—one that recognizes the interdependencies of mental and physical health—is needed to guide practice, research, and policy development. The need for such a perspective to gain traction in health care settings, schools, and communities is especially evident in the stories of children, youth, and adults with disabilities who view themselves as competent, creative human beings rather than as broken bodies and minds in need of fixing (King, Cathers, Miller Polgar, MacKinnon, & Havens, 2000). This latter view of disability and personhood, which is assets focused (Lerner & Benson, 2003), is congruent with the science of positive psychology, an area of study concerned with the positive aspects of life that make it worth living (Seligman & Csikszentmihalyi, 2000).

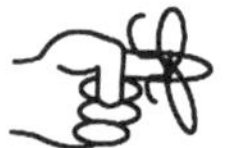

Remember this. . . .
***Mental health promotion* includes efforts to enhance a person's ability to achieve developmentally appropriate tasks (competence); to strengthen his or her ability to cope with adversity; and to promote a positive sense of self-esteem, mastery, well-being, and social inclusion.**

This chapter discusses the topics of child mental health, risk and resilience, and out-of-school participation as they relate to children and youth with disabilities. These discussions broaden the criteria for mental health and adjustment to include positive aspects of mental health such as personal happiness; life satisfaction; creative expression; and a sense of enjoyment, relatedness, and optimism (Cicchetti, Rappaport, Sandler, & Weissberg, 2000; Moore & Lippman, 2005; Seligman & Csikszentmihalyi, 2000). The chapter also describes a full spectrum of mental health interventions, which include mental health promotion and prevention in addition to interventions that respond to the needs of children and youth with disabilities who also have diagnosable MEB disorders.

Childhood Disability and Mental Health

This section begins with a definition of childhood disability and then discusses the topic of MEB disorders in children with disabilities. It includes an introduction to risk mechanisms and protective factors, and it describes the ways in which a disability puts a child at greater risk for adverse life experiences, including poverty, marginalization, and victimization.

Defining Childhood Disability

Childhood disability encompasses a broad spectrum of conditions. The Individuals With Disabilities Education Improvement Act of 2004 (IDEA), federal legislation that mandates early intervention and special education services for children and youth with special needs, includes 13 categories of disability: (1) autism; (2) deaf–blindness; (3) deafness; (4) emotional disturbance; (5) hearing impairment; (6) mental retardation (commonly referred to as *intellectual disability*); (7) multiple disabilities; (8) orthopedic impairment; (9) other health impairment; (10) specific learning disability; (11) speech or language impairment; (12) traumatic brain injury; and (13) visual impairment, including blindness. See Resource 9.1 for a list of resources concerning childhood disability.

Resource 9.1. Childhood Disability, Mental Health, and Development

Following is a short list of resources pertaining to childhood disability, mental health, and development:

- *CanChild Centre for Childhood Disability Research (www.canchild.ca):* CanChild is a research and educational center that provides evidence-based information to improve the lives of children and youth with disabilities and their families.
- *Frank Porter Graham Child Development Institute (www.fpg.unc.edu):* The Frank Porter Graham Institute is one of the nation's largest multidisciplinary centers for studying young children and their families, including children with disabilities.
- *Georgetown University Center for Child and Human Development (http://gucchd.georgetown.edu):* The GUCCHD's mission is to improve the quality of life of all children and youth, including children with special needs, adults with developmental and other disabilities, and their families.
- *National Dissemination Center for Children With Disabilities (www.nichcy.org):* NICHCY provides a breadth of general information about disabilities in infants, toddlers, children, and youth with disabilities.

Childhood disability can be defined as the gap between a child's functional abilities and the demands of the child's social and physical environments (Brandt & Pope, 1997). This definition is functional rather than diagnostic or categorical; it emphasizes the fit between a child's abilities and environmental opportunities to engage in everyday activities at home, in the neighborhood, at school, and in the larger community. In this view, disability is seen as a person-in-environment construction resulting from a suboptimal fit between a child's functional abilities and environmental factors (i.e., accessibility of services and built environments, societal attitudes, availability of appropriate resources).

Childhood Disability and Mental Health Conditions

Prevalence estimates of childhood disability, and the occurrence of MEB disorders within this population, differ depending on how the disabilities and disorders are defined and measured and depending on which populations and diagnostic groups are included in the surveys. Nationally representative prevalence estimates of the full range of childhood disabilities—and of the full range of MEB disorders within this population—are not available in the United States (National Research Council [NRC] & Institute of Medicine [IOM], 2009). Between 2006 and 2007, however, 9% of children and youth ages 3 to 21 (6.7 million) met the IDEA definition of disability and received IDEA services (Planty et al., 2009).

Population-based surveys have shown that children and youth with disabilities are 2.5 to 5 times more likely to experience psychiatric or adjustment problems than their peers (Cadman, Boyle, Szatmari, & Offord, 1987). Results of the National Health Interview Survey on Disability (NHIS–D) hint at the potential scope of the problem: Nearly 1 in 3 children with developmental disabilities were identified as having co-occurring mental conditions (Schwartz et al., 2006). On the basis of the NHIS–D sample and definition of disability, an estimated 54% of children with disabilities have functional behavioral limitations, nearly 33% have functional behavioral limitations in combination with mental or emotional problems, and nearly 13% have mental or emotional problems alone.

Disability and Vulnerability

Children with disabilities are considered a vulnerable population because they are at increased risk for developing MEB difficulties (NRC & IOM, 2009; Wolraich, Drotar, Dworkin, & Perrin, 2008). The reasons for a child's vulnerability to mental illness are complex and involve a combination of genetic and environmental factors. Recent research has shown that most MEB disorders are not biologically predetermined by a small number of genes. Rather, a child's social and physical environment exerts a powerful influence on the expression of a specific gene or set of genes. This process is known as *epigenetic modification* of gene expression by experience. The extent to which genetic inheritance plays a role in the expression of MEB conditions among children and youth with various disabilities has yet to be untangled. It is clear, however, that environmental experiences shape the expression of genetic predispositions to illness (NRC & IOM, 2009), and children with disabilities are more likely than their peers to encounter negative social environments and experiences across childhood and adolescence. It cannot be assumed, however, that all children with disabilities will experience MEB disorders, just as not every child growing up in poverty will fall behind developmentally. It does mean that children with disabilities are more likely to experience poorer mental health outcomes than children who experience fewer life adversities. Because children do not outgrow developmental conditions such as autism or physical impairments such as blindness, the associated challenges are lifelong.

Role of Risk and Protective Factors in Child Mental Health

The study of *resilience,* defined as "the manifestation of positive adaptation despite significant life adversity" (Luthar, 2003, p. xxix), involves the identification of risk and protective factors. Risk factors increase a child's chances of developing psychological, emotional, and behavioral problems, and protective factors serve to insulate a child from potentially harmful experiences (Masten, 2001). The development of MEB disorders involves multiple risk factors and complex interactions among various levels of risk and protection ranging from intrapersonal (e.g., intellectual ability, brain development) to familial (e.g., parent mental health) to educational (e.g., school connectedness) and beyond.

Risk and protective factors are thought to operate in two major ways: magnitude of risk exposure and developmental timing (NRC & IOM, 2009). *Risk exposure* is the number of risk factors experienced by a child at any point in time. *Total risk exposure,* the number of risk factors operating in a child's life (e.g., maternal depression, parental unemployment, poverty, residential instability), increases a child's vulnerability to an emotional or behavioral disorder and is associated with higher rates of MEB disorders regardless of the type of risk (NRC & IOM, 2009). In other words, accumulated risk, rather than exposure to a single risk factor, is most predictive of a child developing an MEB disorder. The analogy of juggling helps to illustrate this point. Every juggler, regardless of his or her juggling proficiencies, reaches a point at which the sheer number of objects to be juggled overwhelms his or her abilities. Likewise, with risk exposure, everyone has a personal tipping point—a threshold beyond which the number of life adversities to be juggled overwhelms his or her adaptive capacities to do so.

The development of MEB disorders is also developmentally and contextually sensitive. That is, the timing of exposures to general and condition-specific risk and protective factors at different developmental stages and in various developmental contexts matters a great deal. For example, poverty experiences in infancy and early childhood have been shown to be particularly damaging, adversely affecting a child's development (Shonkoff & Phillips, 2000; Zeanah, 2000). Also, some risk factors are condition specific, meaning that certain factors are more strongly correlated with the expression of specific MEB disorders, such as depression, behavioral disorders, or schizophrenia (see NRC & IOM, 2009, for further reading).

The search for *universal protective factors,* conditions and experiences that insulate a child from potentially harmful experiences irrespective of the type of risk exposure, has led to the development of a short list of personal attributes and protective factors associated with resilience. The list includes a range of personal attributes (e.g., cognitive abilities, temperament, self-regulation skills, self-efficacy, outlook on life) in combination with healthy, reliable relationships with peers and competent, caring adults (Masten, Best, & Garmezy, 2008). King and colleagues (King, Brown, & Smith, 2003; King et al., 2000) have identified similar protective factors for children, youth, and adults with disabilities. Those factors include meaning in life, which is acquired through the paths of belonging (relationships), doing (meaningful engagement in activities), and understanding (self or the world). Other protective factors involve the importance of beliefs: being believed in (social support), believing in oneself (perseverance and determination), and spiritual beliefs. Protective processes include transcending (replacing losses with gains), self-understanding (realizing new things about oneself, accepting disability, and transcending or rising above limitations), and accommodating (making decisions about relinquishing something in life).

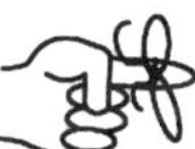

Remember this. . . .
I had people in my life who let me prove things to myself. . . . That's probably the biggest thing, [the belief] that you can do anything, because once somebody tells you that you can do anything and once somebody believes and has you believing that you can do anything, your whole world is wide open. You have so many more opportunities to make something out of your life if somebody says, "Yeah, you can do it." Well, I'm going to set myself up a goal and I'm going to say, "I'm going to get there." (King et al., 2000, p. 742)

Linkages Between Participation and Resilience

Participation, or involvement in life situations (World Health Organization [WHO], 2001), includes the concepts of doing (performance) and belonging (involvement). The doing aspects of participation are considered engines of human development (Bronfenbrenner, 1999); under ideal circumstances, they fuel a child's sense of mastery motivation, identity development, and sense of self-efficacy and self-esteem (Masten, 2001). Participation in shared activities and experiences, or *social involvement,* is a vehicle by which children and youth gain experiences of belonging, taking part, being included in life, and being accepted, all of which are powerful protective factors. Although positive participatory experiences are not an antidote to negative life experiences, they do buffer the effects of significant life adversities, and they provide avenues for promoting child mental health and for preventing secondary MEB problems.

Childhood Disability and Life Adversities

The link between exposure to childhood adversities, conceptualized as circumstances and conditions that severely challenge or threaten a child's coping mechanisms and adaptive capacities (Luthar, 2003), and the development of MEB disorders is well established. In general, the odds of negative mental health outcomes in both childhood and adulthood increase significantly with exposure to multiple childhood adversities (Furstenberg, Cook, Eccles, Elder, & Sameroff, 1999). A disability puts a child at greater risk for adverse experiences, including poverty, marginalization, and victimization—an amalgamation of risk that poses a considerable threat to a developing child's mental health. Children with disabilities also experience higher-than-average rates of comorbid mental health conditions (Emerson, 2003; Jans, Stoddard, & Kraus, 2004; Simeonsson, McMillen, & Huntington, 2002); as a result, MEB issues can further complicate or exacerbate existing activity limitations and participation restrictions.

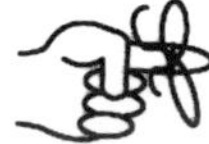

Remember this. . . .
"One factor lurks in the background of every discussion of the risks for mental, emotional, and behavioral disorders and antisocial behavior: poverty. . . . We are persuaded that the future mental health of the nation depends crucially on how, collectively, the costly legacy of poverty is dealt with" (NRC & IOM, 2009, p. xv).

Poverty

The interconnection between poverty and childhood disability is complex and multidirectional. Children living in poverty are at greater risk for a disability or developmental delay (Emerson & Hatton, 2005), and disability increases the odds of a family living in poverty (Brehaut et al., 2004; Emerson & Hatton, 2005; Hanvey, 2002). The life adversities associated with poverty (e.g., unsafe and stressful environments, residential instability, inadequate nutrition, material deprivation, maternal depression, parental unemployment, poor schools, limited access to health care)

Resource 9.2. Poverty and Family Economic Hardship

To learn more about child poverty and family economic hardship, visit the National Center for Children in Poverty Web site (www.nccp.org/pages/pdf/page_131.pdf) to learn the answers to the following important questions:

1. What is the nature of poverty and economic hardship in the United States?
2. How serious is the problem of economic hardship for American families?
3. Is it possible to reduce economic hardship among American families?

Source. Cauthen and Fass (2008).

increase the odds that a child's developmental needs will go unmet. It also increases the likelihood that a child's opportunities to engage in a range of developmentally enriching experiences will remain out of reach (Masten, 2001). Poverty often stresses family interactions and, in some cases, makes it impossible for caregivers to engage in parenting behaviors that support a child's optimal development.

Childhood disability in the context of poverty means that children and families must cope not only with the disability itself but also with the added burdens of poverty-related health disparities, social disadvantage, inadequate health-related services, and the extra direct costs (time, money, and resources) associated with a child's disability (Hanvey, 2002; Petrenchik, 2008). Children living in poverty are far less likely to receive appropriate services, including routine health care and specialty care, than are other children (Mayer, Skinner, & Slifkin, 2004); this inadequate access to care contributes to medical complications and secondary disabilities and increases financial burdens and family distress (Gerhardt, Walders, Rosenthal, & Drotar, 2004; Zipper & Simeonsson, 2004). See Resource 9.2 to learn more about the impact of economic hardship on American families.

Marginalization and Victimization

Children and youth with disabilities often feel socially isolated, stigmatized, and marginalized from society (Baker & Donelly, 2001; Davis & Watson, 2001). Being bullied and socially excluded, which are more common among children with disabilities than among their peers (Hanvey, 2002), can lead to feelings of friendlessness and social separation (Ladd & Troop-Gordon, 2003). When peer relation problems are chronic, children are at greater risk for depression, conduct problems, negative self-perceptions, and long-term adjustment problems (Ladd & Troop-Gordon, 2003).

Children with disabilities and special health care needs experience higher levels of social isolation and victimization than their same-aged peers. They are more likely to be excluded from peer activities and to have fewer reciprocated friendships (Nadeau & Tessier, 2006), and they tend to be less accepted by classmates (Crothers, Linden, & Kennedy, 2007; Nowicki & Sandieson, 2002). Children with disabilities are also more likely to believe that peers and friends do not care about them to a great extent (Minnesota Department of Health, 2004). Often perceived as "different" by peers, these children are more likely than their counterparts without disabilities to be bullied (Flynt & Collins Morton, 2004; Luciano & Savage, 2007). Factors associated with victimization include communication difficulties and social skill deficits (Luciano & Savage, 2007) as well as slower movements and reduced stamina, all of which predispose children with disabilities to being viewed as weak (Flynt & Collins Morton, 2004). Children with disabilities are also more likely than children without disabilities to experience sexual abuse and maltreatment (Sullivan & Knuston, 2000).

Childhood experiences of marginalization and victimization operate in a cumulative fashion on a child's mental health. In a cascading effect, the presence of a disability predisposes children to experiences of discrimination (Green, Davis, Karshmer, Marsh, & Straight, 2005), maltreatment (Sullivan & Knuston, 2000), bullying (Flynt & Collins Morton, 2004), and social exclusion (Crothers et al., 2007; Nadeau & Tessier, 2006; Nowicki & Sandieson, 2002). These experiences negatively affect a child's emotional well-being and place him or her at increased risk for the development of secondary mental health conditions (Emerson & Hatton, 2007).

Children with disabilities and comorbid mental health problems tend to have poorer developmental outcomes, with mental health issues often interfering with the achievement of various developmental milestones, including completion of formal education (Jans et al., 2004) and establishment of healthy, enduring friendships (Cadman et al., 1987; Crothers et al., 2007). The experience of chronic social isolation is considered a key factor in the development of MEB disorders in children with disabilities (Emerson & Hatton, 2007), as well as in the exacerbation of existing mental health problems.

Caregivers of Children With a Disability

Providing for the physical, social, emotional, and developmental needs of a child with a disability can be overwhelming for families, particularly in the absence of adequate resources and social supports. The caregiving demands of parents of children with disabilities have been shown to directly and negatively affect both their psychological well-being and their physical health (Brehaut et al., 2004; Raina et al., 2005). Caregivers (principally mothers) have reported spending between 50 and 60 hours per week above and beyond household responsibilities and paid work on their child's personal care needs, advocacy and service coordination activities, and transportation (Hanvey, 2002). In addition, parents often work to create peer relationships for their child, lobby for needed services and supports, and work to ensure their child's acceptance and participation in the community. Such demands often result in parental exhaustion and can lead to isolation from family and social networks because of the demands of caregiving (Green, 2003; Minnesota Department of Health, 2004).

Parental mental health difficulties, which can develop as a result of caregiving demands, have a clear influence on family home life as well as children's behavior and emotional adjustment, and studies have consistently reported a strong association between parent–caregiver psychological well-being and child behavior problems. Parents' distress and depression have been linked to behavioral problems in children in general (Shonkoff & Phillips, 2000) and in children with disabilities (King, King, Rosenbaum, & Goffin, 1999).

Paradoxically, although the professional literature emphasizes the emotional, physical, and financial costs of raising a child with a disability, the parenting literature often focuses on the joys that a child with disabilities brings (Darling, 1987; Summers, Behr, & Turnbull, 1989). Raising a child with a disability can be a life-changing experience that spurs families to examine their belief systems. Parents can come to gain a sense of coherence and control through changes in their worldviews, values, and priorities that involve different ways of thinking about their child, their parenting role, and the role of the family (King, Baxter, Rosenbaum, Zwaigenbaum, & Bates, 2009). Although parents may grapple with lost dreams, positive adaptations can occur, including changed worldviews concerning life and disability and appreciation of the positive contributions made by children to family members and society as a whole. As a result of their experiences, parents adopt perspectives of optimism, acceptance, and appreciation, and strive to change the environment or to meet their child's needs as well as possible (King, Baxter, et al., 2009). These perspectives provide parents with a sense of hope and control over their situation and an appreciation for what they have in life, and they may become more certain about what matters. This work, like studies on the meaning of activity, occupation, or life experience, points to the importance of choice and control in adjustment to life events (e.g., Hammell, 2004).

Participation in Out-of-School Activities: A Critical Nutrient of Child Mental Health

Children spend approximately 40% to 50% of their waking hours engaged in out-of-school activities (Larson & Verma, 1999). How children spend nonschool hours affects their mental health, well-being, and development. Although few studies have specifically examined the mental health benefits of participation for children with disabilities, activity participation—specifically, sustained participation in organized out-of-school activities—is positively associated with positive health and developmental outcomes for children and youth. The psychosocial benefits of participation in structured out-of-school activities and physical activity include an improved sense of well-being, decreased incidence of depression, improved self-esteem and self-image, and greater life satisfaction (Mahoney, Larson, & Eccles, 2005). The benefits of these experiences appear to be particularly potent for children facing significant life adversities (Sandler, Ayers, Suter, Schultz, & Twohey-Jacobs, 2004).

Involvement in neighborhood- and community-based out-of-school activities provides children with disabilities with important opportunities for social participation and connection with peers and adults. The social context in which these activities occur is highly relevant to children's physical and mental health and to their perceived quality of life. A recent study found noteworthy developmental trends with respect to the intensity, enjoyment, and "with-whom" aspects of social activities for children with and without disabilities (King, Law, Hurley, Petrenchik, & Schwellnus, 2010). Compared with 12- to 14-year-olds without disabilities, 12- to 14-year-olds with disabilities took part in social activities less intensely and were more likely to take part in social activities with relatives (vs. friends) and to enjoy those activities less. Thus, whereas children without disabilities engaged in a widening social world characterized by more intense social participation, greater participation with nonfamily members, and stable levels of enjoyment across age groups, children with disabilities reported only modest changes in social participation intensity. These youngsters also had smaller networks of activity companions outside of the family and reported less enjoyment of social activities.

School-age children with disabilities have been found to participate in significantly fewer organized and informal activities and to participate in those activities less intensely than children without disabilities (King, Petrenchik, Law, & Hurley, 2009). They also participate in significantly fewer active physical, social, and skill-based activities (King, Petrenchik, et al., 2009). Children without disabilities have been found to report significantly greater enjoyment of organized than informal activities, whereas this was not the case for children with disabilities (King, Petrenchik, et al., 2010). The lower average enjoyment of organized activities by children with disabilities may reflect a series of cascading processes underlying lack of psychological engagement in activity: fewer perceived choices, lower intrinsic motivation, lack of opportunities for meaningful experiences within the activity setting, feelings of social awkwardness or exclusion, and lack of physical and emotional support to encourage involvement.

Not all children with disabilities are alike. Studies have repeatedly shown that children experience disability differently with respect to their participation in social roles and activities. Some, depending on inner resources and environmental supports and opportunities, are resilient and do well. Others, because of greater risk, fewer protective factors, or some combination of the two, experience social exclusion and psychosocial difficulties. A recent study of school-age children with disabilities (King, Petrenchik, et al., 2010) revealed four types of participators:

1. *Social participators:* A highly social and neighborhood-focused group
2. *Broad participators:* A group of high participators who enjoy participation
3. *Low participators:* A group with low activity enjoyment and weak activity preferences
4. *Recreational participators:* A group of younger children who participate in recreational activities with family members.

The significant predictors of group membership were a mix of sociodemographic factors (child age, parent ethnicity), child psychosocial factors (peer problems and prosocial behavior difficulties), parent and family factors (parent physical health, family intellectual and cultural orientation), and environmental factors (parent perceptions of barriers in the work and school environment, unsupportive attitudes, and absence of support in the community). Above all, the groups were significantly different on the basis of children's levels of psychosocial functioning. For example, the low participators had significantly greater levels of emotional difficulties, greater peer problems, and lower levels of prosocial behavior. Social participators displayed the lowest level of peer problems. These findings correspond to previous research linking better emotional, behavioral, and social functioning to greater child participation (Bartko & Eccles, 2003; Byrne, Cunningham, & Sloper, 1988; Rae-Grant, Thomas, Offord, & Boyle, 1989). These relationships may be bidirectional rather than causal. For example, psychosocial difficulties may make children less motivated to participate in activities, and lower levels of participation may in turn result in psychosocial difficulties.

That the severity of children's physical impairment was not associated with differences in group membership is noteworthy. Meta-analyses and literature reviews have consistently indicated that chronic physical health status per se has little effect on adaptation (e.g., Lavigne & Faier-Routman, 1992) and that psychosocial factors are relatively more important with respect to children's outcomes (Wallander & Varni, 1989).

Resource 9.3. Evidence-Based Approaches

Download and read *A Public Health Approach to Children's Mental Health: A Conceptual Framework,* available through the Georgetown University Center for Child and Human Development Web site at http://gucchdtacenter.georgetown.edu/public_health.html. Are you interested in learning about an evidence-informed consultative approach to providing early childhood mental health programming? If so, download and read *What Works? A Study of Effective Early Childhood Mental Health Consultation Programs* from http://gucchd.georgetown.edu/78358.html to learn

- The essential components of effective mental health consultation programs;
- The skills, competencies, and credentials of effective consultants;
- The training, supervision, and support needs of consultants;
- The level of intervention intensity (i.e., frequency and duration) needed to produce good outcomes; and
- Which outcomes should be targeted and how they should be measured.

Mental Health Promotion and Prevention Interventions in Childhood Disability

Mental health promotion and prevention interventions for children with disabilities can be organized into three major tiers of service: (1) universal, (2) targeted, and (3) individualized (see Chapter 1). Mental health promotion involves all children and is characterized by a focus on well-being rather than on prevention of illness and disorder, although it may also decrease the likelihood of disorder. Prevention interventions are targeted efforts involving children at imminent risk or at elevated risk and those who currently appear risk free but for whom specific interventions have been demonstrated to reduce future risk (NRC & IOM, 2009). See Resource 9.3 for additional reading on mental health promotion and prevention approaches.

Within the mental health intervention spectrum, the appropriate level of intervention (i.e., universal, targeted, or individualized) for enhancing mental health and resilience in children with disabilities is determined by assessing a child's degree of risk for developing MEB disorders. For example, participation in an activity-based out-of-school program intentionally designed to teach coping strategies to a child showing elevated but subclinical levels of anxiety would be considered an individualized preventive intervention. For a child who has not been identified on the basis of individual risk for developing mental health problems, out-of-school participation in a community-based theater troupe for the purpose of promoting a sense of well-being and socioemotional competence is considered a universal mental health promotion intervention.

Currently, a lack of research evidence exists on which configurations of participation, at which points in time, and in which contexts are most effective for promoting MEB health and preventing mental illness among groups of children with particular disabilities. In the absence of such an evidence base, therapists must draw on robust research findings in the areas of child mental health and resilience, developmental science, and neuroscience to guide the development of participation-based interventions.

Two issues are particularly important in the promotion of mental health for children and youth with disabilities. First, services and interventions must expand to include an explicit focus on the psychosocial implications of reduced physical functioning, impaired social interaction, and disrupted sensory processing. Second, mental health promotion requires involvement in chains of positive experiences (Rutter, 1999) that provide children and youth with disabilities ample opportunities to "realize aspirations, to satisfy needs, and to change or cope with the environment" (WHO, 1986). Effective mental health promotion interventions should, therefore, reorient services to include a focus on the hopes, needs, and preferences of the child or youth as a whole person, including the developmental imperative

Box 9.1. Guiding Principles of Mental Health Promotion

Mental health promotion interventions include

- The promotion of social inclusion and the prevention of marginalizing experiences and victimization (World Health Organization [WHO], 1986);
- The creation of supportive environments that are safe, stimulating, satisfying, and enjoyable (WHO, 1986); and
- Sustained opportunities to participate in developmentally enriching activities that foster resilience and promote mental health by cultivating children's skills, competencies, talents, strengths, and social relationships (Masten, 2001).

for participation and social inclusion. These mental health promotion principles are described more fully in Box 9.1.

The case example in Box 9.2, which involves a school-age child with a disability, demonstrates these principles in action. It is based on actual clinical experiences and reflects many of the common issues faced by children with physical disabilities whose mental, emotional, and social needs are often overshadowed by the attention given to their physical care and functional independence.

Summary

Children and youth with disabilities have higher rates of MEB disorders than their peers without disabilities. The extent to which a child's genes play a role in these disparities is unclear. It is apparent, however, that children and youth with disabilities often face significant life adversities in the form of social isolation, marginalization, victimization, and poverty. Still, the promotion of mental health and the prevention of secondary MEB problems for children and youth with disabilities are often overshadowed by the use of therapies designed to address underlying impairments in body structures and functions, including mental and sensory functions. Adequately addressing the mental health needs of these children and youth will require creating a better balance among the time and attention given to promoting health in body, mind, and spirit.

The statement *risk accumulates, opportunity ameliorates* (Garbarino, 1995, p. 149) serves as a reminder that child mental health requires more than the absence of risk. Healthy development hinges, in large measure, on environmental opportunities that cultivate a child's skills, competencies, talents, strengths, and social relationships. Positive experiences of doing and belonging, or optimal participatory experiences, have been shown to buffer the effects of significant life adversities. They provide important avenues for promoting mental health and for preventing secondary MEB problems in children with disabilities by promoting a sense of personal competence and social connection.

Five decades of resilience research converges on this point: Children and youth with an internalized sense of competence and feelings of self-worth tend to persist in the face of life challenges and difficulties and grow because of them. Occupational therapy's work, then, is providing enriching opportunities for doing and belonging that cultivate a child's talents and abilities and fosters a positive sense of self-worth and personhood.

Box 9.2. Case Example: Anna

Anna, age 10, was diagnosed with nemaline rod myopathy. She is considered medically fragile, is fed by G-tube, has a tracheotomy, and requires frequent suctioning and the occasional support of a ventilator. Anna does not speak and experiences significant physical limitations. She can only move her head, eyes, and two index fingers. Despite her physical challenges, she drives a wheelchair and uses an augmentative and alternative communication (AAC) system independently, which she operates by switches.

Anna's receptive language skills are age appropriate in two languages, Slovakian and English. Her expressive language skills in English are at the Grade 2 level. She is bright and academically competitive. Anna lives in a small house with her older brother and parents, who emigrated from Slovakia 10 years ago. Her parents speak little English. Anna attends a Grade 4 mainstream class, where she receives the full-time support of an educational assistant. Anna attends most classes, except gym. After school, she stays at home, where she watches TV or plays on the computer, which has been adapted to her physical needs. The occupational therapist has been asked to adapt the school's written tests for Anna so that she can complete them independently and to troubleshoot the computer access at home so that she can write her homework. During the occupational therapist's school visit, the therapist notices that Anna sits at the back of the classroom and only interacts with her educational assistant. When the therapist visits Anna at home, Anna tells her that she would like to use e-mail and asks whether she could correspond with her. When the occupational therapist inquires about her friends, Anna tells the therapist that she has two friends at school who talk to her, but she has not seen them outside of the school setting. She confides that she often feels lonely and disconnected from her peers.

Assessment and Intervention Planning

Assessment and intervention will address Anna's psychosocial well-being, social inclusion, and meaningful participation in school, at home, and in community-based out-of-school activities. The assessment will focus on Anna's interests and her social networks and on the qualities of her environmental settings. The occupational therapist will identify participation barriers, including (1) policies, practices, attitudes, and lack of appropriate resources and supports and (2) communication-relevant barriers.

The intervention will involve creating optimal environmental settings that offer choice and opportunity and support growth-enhancing experiences for Anna. The focus will be on supporting meaningful engagement and social interactions in Anna's natural environments with a variety of people, especially her peers. The goal for Anna is to promote her mental health and prevent secondary MEB disorders through positive experiences of doing and belonging, which will be achieved by using multifaceted intervention strategies with a focus on enhancing participation and social inclusion in a variety of settings.

Participation and Inclusion at School

Anna is a competitive student; therefore, she will be supported to participate in the same activities as her peers and should be expected to meet the same educational standards. The occupational therapist's role is to assist teachers in modifying Anna's workloads, providing her with adequate time to complete tasks and maximizing her level of physical independence, thereby allowing her to focus on the same curricular content as her peers. This intervention should focus not only on Anna's independent (and solitary) participation in curriculum through adaptations but also on optimizing her environment to support meaningful engagement in academic activities and to encourage a sense of belonging in the classroom and school community, which will be achieved by enabling and supporting social interactions with peers and school personnel in classroom settings and during informal recess interactions. Examples of specific strategies include (1) providing structured ongoing opportunities for peer interactions, such as group projects; (2) supporting Anna's inclusion in school trips and gym class, which are fun activities offering natural opportunities for peer interaction; and (3) creating social environments that support the successful fulfillment of these opportunities (e.g., teaching school personnel and peers about communicating using AAC strategies or use of peer instruction and support by forming collaborative learning groups).

Participation and Inclusion in Community-Based After-School Activities

During her occupational therapy assessment, Anna identifies the following interests: going to the library, dancing, participating in dramatic arts, and going for walks in the neighborhood. The occupational therapist's role is to offer choices, create opportunities, and provide supports, both directly and by serving as an intermediary and advocate. Offering choices involves inviting Anna to identify and select specific community-based programs of interest to her. Creating opportunities involves supporting Anna and her family in their advocacy efforts with community organizations and agencies such as the local library, children's theater, and dance studios to support Anna's participation in programs offered to all children. Providing supports directly and as an intermediary involves coordinating organizational and

Box 9.2 (*cont.*)

social supports, collaborating with community partners and the family to enable Anna's meaningful participation, and creating a community of informed and sensitive peers. Participation in programs of Anna's choosing will provide her with opportunities to meet peers and to gain group membership.

Anna has also expressed an interest in walking in her neighborhood. Anna's family will be encouraged to invite neighborhood children of Anna's age to join them for walks in the neighborhood and to create opportunities for them to visit Anna at home, providing further opportunities to build meaningful relationships. Because of her strong computing abilities, Anna can maintain her new peer relationships through social media such as e-mail, instant messaging, Facebook, and interactive online games, all of which would allow her stay connected with her peers outside of school.

Participation at Home

Anna expresses an interest in helping her mother with cooking. The occupational therapist will discuss with Anna and her mother the tasks that interest Anna and strategies for involving her on a regular basis. For example, Anna can read recipes aloud to her mother as she is cooking, she can become involved in cooking decisions (e.g., selecting pizza toppings or cake decorations), and she can be responsible for creating shopping lists and participating in grocery shopping. The latter will offer Anna opportunities to get out of the house, to meet and talk with people in her community, and to expand her social networks.

Participation in Special Events

Anna enjoys writing poetry, and the occupational therapist can encourage her to share her expressive work with others. For example, the occupational therapist can assist Anna in arranging a poetry reading at her school or local library or encourage her to join or form a poetry club. The therapist can also play a role in enabling Anna to publish her poems through the International Society for Augmentative and Alternative Communication (ISAAC) and to present her work at conferences for people who use AAC or health care professionals (e.g., ISAAC conference or Independence, Community, and Empowerment conference). Participation in such events will provide opportunities for Anna to meet others who use AAC strategies, to expand her social networks, and to develop greater confidence in herself and her creative abilities.

Models of Service Provision

In keeping with best practice principles (Dunn, 2000), the occupational therapist provides direct and indirect services in Anna's natural activity settings.

Child- and Family-Centered Interventions

Direct intervention with Anna focuses on adapting Anna's communication system so it is most effective for social interaction and participation in specific activity settings. The goal is to create effective AAC systems to provide opportunities for Anna to easily interact with people in different environments. Collaboration with a speech–language pathologist is important to adjust the AAC system to specific emerging needs (e.g., programming new vocabulary that is setting specific or reorganize existing vocabulary for targeted efficient access). For example, Anna identifies that she would like to interact with her non–English-speaking grandmother, who will be visiting soon. Collaboration with a computer technician or vendor may be needed to add a second language to Anna's AAC system. Also, the occupational therapist can help Anna prepare an "about me" speech so she can introduce herself to new peers and instructors in community programs.

Home-based interventions with the family focus on (1) caregiving strategies for a child with complex needs; (2) balancing family needs and routines; and (3) developing strategies for supporting Anna's participation at home, at school, and in the community. In the area of participation, Anna's parents are provided with information on specific community-based opportunities available to Anna and her family. Together, the family and the occupational therapist explore and discuss the available options and develop a plan for enabling Anna's participation in a setting of her choosing. For her participation in this area to be sustainable, the occupational therapist must make certain that the opportunities Anna chooses fit with the needs and resources of the entire family (e.g., time, money, transportation).

Community-Based Interventions

Community-based interventions involve accompanying Anna during her initial participation in various community programs and settings (i.e., dance studio, library, theater) to help ensure that her

(Continued)

Box 9.2 (*cont.*)

initial interactions with unfamiliar people are successful. Positive interaction experiences are crucial in developing positive peer relationships, and repeated unsuccessful interaction experiences produce negative peer attitudes and low motivation for future contacts.

Systems-Level Interventions

Systems-level interventions involve collaborations with and coordination among school personnel and key stakeholders from the community agencies, including administrators and instructors. The purpose is to secure services and resources for Anna; to modify policies, procedures, or practices that pose barriers to Anna's participation; and to promote the adoption of new procedures and policies that will result in sustainable participation and social inclusion. All such strategies are important for optimizing Anna's chances of achieving her full health potential. The strategies involved will include educational and consultative activities.

Educational activities include providing general education about principles of communicating using AAC and educating Anna's peers and teachers about how they can become effective communication partners, which is done through a series of structured interactive activities and by the occupational therapist's modeling positive, respectful interactions. In these sessions with peers and school personnel, Anna serves as an educator and advocates for herself by talking about her interests, strengths, challenges, and goals.

Such educational sessions are important for creating a more welcoming school climate by increasing participants' knowledge and understanding of children with disabilities. They are also important for educating others about Anna's abilities and for exploring possibilities for including Anna in school- and community-based activities. For example, the occupational therapist can help others understand how Anna can safely and successfully participate in dance using her wheelchair, thereby creating new opportunities for Anna to be involved in dance lessons and performances with her peers.

Consultations are time limited and task specific. Case consultations involve a series of meetings with Anna's teacher to explore ways in which the teacher can enhance Anna's participation in classroom activities and field trips. Consultations may also be provided during times of school transition, for example, when Anna changes a grade level, homeroom teacher, classroom, or school. Other areas of consultation involve a variety of community agencies and include issues of personal safety, accessibility of the built environment, and modification of tasks and the sensory environment to enable Anna's successful participation.

References

Baker, K., & Donelly, M. (2001). The social experiences of children with disability and the influence of the environment: A framework for intervention. *Disability and Society, 16,* 71–85.

Bartko, W. T., & Eccles, J. S. (2003) Adolescent participation in structured and unstructured activities: A person-oriented analysis. *Journal of Youth and Adolescence, 32,* 233–241.

Brandt, E., & Pope, A. M. (1997). *Enabling America: Assessing the role of rehabilitation science and engineering.* Washington, DC: National Academies Press.

Brehaut, J. C., Kohen, D. E., Raina, P., Walter, S. D., Russell, D., Swinton, M., et al. (2004). The health of primary caregivers of children with cerebral palsy: How does it compare with that of other Canadian caregivers? *Pediatrics, 114*(2), e181–e191.

Bronfenbrenner, U. (1999). Environments in developmental perspective: Theoretical and operational models. In S. L. Friedman & T. D. Wachs (Eds.), *Measuring environment across the life span: Emerging methods and concepts* (pp. 3–30). Washington, DC: American Psychological Association.

Byrne, E. A., Cunningham, C. C., & Sloper, P. (1988) *Families and their children with Down's syndrome: One feature in common.* London: Routledge.

Cadman, D., Boyle, M., Szatmari, P., & Offord, D. R. (1987). Chronic illness, disability, and mental and social well-being: Findings of the Ontario Child Health Study. *Pediatrics, 79*(5), 805–813.

Cauthen, N. K., & Fass, S. (2008). *Child poverty and family economic hardship.* New York: National Center for Children in Poverty. Retrieved July 10, 2009, from www.nccp.org/pages/pdf/page_131.pdf

Cicchetti, D., Rappaport, J., Sandler, I., & Weissberg, R. P. (Eds.). (2000). *The promotion of wellness in children and adolescents.* Washington, DC: CWLA Press.

Crothers, I. R., Linden, M. A., & Kennedy, N. (2007). Attitudes of children towards peers with acquired brain injury (ABI). *Brain Injury, 21*(1), 47–52.

Darling, R. B. (1987). The economic and psychosocial consequences of disability: Family–society relationships. *Marriage and Family Review, 11*(1–2), 45–61.

Davis, J. M., & Watson, N. (2001). Where are the children's experiences? Analyzing social and cultural exclusion in "special" and "mainstream" schools. *Disability and Society, 16*(5), 671–687.

Dunn, W. (2000). *Best practice occupational therapy: In community service with children and families.* Thorofare, NJ: Slack.

Emerson, E. (2003). Prevalence of psychiatric disorders in children and adolescents with and without intellectual disability. *Journal of Intellectual Disability Research, 47*(1), 51–58.

Emerson, E., & Hatton, C. (2005). *The socio-economic circumstances of families with disabled children.* Lancaster, England: Lancaster University, Institute for Health Research. Retrieved July 13, 2009, from www.lancs.ac.uk/shm/dhr/publications/ericemerson/sec childdisability.pdf

Emerson, E., & Hatton, C. (2007). Mental health of children and adolescents with intellectual disabilities in Britain. *British Journal of Psychiatry, 191*(6), 493–499.

Flynt, S. W., & Collins Morton, R. (2004). Bullying and children with disabilities. *Journal of Instructional Psychology, 31*(4), 330–333.

Furstenberg, F., Cook, T., Eccles, J., Elder, G., & Sameroff, A. (1999). *Managing to make it: Urban families and adolescent success.* Chicago: University of Chicago Press.

Garbarino, J. (1995). *Raising children in a socially toxic environment.* San Francisco: Jossey-Bass.

Gerhardt, C., Walders, N., Rosenthal, S., & Drotar, D. (2004). Children and families coping with pediatric chronic illness. In K. Maton, C. Schellenbach, B. Leadbeater, & A. Solarz (Eds.), *Investing in children, youth, families, and communities: Strengths-based research and policy* (pp. 173–189). Washington, DC: American Psychological Association.

Green, S. E. (2003). "What do you mean 'what's wrong with her?'" Stigma and the lives of families of children with disabilities. *Social Science and Medicine, 57,* 1361–1374.

Green, S., Davis, C., Karshmer, E., Marsh, P., & Straight, B. (2005). Living stigma: The impact of labeling, stereotyping, separation, status loss, and discrimination in the lives of individuals with disabilities and their families. *Sociological Inquiry, 75*(2), 197–215.

Hammell, K. W. (2004). Dimensions of meaning in the occupations of daily life. *Canadian Journal of Occupational Therapy, 71*(5), 296–305.

Hanvey, L. (2002). *Children with disabilities and their families in Canada* (Discussion paper). Washington, DC: National Children's Alliance.

Individuals With Disabilities Education Improvement Act of 2004, Pub. L. 108–446, 20 U.S.C § 1400 *et seq.*

Jans, L., Stoddard, S., & Kraus, L. (2004). *Chartbook on mental health and disability in the United States* (InfoUse Report). Washington, DC: National Institute on Disability and Rehabilitation Research.

King, G., Baxter, D., Rosenbaum, P., Zwaigenbaum, L., & Bates, A. (2009). Belief systems of families of children with autism spectrum disorders or Down syndrome. *Focus on Autism and Other Developmental Disabilities, 24,* 50–64.

King, G. A., Brown, E. G., & Smith, L. K. (2003). *Resilience: Learning from people with disabilities and the turning points in their lives.* Westport, CT: Praeger.

King, G., Cathers, T., Miller Polgar, J., MacKinnon, E., & Havens, L. (2000). Success in life for older adolescents with cerebral palsy. *Qualitative Health Research, 10*(6), 734–749.

King, G., King, S., Rosenbaum, P., & Goffin, R. (1999). Family-centered caregiving and well-being of parents of children with disabilities: Linking process with outcome. *Journal of Pediatric Psychology, 24*(1), 41–53.

King, G., Law, M., Hurley, P., Petrenchik, T., & Schwellnus, H. (2010). A developmental comparison of the out-of-school recreation and leisure activity participation of boys and girls with and without physical disabilities. *International Journal of Disability, Development and Education, 57*(1), 77–107.

King, G., Petrenchik, T., DeWit, D., McDougall, J., Hurley, P., & Law, M. (2010). Out-of-school time activity participation profiles of children with physical disabilities: A cluster analysis. *Child: Care, Health, Development, 36,* 726–741.

King, G., Petrenchik, T., Law, M., & Hurley, P. (2009). The enjoyment of formal and informal recreation and leisure activities: A comparison of school-aged children with and without physical disabilities. *International Journal of Disability, Development and Education, 56*(2), 109–130.

Ladd, G. W., & Troop-Gordon, W. (2003). The role of chronic peer difficulties in the development of children's psychological adjustment problems. *Child Development, 74*(5), 1344–1367.

Larson, R. W., & Verma, S. (1999). How children and adolescents spend time across the world: Work, play, and developmental opportunities. *Psychological Bulletin, 125*(6), 701–736.

Lavigne, J. V., & Faier-Routman, J. (1992). Psychological adjustment to pediatric physical disorders: A meta-analytic review. *Journal of Pediatric Psychology, 17*(2), 133–157.

Lerner, R. M., & Benson, P. I. (Eds.). (2003). *Developmental assets and asset-building communities*. New York: Kluwer Academic.

Luciano, S., & Savage, R. S. (2007). Bullying risk in children with learning difficulties in inclusive educational settings. *Canadian Journal of School Psychology, 22*(1), 14–31.

Luthar, S. S. (Ed.). (2003). *Resilience and vulnerabilty: Adaptation in the context of childhood adversities*. Cambridge, England: Cambridge University Press.

Mahoney, J. L., Larson, R. W., & Eccles, J. S. (Eds.). (2005). *Organized activities as contexts of development: Extracurricular activities, after-school and community programs*. Mahwah, NJ: Lawrence Erlbaum.

Masten, A. S. (2001). Ordinary magic: Resilience processes in development. *American Psychologist, 56,* 227–238.

Masten, A. S., Best, K. M., & Garmezy, N. (2008). Resilience and development: Contributions from the study of children who overcome adversity. *Development and Psychopathology, 2*(4), 425–444.

Mayer, M. L., Skinner, A., & Slifkin, R. T. (2004). Unmet need for routine and specialty care: Data from the National Survey of Children With Special Health Care Needs. *Pediatrics, 113*(2), e109–e115.

Minnesota Department of Health. (2004). *Children with special health needs: Social isolation of children and families* (Minnesota Department of Health Fact Sheet). St. Paul: Minnesota Department of Health, Minnesota Children With Special Health Needs.

Moore, K. A., & Lippman, L. H. (Eds.). (2005). *What do children need to flourish? Conceptualizing and measuring indicators of positive development.* New York: Springer.

Nadeau, L., & Tessier, R. (2006). Social adjustment of children with cerebral palsy in mainstream classes: Peer perception. *Developmental Medicine and Child Neurology, 48,* 331–336.

National Research Council, & Institute of Medicine. (2009). *Preventing mental, emotional, and behavioral disorders among young people: Progress and possibilities*. Washington, DC: National Academies Press

Nowicki, E. A., & Sandieson, R. (2002). A meta-analysis of school-age children's attitudes towards persons with physical or intellectual disabilities. *International Journal of Disability, Development and Education, 49*(3), 243–265.

Petrenchik, T. (2008). *Childhood disability in the context of poverty.* Commissioned paper for the Ontario Ministry of Children and Youth Services, Policy Development and Program Design Division, Children and Youth at Risk Branch. Hamilton, ON: McMaster University, CanChild Centre for Childhood Disability Research.

Planty, M., Hussar, W., Snyder, T., Kena, G., KewalRamani, A., Kemp, J., et al. (2009). *The condition of education* (NCES 2009-081). Washington, DC: National Center for Educational Statistics.

Rae-Grant, N., Thomas, B. H., Offord, D. R., & Boyle, M. H. (1989). Risk, protective factors, and the prevalence of behavioral and emotional disorders in children and adolescents. *Journal of the American Academy of Child and Adolescent Psychiatry, 28,* 262–268.

Raina, P., O'Donnell, M., Rosenbaum, P., Brehaut, J., Walter, S. D., Russell, D., et al. (2005). The health and well-being of caregivers of children with cerebral palsy. *Pediatrics, 115*(6), e626–e636.

Rutter, M. (1999). Resilience concepts and findings: Implications for family therapy. *Journal of Family Therapy, 21,* 119–144.

Sandler, I. N., Ayers, T. S., Suter, J. C., Schultz, A., & Twohey-Jacobs, J. (2004). Adversities, strengths, and public policy. In K. I. Maton, C. J. Schellenbach, B. J. Leadbeater, & A. L.

Solarz (Eds.), *Investing in children, youth, families, and communities: Strengths-based research and policy* (pp. 31–49). Washington, DC: American Psychological Association.

Schwartz, C., Garland, O., Waddell, C., & Harrison, E. (2006). *Mental health and developmental disabilities in children.* Research report prepared for Child and Youth Mental Health. Vancouver: British Columbia Ministry of Children and Family Development, Children's Health Policy Centre.

Seligman, M., & Csikszentmihalyi, M. (2000). Positive psychology: An introduction. *American Psychologist, 55*(1), 5–14.

Shonkoff, J. P., & Phillips, D. A. (Eds.). (2000). *From neurons to neighborhoods: The science of early childhood development.* Washington, DC: National Academies Press.

Simeonsson, R. J., McMillen, J. S., & Huntington, G. S. (2002). Secondary conditions in children with disabilities: Spina bifida as a case example. *Mental Retardation and Developmental Disabilities Research Reviews, 8,* 198–205.

Sullivan, P. M., & Knutson, J. F. (2000). Maltreatment and disabilities: A population-based epidemiological study. *Child Abuse and Neglect, 24*(10), 1257–1273.

Summers, J. A., Behr, S. K., & Turnbull, A. P. (1989). Positive adaptation and coping strengths of families who have children with disabilities. In G. H. S. Singer & L. K. Irvin (Eds.), *Support for caregiving families: Enabling positive adaptations to disability* (pp. 27–40). Baltimore: Paul H. Brookes.

Wallander, J. L., & Varni, J. W. (1989). Social support and adjustment in chronically ill and handicapped children. *American Journal of Community Psychology, 17*(2), 185–201.

Wolraich, M., Drotar, D., Dworkin, P., & Perrin, E. (2008). *Developmental–behavior pediatrics: Evidence and practice.* Philadelphia: Elsevier.

World Health Organization. (1986). *Ottawa Charter for health promotion.* Geneva: Author.

World Health Organization. (2001). *International classification of functioning, disability and health.* Geneva: Author.

World Health Organization. (2010). *Mental health: Strengthening our response* (Fact sheet 220). Geneva: Author. Retrieved October 28, 2010, from www.who.int/mediacentre/factsheets/fs220/en/print.html

Zeanah, C. H. (Ed.). (2000). *Handbook of infant mental health.* New York: Guilford Press.

Zipper, I., & Simeonsson, R. (2004). Developmental vulnerability in young children with disabilities. In M. Fraser (Ed.), *Risk and resilience in childhood: An ecological perspective* (pp. 161–181). Washington, DC: NASW Press.

CHAPTER 10

Occupational Therapy for Children With Severe Emotional Disturbance in Alternative Educational Settings

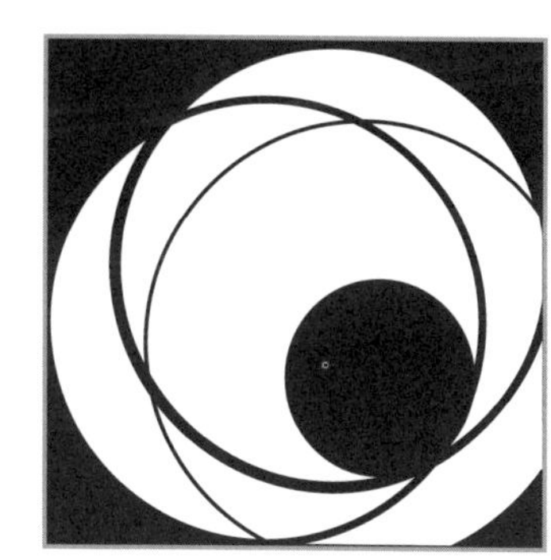

Karin Barnes, PhD, OTR; Kimberly Vogel, EdD, OTR; and Alison Beck, PhD, OTR

Learning Objectives

After reading this material and completing the examination, readers will be able to

- Identify the medical, physical, and social factors associated with students with severe emotional disturbance (SED);
- Recognize features of the Re–ED ("reeducation of emotionally disturbed children") approach developed by Nicholas Hobbs for youth with SED attending alternative schools;
- Identify examples of occupational therapy groups for youth with SED;
- Recognize strategies for increasing occupational therapy services for youth with SED;
- Recognize elements of a functional behavioral assessment and contributions that could be made by occupational therapists;
- Identify strategies for avoiding behavioral outbursts, dealing with them if they occur, and teaching anger management to children and youth;
- Differentiate social skills training and social and emotional learning; and
- Identify how occupational therapists could modify sensory aspects of the environment to decrease severe emotional outbursts and the use of seclusion and restraints.

When working with children and youth with severe emotional disturbance (SED), occupational therapists can provide services to promote successful school and community participation. Although the terms *severe* and *serious* are frequently used interchangeably, "severe" is used in this chapter because of its descriptive nature. The term *severe* is used to describe children who have behaviors that are "highly disruptive, dangerous, or prevent learning" (American Occupational Therapy Association [AOTA], 2008a, p. 2). Few occupational therapists work with this population

(Barnes, Beck, Vogel, Grice, & Murphy, 2003), and even fewer work in alternative education settings (Dirette & Kolak, 2004). In collaboration with educational staff, families, and community leaders, however, interventions emphasizing mental health and well-being and symptom reduction can be used to improve the occupational performance of children with SED.

Definition of *Severe Emotional Disturbance*

Children and youth with SED make up from 1% to 5% of the U.S. school population (Cheney, Flower, & Templeton, 2008). Severe emotional difficulties often result in problems such as violent behaviors, attempted suicide, and depression. Definitions of *SED* vary among agencies (Narrow et al., 1998; Vernberg, Roberts, & Nyre, 2008), thus making prevalence difficult to determine. As reported in Simpson, Bloom, Cohen, and Blumberg (2005), however, researchers have agreed that the percentage of children with serious emotional and behavioral disorders ranges from 4% to 13% of the U.S. population of children ages 4 to 17.

The classification of childhood emotional disturbance differs in medical (psychiatric) and educational (school) systems. In the medical system, the *Diagnostic and Statistical Manual of Mental Disorders* (4th ed., text rev.; *DSM–IV–TR;* American Psychiatric Association, 2000) and the *International Statistical Classification of Disease and Health-Related Problems* (World Health Organization, 2008) systems are used to categorize diagnoses. Diagnoses are based on specific classifications, such as mood disorder, oppositional defiant disorder, and anxiety disorder. The psychiatric community has debated the need for a more flexible classification system than the one currently in use (Carrey & Gregson, 2008).

In contrast, public school systems operate under the legal definitions found in the Individuals With Disabilities Education Improvement Act of 2004 (IDEA; Center for Effective Collaboration and Practice, 2010):

> a condition exhibiting one or more of the following characteristics over a long period of time and to a marked degree, which adversely affects a child's educational performance: (A) An inability to learn that cannot be explained by intellectual, sensory, or health factors; (B) An inability to build or maintain satisfactory interpersonal relationships with peers and teacher; (C) Inappropriate types of behavior or feelings under normal circumstances; (D) A general pervasive mood of unhappiness or depression; (E) A tendency to develop physical symptoms or fears associated with personal or school problems. (p. 1)

The classification used in schools is designed to take into account the impact of emotional disturbance on the child's ability to learn, participate, and benefit from the general or special education services provided to the child. Thus, the focus is related to the ability to participate in school activities, not the disease or disorder requiring medical intervention.

Different terms have been used to refer to the serious emotional problems and behaviors that children with SED demonstrate. IDEA (2004) now uses *emotional disturbance (ED)* for students regardless of the severity of the problems. The U.S. Department of Health and Human Services (2000) uses SED as a legal term to refer to children with disruption in social, emotional, and academic areas. This chapter uses SED because it is used frequently in the literature and is descriptive of the children's difficulties.

Characteristics of Children With Severe Emotional Disturbance

Many factors have been associated with SED, including those residing within the person and within the environment. Repie (2005) reported findings from a national survey of teachers, special education teachers, counselors, and psychologists that indicated that the top four emotional and behavioral problems of this group of students were (1) impaired self-esteem, (2) attention deficit and hyperactivity, (3) difficulty with peer relationships, and (4) classroom disruptiveness. Those challenges may lead to poor academic performance, involvement with the juvenile justice system (Vernberg et al., 2008), and outcomes that are the poorest of any disability group (Heathfield & Clark, 2004). A National Health Interview Survey (Simpson et al., 2005) also reported that activities of daily living (ADLs) were disrupted in 4 of 5 children with definite or severe difficulties. Participants in the survey consisted of 5% of the noninstitutionalized population of children with SED in the United States.

Poverty has also been associated with SED. In the National Adolescent and Child Treatment Study, more than 25% of the respondents with SED lived below the poverty line and were dependent on public assistance (Silver et al., 1992).

Students with SED are represented in higher numbers in alternative settings than are students with other disabilities (Reddy, 2001). Leone and McLaughlin (1995) reported that 5% of children with SED are placed in residential, hospital, and foster care settings compared with 1% of children with other disabilities. Children and youth with SED who receive services in residential treatment demonstrate multiple and complex needs. According to a recent survey by Abt Associates (2008), the diagnoses of children and youth in residential treatment programs include mood disorders (91%), posttraumatic stress disorder (84%), anxiety disorders (80%), alcohol or substance use disorder (70%), psychotic disorders (63%), and eating disorder (34%). Comorbidity of two or more diagnoses occurs frequently. The most common conditions reported along with SED include, in descending order, attention deficit hyperactivity disorder or impulse control problems, aggression or oppositional defiant disorder, conduct disorder, learning disorders, communication disorders, pervasive developmental disorder or autism, and sleep disorders. Another significant finding of the survey was that 25% of respondents reported that children and youth admitted to their programs have other medical complications and physical disabilities.

As a group, children with SED have difficulty achieving educational goals, whether in the public school system or in residential settings (Silver et al., 1992). Students with SED have problems that negatively affect academic performance and require intervention, including internalizing symptoms and externalizing and disruptive behavior problems. *Externalizing symptoms* include negative verbal interactions, aggression, and antagonizing of peers (Reddy, De Thomas, Newman, & Chun, 2009). *Internalizing symptoms* include somatic complaints, social isolation, hopelessness, and depression. Externalizing and internalizing characteristics are often seen together, as with students who demonstrate both aggression and depression. These severe behavior problems have a drastic impact on a child's occupational performance at school, at home, and in the community.

Students with SED are at risk for school dropout, incarceration, and hospitalization (Heathfield & Clark, 2004). Failure to complete high school is high, as is subsequent failure to attain and maintain employment (Zigmond, 2006). Adolescents with SED report that persisting either in school or at a job provides them with few rewards (Zigmond, 2006). Zigmond also suggested that because life can be unpredictable, adolescents and young adults with SED readily become unstable in the community, especially if supports are not available. Box 10.1 summarizes the characteristics of SED.

Challenges to Participation

In a national survey, Repie (2005) found that teachers, special education teachers, counselors, and psychologists listed barriers to the access and use of mental health services by youth with SED, including family stressors, family financial problems, stigma, long waiting lists, managed care, and insurance issues. In the school setting, evaluation of emotional and behavioral problems was the service most frequently available; however, the survey respondents reported that when services were available they were generally ineffective (Repie, 2005). Lack of services within the school can lead to high dropout rates, unhealthy choices by students, aggression, defiance, and social isolation, among other problems (Repie, 2005). Formal training for teachers in how to effectively serve students with SED is often lacking (Reddy et al., 2009). Services tend to be fragmented and uncoordinated, making meeting the complex needs of this population difficult to achieve (Heathfield & Clark, 2004).

Difficulties related to client factors and performance skills can impair a child's ability to achieve success in school. For example, limited social–emotional skills have been found to be a greater barrier to participation in learning than limited cognitive skills (Koller & Bertel, 2006). Correspondingly, school personnel view impaired self-esteem as the most serious barrier to learning (Repie, 2005). Dirette

Box 10.1. Characteristics of Severe Emotional Disturbance

Multiple Factors Associated With SED

- High incidence of mental health diagnoses, medical problems, physical disabilities, or all of these
- Attention deficit hyperactivity disorders and learning disorders
- Oppositional defiant disorder.

Functional Limitations

- Poor self-esteem and limited social and emotional skills
- ADL limitations (sleep issues)
- Limited peer relationships
- Severe behavior problems.

At Risk for Limited Outcomes

- School dropout
- Social isolation
- Incarceration
- Difficulty maintaining employment.

and Kolak (2004) found that alternative school staff reported that most of their students had poor time management skills, lack of coping skills, limited attention span, and anger management difficulty.

Family characteristics can also be a barrier to participation. Children of parents with less education have lower levels of participation in after-school youth programs for a variety of familial, social, and economic reasons (Keller, Bost, Lock, & Marcenko, 2005). Environmental and contextual factors that support the positive development of children include physical and psychological safety, appropriate structure, supportive relationships, opportunities for belonging, and positive social norms (Mahoney, Eccles, & Larson, 2004). The prevalence of unstable families, frequent and prolonged institutionalization, and difficulty being accepted in society among children with SED often compromise the positive effects of supportive factors.

Alternative Educational Environments

Children who have the most severe behavioral or emotional disturbance are frequently educated in settings away from the regular education classroom and from the public school setting. In 2004, 17.4% of students with the disability classification of ED were educated outside of regular schools (National Center for Education Statistics [NCES], 2006). Of those students who participated in regular education, 28.4% were away from their regular classroom for 60% or more of the school day (NCES, 2006).

The U.S. Department of Education defines an *alternative education school* as

> a public elementary/secondary school that addresses the needs of students which typically cannot be met in a regular school and provides nontraditional education which is not categorized solely as regular education, special education, vocational education, gifted and talented or magnet school programs. (NCES, 2002, p. 55)

Individual states and school districts, however, may influence the characteristics of alternative schools. Generally, alternative education includes schools or programs that are in nontraditional settings separate from the general education classroom and serve students who are at risk of school failure, are disruptive or have behavior problems, and have been suspended or expelled (Lehr, Lanners, & Lange, 2003).

The number of alternative education settings (and of youth served in such settings) has increased dramatically over the past 15 years. In 2000 to 2001, 10,900 alternative schools provided educational services to 612,000 students in the United States, or about 1.3% of public school students (Kleiner, Porch, & Farris, 2002). Alternative education settings include "public alternative schools, charter schools for at-risk youths, programs within juvenile detention centers, community-based schools operated by districts, and alternative schools with evening and weekend formats" (Foley & Pang, 2006, p. 10).

Characteristics of students attending alternative education programs vary across types of programs and by state (Foley & Pang, 2006; Reddy, 2001). The Alternative Schools Research Project (Lehr, Tan, & Ysseldyke, 2009) collected data about alternative schools and students through a nationwide survey and found that "students with an [individualized education program] attending alternative schools were most often students with emotional/behavior disorders, learning disabilities, and other health impairments" (p. 29). Foley and Pang (2006) cited the most common reasons children were transferred to an alternative education setting as history of social–emotional problems, physical aggression, chronic truancy problems, and verbally disruptive behavior.

Because of the severity of behavior problems and complex emotional needs of youth attending alternative education settings, school staff must have specialized skills and work together in a unified manner to foster student success. The Positive Education Program (PEP), which was established in 1971, is an example of an alternative special education and mental health program designed for students with SED in Cleveland, Ohio (Fecser, 2003). PEP programs are grounded in the principles of Re–ED (reeducation of emotionally disturbed children) "to help troubled and troubling children and youth successfully learn and grow by blending high-quality education and mental health services in partnership with families, schools, and communities" (PEP, 2008). Re–ED was developed by Hobbs (1966) as a new way to help youth with SED (Cantrell & Cantrell, 2007). The overriding philosophy of this approach is *success:* "Successful living is healing" (Cantrell & Cantrell, 2007, p. 134). Three beliefs lay the foundation for how to help young people and families: "We are emotional beings who need each other. Growth can be enhanced. Today can be used to build health" (Cantrell & Cantrell, 2007, pp. 5–7). The Re–ED strengths-based model applies 12 guiding principles developed by Hobbs (1966; Box 10.2). All

Box 10.2. Twelve Principles of Re–ED

Hobbs (1966) identified the following 12 Re–ED principles:

1. Life is to be lived now, not in the past, and lived in the future only as a present challenge.
2. Trust between the child and adult is essential, the foundation on which all other principles rest, the glue that holds teaching and learning together; the beginning point for reeducation.
3. Time is an ally, working on the side of growth in a period of development when life has a tremendous forward thrust.
4. Competence makes a difference; children and adolescents should be helped to be good at something, and especially at schoolwork.
5. Self-control can be taught and children and adolescents helped to manage their behavior without the development of psychodynamic insight; symptoms can and should be controlled by direct address, not necessarily by an uncovering therapy.
6. The cognitive competence of children and adolescents can be considerably enhanced; they can be taught generic skills in the management of their lives and strategies for coping with the complex array of demands placed on them by family, school, community, or job; in other words, intelligence can be taught.
7. Feelings should be nurtured, shared spontaneously, controlled when necessary, expressed when too long repressed, and explored with trusted others.
8. The group is very important to young people; it can be a major source of instruction in growing up.
9. Ceremony and ritual give order, stability, and confidence to troubled children and adolescents, whose lives are often in considerable disarray.
10. The body is the armature of the self, the physical self around which the psychological self is constructed.
11. Communities are important for young children and youth, but the uses and benefits of community must be experienced to be learned.
12. In growing up, a child should know some joy in each day, and look forward to some joyous event for the morrow.

staff participate in ongoing education and development to internalize and practice these principles in day-to-day activities. Teaching and related services staff are considered teacher–counselors, recognizing that the therapeutic alliance between the adult and child is key to personal growth (Fecser, 2003; Box 10.3).

Re–ED also emphasizes ecological perspectives and the importance of working closely with everyone in the child's home, school, and community environments. Occupational therapists working in an alternative school such as PEP are trained, along with other professionals, to become skilled in developing trust and positive interaction, managing behavior, and facilitating group work. Examples of occupation-based groups developed and facilitated by an occupational therapist within a PEP program are described in Box 10.4.

Intensive Coordinated Services

National agendas are in place to deliver mental health services that aim for prevention of mental illness and promotion of mental health, emphasizing the need for prevention and intervention to go hand in hand (Dwyer, 2002). Implementation of these ideas includes a complete array of comprehensive, organized services that have an impact at home, at school, and in the community (Dodge, Keenan, & Lattanzi, 2002; Dwyer, 2002). Occupational therapy's support of family-centered care and children's successful occupational performance can make important contributions to such preventive and intervention efforts. However, systemwide initiatives do not typically incorporate occupational therapy. It is critical that occupational therapists advocate for their services to be included in these agendas.

Remember this. . . .
Systemwide initiatives focus on

- **Promotion of mental health;**
- **Prevention of mental illness; and**
- **Comprehensive, organized services linking home, school, and community.**

Comprehensive services to address behaviors that are highly unmanageable and unsafe and that interfere with learning may be provided in settings outside the public school system, such as juvenile detention centers and charter schools. The occupational therapist may evaluate and provide services in those settings,

Special educators, psychologists, and occupational therapists have recognized the value of using the public health model of service delivery for students with mental health difficulties. This three-tiered model depicts Tier 1 as preventive and proactive strategies, Tier 2 as targeted interventions for at-risk students, and Tier 3 as intensive coordinated interventions for students identified with significant difficulties (American Occupational Therapy Association [AOTA], 2008a). Occupational therapists can participate in all aspects of this process and provide interventions that

Box 10.3. Qualities of the Teacher–Counselor (Re–ED Approach)

- *One must have an attitude of "We never give up on kids."* Even with the most challenging behaviors, teachers are effective in dealing with them and in forgiveness.
- *A teacher–counselor will go the extra mile.* Staff will go to extremes to help children be successful.
- *Teacher–counselors know the power of kindness.* Time spent supporting a child through a crisis by giving a kind word or pat on the back helps create a bond of trust.
- *Teacher–counselors know the importance of joy in the life of a child.* Joy is demonstrated by helping children participate in enjoyable activities.
- *Teacher–counselors take care of each other.* The staff become sources of support for one another, which helps sustain quality interactions among all adults and children.

Source. Fecser (2003).

Box 10.4. Occupation-Based Groups Embedded in a Therapeutic Day School, Positive Education Program

Occupational Therapy Hobby Shop

Goal: Expose students to a variety of hobby activities that can be done at home during out-of-school time for recreation and leisure (skill development and reflection on personal interests).

Secondary goals:

- Work or socialize with peers
- Develop frustration tolerance and coping abilities
- Foster creativity
- Encourage persistence and time management
- Experience enjoyment with health-promoting activities.

Occupational Therapy Relaxation Group

Goals: (1) Teach and practice the relaxation methods of deep breathing, progressive relaxation, and guided imagery–meditation and (2) promote the use of these strategies to increase self-control and good decisions.

Secondary goals: Practice skills when experiencing a crisis cycle, and regulate arousal throughout the day.

Project Magic

Goals: By learning independent magic tricks, students develop hand skills, visual and cognitive sequencing, social and communication skills, frustration tolerance, acceptance of instruction from guest magician, and functional work skills.

Community Transportation Group

Goal: Teach practical living and social skills required for riding public transportation to various community destinations. Students must learn the following skills:

- Use bus schedules and purchase tickets
- Find bus stops; respond appropriately to strangers
- Interact appropriately with peers
- Make simple purchases at stores and interact appropriately with store employees
- Demonstrate problem-solving, good judgment, and frustration tolerance
- Ask for help, if needed, from an appropriate adult.

PAL Chess Club

Local police officers come in to play chess with the students.

Goals: (1) Foster positive relationships between the students and police officers and (2) practice playing chess in a social situation.

—Developed and implemented by Diane Ventura, OTR/L
Positive Education Program, Cleveland, OH

address positive mental health, environmental and social contextual issues, coping, resilience, development of meaningful interests, and reduction of problem behaviors. Examples of prevention of mental illness and promotion of positive mental health interventions by occupational therapists include encouraging students' success in multiple school contexts by consulting with educational staff to make useful modifications, fostering participation in extracurricular activities and the development of friends, and assisting in screening and early identification of mental health challenges.

Students who are placed in alternative settings are also in need of individualized (Tier 3) interventions because they have been placed away from the regular

Box 10.5. Barriers to Occupational Therapists Serving Students With Severe Emotional Disturbance

Team Member Issues

- Team members do not understand the role of occupational therapy with students with SED.
- Team members view the promotion of mental health as being the role of psychologists and counselors.

Occupational Therapist Issues

- Therapists lack time to collaborate.
- Therapists lack knowledge and skills to handle disruptive behaviors.
- Caseloads are high.

education settings as a result of behavior, emotional difficulties, or both. This group of children demonstrates difficulty in most areas of occupation at school, such as sitting in class, refraining from using loud voices, and taking turns. Students may require frequent removal from the classroom because of severe behavioral outbursts (e.g., fighting and arguing, striking others, throwing objects) resulting from environmental and contextual triggers. Triggers may include bright lights, ambient noises, personal space problems, and schedule irregularities. In the school mental health model, intensive interventions require a comprehensive approach involving all school personnel, families, and community providers.

Providing Occupational Therapy Services: Concerns and Solutions

Although the need for occupational therapy services for children with SED has been identified as an important practice area (Bazyk, 2007; Dirette & Kolak, 2004; Jackson & Arbesman, 2005), barriers to service provision have been noted (Barnes et al., 2003; Beck, Barnes, Vogel, & Grice, 2006; Case-Smith & Archer, 2008; Box 10.5). Barnes et al. (2003) reported that students with SED formed the smallest percentage of the school occupational therapist's caseload. Children with SED are underserved and can benefit greatly from occupational therapy. Strategies for increasing occupational therapy's role in serving students with SED involve obtaining specialized knowledge and skills about SED, articulating the roles of occupational therapy, fostering team collaboration, articulating how occupational therapy services will affect the students' goals, and incorporating intervention strategies in the school settings to enhance student participation. Box 10.6 presents an example of how one school occupational therapist worked with team members to address the psychosocial and classroom behavioral needs of a group of students.

Occupational therapists often have high caseloads, limiting their time for service delivery to all students, including those with SED. One possible solution to the high caseload and time limitations is to apply a workload model instead of caseload model. A *workload model* includes all work activities that benefit students directly and indirectly, such as teacher training, environmental assessment, and advocacy, as a part of occupational therapy services—not just the students on one's caseload (AOTA, 2006). A workload analysis can illustrate how direct and indirect services contribute to promotion, prevention, and intervention strategies with children and youth with and without SED. This analysis may provide a means to illustrate how schedules and

Box 10.6. School Occupational Therapist's Psychosocial Support for Classroom Participation

Although children are frequently referred to occupational therapy for handwriting, self-care, and feeding difficulties, occupational therapy is a profession that takes a holistic view of children's school performance. Occupational therapists advocate for students' participation in such seemingly ordinary yet easily overlooked areas as access to recess and lunchroom routines with peers. In my school district, the occupational therapist who serves children in a particular school building also functions as a general resource for that school. In the process of serving students with individualized education programs, we develop relationships with teachers in the school and make ourselves available to provide support directly to other teachers who may not be teaching students directly served through IDEA.

For example, when a resource teacher was having difficulty with the students' undesirable behaviors in her small reading group, she asked me for help. I observed her group, and I affirmed her successful strategies, which included having the students work in dyads and creating an activity that embedded the lesson into a game. I provided her with suggestions to help restructure the physical, social, and cognitive demands of the task for individual students in the group. Also, I suggested other strategies, including using a T-stool for a boy who needed lots of movement, shifting the pairing of the student dyads to encourage emerging leadership strengths, and enabling students who tended to respond passively to have more opportunity to initiate. I encouraged her to facilitate student initiation by suggesting ways to structure activities for specific behavioral responses for each of the children. As I visited the school each week, I checked in with the teacher and helped her brainstorm through other issues as they arose.

Later, the teacher decided to form a small social skills training group with six students in her class. She obtained behavioral support teaching materials from the school district but realized that she did not feel equipped to manage what could become a mental health group. The teacher approached me as her school occupational therapist, and we then met with the school psychologist. As a team, we decided that I would provide support for her in group facilitation and in grading activities to support the practice of the group skills. We met a few times and exchanged e-mails as she narrowed the target skills that she wished to teach, and I helped her arrange them into a logical sequence. I developed activities to practice the behaviors and then co-led the initial groups to help model group facilitation skills. She was able to teach this small group of six students some very specific skills to support their social participation within the school with the support of occupational therapy. Of the six students in the group, one was eventually referred to occupational therapy for specific support in developing adaptive behaviors to enable increased effectiveness in his role as a student. Another received response to intervention support from occupational therapy concerning the use of a less restrictive level of intervention.

—Claudette Fette, OTR
Texas public school occupational therapist

methods can be changed to allow more time for new roles and responsibilities, such as including students with SED in workloads (Box 10.7).

Occupational Therapy Services for Children and Youth With Severe Emotional Disturbance

Occupational therapy's domain of practice is designed to support participation through engagement in occupation. As such, its unique contribution is the use of meaningful occupations in evaluation and intervention to help children participate in ADLs, instrumental activities of daily living (IADLs), education, play, leisure, rest or sleep, and social participation. Occupational therapy services emphasize building competencies and feelings of well-being by helping children engage in the activities they need or want to do. In addition, when working with children and youth with SED, it is essential that therapists have knowledge and skill in reducing problem behavior. The following approaches relevant to the promotion of mental health and

Box 10.7. Increasing Occupational Therapy Services for Students With Severe Emotional Disturbance

- Obtain knowledge about intervention approaches specific to students with severe emotional disturbance and relevant to occupational therapy (e.g., through workshops, Internet resources):
  - Positive behavioral interventions and support and other behavioral approaches to promote positive behavior and manage behavior outbursts
  - Social and emotional learning
  - Sensory-based approaches.
- Communicate the scope of occupational therapy services, including mental health promotion, prevention, and intervention during team meetings and in-service presentations.
- Collaborate effectively with all team members.
- Create opportunities to embed occupational therapy services in a variety of school contexts (classroom, cafeteria, recess, art):
  - Contribute to the functional behavioral assessment and behavior intervention plan
  - Attend schoolwide programs related to behavioral intervention and contribute to committee work
  - Integrate sensory-based strategies in practical ways to enhance teacher carryover.

reduction of problem behaviors in children with SED include (1) occupation-based group interventions, (2) behavioral approaches, (3) strategies for promoting social participation, and (4) sensory-based approaches.

Occupation-Based Group Interventions

To promote successful participation in a range of meaningful occupations, occupational therapists may use occupation-based groups. Although the focus of such task-oriented groups is engagement in meaningful occupation, multiple goals can be targeted. Dirette and Kolak (2004) reported that most students in alternative schools demonstrated limitations in healthy lifestyle behaviors (e.g., healthy nutrition, physical fitness) and participation in play or leisure activities. Occupation-based groups, which place as much emphasis on psychosocial skills as on the development of life skills, such as cooking and budgeting, and the development of hobbies and leisure activities, could easily be implemented in residential settings and schools. The formation of after-school clubs or groups, led by occupational therapists in alternative schools, can further encourage leisure participation and foster the development of friendships.

Occupation-based groups allow for the exploration and development of personal interests by promoting participation in a variety of age-appropriate occupations such as craft activities, cooking and baking, board games, and community outings. As the student participates in various activities, the occupational therapist should identify innate talents and skills (e.g., artistic abilities, creativity, attention to detail). Such awareness may help the student pursue a serious leisure activity or hobby.

Occupation-based groups also provide multiple opportunities to foster a variety of social, emotional, and cognitive skills. Social skills are learned behaviors, such as cooperation and empathy. *Sociocognitive skills* refer to the ability to comprehend social interchange and know what to do in light of others' responses. *Emotional regulation* is the awareness and control of one's feelings. Occupation-based groups give children opportunities to learn and practice these skills in the process of participating in activities and interacting with other children (Olson, Colangelo, & Shaw, 2009). Box 10.8 presents an example of how an occupation-based group could be structured.

Occupational therapists must have a thorough understanding of both content and process in creating occupation-based groups. Thought must be given to the structure, style of leadership, acceptable norms, the activity itself, and the group process (Olson et al., 2009). The tasks of the group leader or coleaders include structuring or guiding how the session runs, giving information and feedback, allowing students to try out different behaviors and reflect on them, encouraging group belonging, and demonstrating desired behaviors (Olson et al., 2009). Various models are described in the literature for organizing group sessions and processing or reflecting on the group dynamics to generalize learning to each member's life. Bazyk (2006) used a three-step process adapted from a model created by Williamson and Dorman (2002) in running occupation-based social skills groups in an after-school program for low-income urban youth. Refer to Box 10.6 for examples of occupation-based groups developed and embedded in an alternative school; Chapter 5 provides a full discussion of occupation-based groups.

Behavioral Approaches

Behavior management or behavior modification strategies are among the most frequently used approaches to reduce problem behaviors and promote positive interaction in children with SED (Ikiugo, 2007; Reddy et al., 2009). Behavioral approaches guide the interdisciplinary process of functional behavioral assessment (FBA) and the development of intervention strategies, which are referred to as *behavioral intervention plans (BIPs)*. Completion of an FBA and a BIP is required in schools when any student's behavior impedes his or her learning or the learning of others.

The FBA is a person-centered, problem-solving process that involves collecting data to analyze and identify the instructional, social, affective, environmental, and contextual variables that appear to lead to and maintain the behavior. An outcome of the FBA should be a hypothesis statement that includes (1) an operational definition of the problem behavior, (2) descriptions of the antecedent events that predict the behavior, and (3) descriptions of consequences that help maintain the behavior. A team that includes family members, school professionals, and community

Box 10.8. Structure of an Occupation-Based Group

Occupational therapy groups for HOPE (Healthy Occupations for Positive Emotions; Bazyk, 2006) are structured as followed:

- *Conversation time (10 minutes):* Leader introduces social–emotional theme (e.g., trust, expression of feeling) and fosters discussion among members and active listening.
- *Project activity (45 minutes):* Children participate in various creative projects or games designed to expose them to possible leisure interests or hobbies. The project activities allow for the development of skills and opportunities to apply the social–emotional theme for the group.
- *Closure (10 minutes):* The social–emotional theme is reviewed, and the children focus on their emotions, thoughts, and actions related to the activity. The children are encouraged to reflect on how participation in occupation influenced their emotions.

members collaborates to complete the FBA. Occupational therapists may contribute to the FBA by analyzing the student's occupational performance in areas such as classroom work, play, leisure, ADLs, IADLs, sleep or rest, and social participation. Resource 10.1 describes a helpful functional assessment tool; Table 10.1 lists additional assessment tools for assessing the performance of children with SED.

Resource 10.1. Functional Assessment Checklist for Teachers and Staff

The Functional Assessment Checklist for Teachers and Staff (FACTS) is a two-page interview used by school personnel and intended to be an efficient strategy for initial functional behavioral assessment. The FACTS is completed by people (teachers, family, clinicians) who know the student best and is used to develop behavior support plans. The FACTS is available on the Office of Special Education Programs' Technical Assistance Center for PBIS Web site at www.pbis.org, under "School Resources."

Results of the FBA are used to develop the BIP, which provides intervention strategies that address four areas: (1) setting events, (2) antecedents, (3) consequences, and (4) teaching appropriate behavior. Occupational therapists can contribute to the development and implementation of the BIP, especially related to areas of function unfamiliar to other team members (e.g., environmental triggers, sensory-based problems, group interaction, ADL/IADL analysis).

Table 10.1. Assessments for Children With Severe Emotional Disturbance

Assessment	Age or Grade Range	Description
Children's Assessment of Participation and Enjoyment; Preferences for Activities of Children (King et al., 2004)	6–21 years	Picture-based questionnaire and rating scale to evaluate participation, enjoyment, and preferences for recreational, physical, social, skill-based, and self-improvement activities
Perceived Efficacy and Goal Setting System (Missiuna, Pollock, & Law, 2004)	5–10 years	Picture-based self-report questionnaire for child, related questionnaires for parent and teacher; measures child's perceived ability in activities at home, in school, and in the community
Child Occupational Self-Assessment (Keller, Kafkes, Basu, Federico, & Kielhofner, 2004)	8–13 years	Self-report questionnaire evaluating child's perceived competence and importance of occupational performance and environmental adaptation
School Function Assessment (Coster, Deeney, Haltiwanger, & Haley, 1998)	K–6th grade	Questionnaire and rating scales completed by school personnel to evaluate student's participation, performance on tasks, and amount of support needed in school setting
Sensory Profile (Dunn, 1999)	3–10 years	Observation-based questionnaire or self-report to assess child's responses to sensory events in daily life that affect functioning
Social Skills Rating System (Gresham & Elliott, 1990)	3–18 years	A standardized assessment that evaluates social skills such as cooperation, assertiveness, responsibility, empathy, and self-control
Behavior Rating Inventory of Executive Functioning–Preschool Version (Gioia, Espy, & Isquith, 2003)	2–5 years	A rating inventory that evaluates a child's self-monitoring, emotional control, ability to inhibit, shift, initiate, play, organize, and attend
Coping Inventory (Zeitlin & Williamson, 1985)	3–16 years	A rating scale based on observation that evaluates a child's coping behavior for use in school and therapy. Self and environmental categories are further divided into dimensions of productive, active, and flexible styles of coping
KidCOTE (Kunz & Brayman, 1999)	5–18 years	Checklist with grid for evaluating 27 behaviors in the areas of general behaviors, cognitive behaviors, psychosocial behaviors, and sensorimotor performance
Adolescent Role Assessment (Black, 1976)	12–17 years	Gathers information on the adolescent's occupational role involvement over time and across domains

Box 10.9. Examples of Behavior Modification Strategies

- *Changing a circumstance preceding a targeted behavior to decrease it:* Beth and Curtis sat together in art class, and Beth frequently made rude comments to the art teacher because she thought these comments impressed Curtis. At the next art class, the teacher moved Beth away from Curtis. With Curtis gone, she will not have a stimulus to make the rude comments.
- *Changing a circumstance preceding a targeted behavior to increase it:* Juan talks too loudly to other children during group games, causing the other children to be afraid of him. Yet Juan wants to play with them. Using a verbal prompt, the therapist says "soft voice" before he speaks to remind him to speak appropriately. This preceding verbal prompt will increase appropriate speaking and will be faded out as his appropriate voice is reinforced naturally by the other children.
- *Positive reinforcement using a continuous reinforcement schedule:* Mark has been a bully. Nearly all his interactions with other students are negative and demanding. Because Mark does enjoy praise from the teacher, on each rare occasion when he says something nice to another student, he is given verbal praise by the teacher. This continuous praise will increase his nice interactions with other students.
- *Positive reinforcement using an intermittent reinforcement schedule:* After Mark has increased his nice interactions with other students, the teacher will reinforce only some of the occurrences of these interactions (perhaps every other time). By reducing the times Mark is given praise, he will start independently interacting in a nice manner.
- *Differential reinforcement of incompatible behavior:* This strategy involves reinforcing a behavior that is incompatible with an undesirable behavior. Marta nervously chews her fingernails throughout the occupational therapy session. Because Marta likes to receive pretty stickers, each time she has her hands engaged in a task and away from her mouth, she receives a sticker. This will help to reduce fingernail chewing.

Source. Lee and Axelrod (2005).

Having a solid understanding of behavioral approaches is important for understanding children's behaviors and contributing to the BIP. Using a behavioral approach, the therapist identifies the behavior needing change, determines situational or antecedent circumstances that contribute to the behavior, and identifies subsequent events (consequences) that increase or reinforce the occurrence of the behavior (Lee & Axelrod, 2005). The occupational therapist can change antecedent circumstances that influence a behavior, provide subsequent events that increase (reinforce) or decrease (reduce) the behavior, or both. For example, in a cooking group designed to promote cooperation, sharing, and appropriate communication, the occupational therapist verbally reinforces a student's turn taking while mixing the cake batter. Additionally, the therapist uses extinction—withholding of verbal reinforcement and attention—when the student calls another student an inappropriate name. Additional examples of the use of behavior modification strategies are provided in Box 10.9, and suggestions for information on behavioral intervention strategies are listed in Resource 10.2.

Occupational therapists are well equipped to modify environmental triggers (antecedents) to promote desired behaviors, such as moving desks around to decrease anxiety, reducing clutter to prevent distractions, altering noise and light levels, providing quiet areas, changing schedules to build in predictability,

Resource 10.2. Behavior Management

The following books provide practical strategies for analyzing problem behaviors and developing behavioral intervention plans:

- Lee, D., & Axelrod, S. (2005). *Behavior modification: Basic principles* (3rd ed.). Austin, TX: Pro-Ed.
- Murray-Slutsky, C., & Paris, B. A. (2005). *Is it sensory or is it behavior? Behavior problem identification, assessment, and intervention.* Austin, TX: Hammill Institute on Disabilities.
- Trott, M. C. (2002). *Oh behave! Sensory processing and behavioral strategies: A practical guide for clinicians, teachers, and parents.* San Antonio, TX: Psychological Corporation.

providing meaningful activities to reduce boredom, changing transitional times, and using sensory modulation equipment to help the child focus. Further strategies for enhancing behavioral performance are summarized in Box 10.10.

Occupational therapists must also know how to deal with tantrums and intense behavioral outbursts when working with children and youth with SED. *Temper tantrums,* or uncontrolled expressions of anger, generally consist of verbal (e.g., screaming, swearing) and physical (e.g., hitting, biting, kicking) outbursts and are the result of intense emotions with which the child is unable to cope (Murray-Slutsky & Paris, 2005). Tantrums may be caused by many factors, including frustration (e.g., unable to communicate wants, complete a task, or obtain something), hunger, fatigue, illness, and wanting attention. Therapists need to develop knowledge and skill in (1) how to avoid tantrums, (2) what to do if a tantrum or behavioral outburst occurs, and (3) how to help the child develop anger management strategies (e.g., self-control and coping with frustration).

Avoid Tantrums and Behavioral Outbursts

The first strategy is to modify the environment and interactions to avoid the problem behavior. Strategies include (1) recognizing warning signs that the child is becoming frustrated and intervening early, (2) sticking to routines, (3) preparing the child for transitions and new situations, and (4) providing developmentally appropriate activities (Murray-Slutsky & Paris, 2005). Children often display warning signs, such as whining, biting nails, fidgeting, or tensing of muscles, before a meltdown. It is important to teach the child how to recognize when he or she is becoming upset, communicate feelings (with words or pictures), and use self-calming strategies. *Self-monitoring* is a positive behavioral support that helps students develop awareness of their own behaviors, consider when and how often the behaviors occur, and give themselves reinforcement for improvement (Ganz, 2008).

Box 10.10. Strategies for Enhancing Behavioral Performance

- *Small rooms:* Use small, enclosed rooms to help contain behavioral expression.
- *Defined boundaries:* Specify rules clearly and concisely to communicate expectations for behavior. Review rules before each session, post the rules, and enforce rules with agreed-on consequences.
- *Sensory input:* Reduce visual and auditory distractions as much as possible. Modify other sensory variables on the basis of the child's sensory processing.
- *Emotional environment:* Interact in a nurturing, positive, and supportive manner.
- *Task presentation:* Carefully organize the session ahead of time—gather supplies in advance; keep supplies out of sight until needed; break tasks down into manageable parts; minimize down time within sessions; make clean-up part of activity when appropriate.
- *Session organization:* Use written or picture schedules (and post them); begin each session with the same first activity; give advance notice of transitions; make transitions as seamless as possible (e.g., use a preferred item to distract through transition); give choices to promote a sense of control.
- *Concise instructions:* Give brief and concise instructions; do not ask whether the child wants to do something unless you are prepared for a "no" answer; limit extraneous verbalizations.
- *Interesting and enjoyable activities:* Keep children engaged in interesting and motivating activities that provide the just-right challenge.

Source. Murray-Slutsky and Paris (2005, p. 107).

Ganz (2008) described seven steps for embedding self-monitoring with students in the classroom:

> [C]hoose a target behavior, talk with the student about self monitoring, determine how to measure the behavior, determine the method of self-monitoring, teach the student to self monitor (role play and teach to count behaviors), begin self-monitoring with student (increase the criteria periodically), fade teacher monitoring. (p. 47)

Self-monitoring is well suited for occupational therapists to implement because it requires the skills of activity analysis and behavior modification, both of which are within an occupational therapist's expertise. Self-monitoring strategies can be used with children with SED to decrease disruptive behavior, improve on-task behavior in the classroom, and improve social interaction skills with peers and teachers. It is an important step in helping children with ED regulate their physical and emotional states.

What to Do During a Behavioral Outburst

The steps in effectively handling a physical or emotional outburst are as follows (Murray-Slutsky & Paris, 2005):

1. Remain calm, and do not react emotionally (monitor voice volume, facial expression, movement).
2. Ignore the behavior.
3. Protect oneself, others, and the child from harm (e.g., unobtrusively move dangerous objects away from the area, hold child firmly to protect him or her from danger, move out of the way of flying arms and legs).

It is critical that occupational therapists obtain information on national, state, and district policies and procedures regarding the use of restraints or seclusion. In September 2009, the Council for Exceptional Children (CEC) released a policy concerning physical restraint and seclusion in school settings. CEC recommended that legislation be created to protect children from the misuse of restraint and seclusion. Key elements of the policy include that restraint and seclusion be implemented only when the student's behavior poses an immediate danger to the student or others; that data concerning seclusion and restraint be reported to outside agencies; that support for the implementation of preventative schoolwide measures like positive behavioral interventions and supports is provided; and that all school staff have mandatory conflict training.

Help Children Develop Anger Management Strategies

Children and adolescents with SED often display inappropriate types of behavior or feelings under typical circumstances (Center for Effective Collaboration and Practice, 2010). Interventions that help children express anger in appropriate ways are essential for the development of social relationships and learning within classroom and community settings (Resource 10.3).

Resource 10.3. Anger Management

Attwood, T. (2004). *Exploring feelings: Cognitive behavior therapy to manage anger.* Arlington, TX: Future Horizons.

Whitehouse, E., & Pudney, W. (1996). *Volcano in my tummy: Helping children to handle anger.* Gabriola Island, British Columbia: New Society.

Kellner and Bry (1999) described an anger management program found to be successful in reducing the incidence of physical aggression in adolescents with SED attending a therapeutic day school. Adolescents participated in sessions led by two social workers for 30 minutes per week for 10 weeks. A major theme of the group was that angry feelings are normal emotions that a person needs to learn how to handle them. During the beginning sessions, students were taught about anger and its physiology and were encouraged to be aware of their own physiological responses to anger. Education then focused on the identification of triggers resulting in anger. Prosocial criteria for handling anger successfully were taught to prevent violent behavior. Students shared the methods they used to control anger and compared them to the prosocial criteria. Specific strategies used to apply learning in day-to-day life included (1) the use of daily logs to self-monitor angry events and successful management, (2) physiological coping skills (e.g., relaxation, deep breathing, counting activities), (3) role playing, and (4) group leadership.

Students in the anger management program demonstrated improvement, as measured by decreased aggressive incidents during school and decreased teacher and parent ratings of the students' aggressive behavior (Kellner & Bry, 1999). The program can be applied to meet individual students' needs, while using a group focus to benefit all the students in the classroom. Because this program involves a variety of activities (e.g., calming techniques, written logs, role playing), it could be used as the foundation for an occupational therapy group. An example of another anger management program combining sensory-based and cognitive–behavioral strategies is described in Box 10.11.

Box 10.11. Anger Management: Combining Sensory-Based and Cognitive–Behavioral Strategies

Strategies used in an anger management and self-regulation group for children with Asperger syndrome and autism spectrum disorders may be applied to children with SED. A team of teachers, a social worker, and an occupational therapist created the program using concepts from a sensory modulation program, The Alert Program (Williams & Shellenberger, 1996), and an anger management program (Exploring Feeling) using cognitive–behavioral principles (Attwood, 2004). Children participated in the program for 30 minutes per week for 15 weeks.

- *First stage:* Students identify the intensity level of their anger about a particular event and associate it with physical body sensations felt at the time. For example, a child felt furious when people laughed at him and felt like his body started to cook. Pencil-and-paper tasks of coloring in a thermometer to rate anger intensity levels and self-drawings to label body sensations were used to increase the children's understanding.
- *Second stage:* In this stage, anger is conceptualized as a natural part of the fight-or-flight response, and children are told that they can control the intensity of their response when they are aware of the relationship among thinking, feelings, and behavior. Role-play situations are used to give the children practice in achieving positive outcomes in potentially negative emotional situations.
- *Third stage:* Engine-level concepts from the Alert Program are tied to previous learning about anger. Children identify their engine level when they experience anger and the most effective sensory strategy used for calming. A picture of a stop sign labeled "stop, think, and choose" is used as a visual reminder of the process. These words remind the children to stop and use a sensory strategy to calm down when feeling angry, to think about their feelings and alternative behaviors available to them, and finally to choose the best course of action. The team felt that the program was easy to use in the classroom and successful in reducing incidents of uncontrolled anger.

Source. Maas, Mason, and Candler (2008).

Strategies for Promoting Social Participation

Social participation involves the "organized patterns of behavior that are characteristic and expected of an individual or a given position within a social system" (AOTA, 2008b, p. 633). Social participation involves the social interactions with family, community, teachers, peers, and friends. Roberts (2008) defined *social skills* as the capacity to relate to others in a manner that is satisfactory to the person and to others. Social skills are the specific behaviors that a child exhibits to perform a social task, such as active listening and reciprocal conversation. When a child is able to perform a social task competently, he or she is said to have *social competence* (Cook et al., 2008).

Social skills affect the development of significant relationships and how others feel about a child (Mori & Piantanida, 2007). Children and adolescents with SED have difficulty demonstrating satisfactory social skills with peers and teachers, often resulting in academic difficulties (Gresham, Cook, & Crews, 2004). Additionally, in a survey of 39 educators of adolescents with SED in alternative schools, 84% of the respondents identified difficulties in play and leisure (Dirette & Kolak, 2004). Without early intervention, social skill limitations may have negative implications long into adulthood (Cook et al., 2008).

Social Skills Training

Social skills training (SST) interventions involve instruction in targeted interpersonal skills designed to allow students to be successful in their social environments and contexts (Cook et al., 2008). A review of the literature indicates that SST can be an effective approach to increasing social competence for children with SED (Amish, Gesen, Smith, Clark, & Stake, 1988; Cook et al., 2008; Reddy et al., 2009; Stemmac & Josefowits, 1985). Typically, SST involves promoting social skill acquisition, improving social performance, decreasing and eliminating problem behaviors, and generalizing and maintaining positive social skills to allow children to be successful in social environments (Cook et al., 2008). Social behaviors typically targeted are cooperation, assertion, responsibility, empathy, and self-control (Olson et al., 2009). Mori and Piantanida (2007) developed a manual called *Every Child Wants to Play: Simple and Effective Strategies for Teaching Social Skills,* which provides specific strategies to apply in social skill interventions. The program uses simulated group interaction, practice of targeted social skills, and strategies to show children the implied rules of social interaction. Issues such as personal space, give and take, eye contact, and appropriate expression of thoughts are addressed in specific lessons included in the manual.

Social and Emotional Learning

Social and emotional learning (SEL) programs are related to but different from SST in that a greater emphasis is placed on becoming aware of (and thinking about) how feelings influence behavior. Learning activities focus on developing an expanded vocabulary of feeling words, recognizing and expressing feelings, responding to others' feelings, and learning how to express anger in appropriate ways.

> Social and emotional learning programming, when implemented with fidelity and integrated into the fabric of the school and community, provides students with the skills they need to be successful within an environment that promotes their physical and emotional safety and well-being. (Collaborative for Academic, Social, and Emotional Learning, 2008, p. 4)

It is important for occupational therapists to determine whether their state has developed SEL standards and helps promote such efforts.

Sensory-Based Approaches

Children and youth with SED often respond to ordinary sensory input in intense ways that may negatively influence emotions (e.g., causing irritability or tantrums) and social interaction (e.g., causing withdrawal or aggression). Occupational therapists can play an important role in helping children, families, and professionals develop a working knowledge of sensory processing to understand children's behaviors and modify everyday interactions and environments to foster success and well-being (Dunn, 1999). The Alert Program (Williams & Shellenberger, 1996), for example, was developed to assist children in recognizing their arousal states throughout the day and using sensorimotor strategies to self-regulate arousal and behavior. This program uses the analogy of a car engine to describe how one's nervous system functions in different environments and affects attending and learning. The child learns strategies to help get his or her car engine at a "just-right" speed. The strategies are sensory based and are designed to help regulate arousal states. They include putting something in the mouth, movement and proprioceptive activities, touching and fidgeting with items, visual regulation, and auditory regulation (Williams & Shellenberger, 1996). With the occupational therapist's guidance, the child selects strategies to help regulate his or her arousal state appropriately for the demands of the task and environment. This approach can be applied in group or individual situations in a classroom and led by an occupational therapist or by the teacher with occupational therapy consultation (Barnes, Vogel, Beck, Schoenfeld, & Owen, 2008).

To encourage carryover of sensory-based strategies by teachers in the classroom for children with SED, occupational therapists must find ways to incorporate the activities in practical and easy ways using readily available materials. Reflection 10.1 encourages readers to think about how their clients with SED might experience sensory input.

Walking in the Client's Shoes

"All health care providers should imagine, for a moment, feeling overwhelmed, unsafe, and bombarded by unfamiliar stimuli, and imagine entering a complex and over stimulating health care setting. How would they feel in this environment (Cmiel, Karr, Gasser, Oliphant, & Neveau, 2004)? What elements of a therapeutic environment would they find comforting, supportive, and responsive if they were in this state?" (Champagne & Stromberg, 2004, p. 36).

Sensory Strategies to Prevent the Use of Seclusion and Restraints

Sensory-based approaches and sensory rooms are valuable resources as cultures of care shift to become more responsive to the needs of consumers in inpatient and residential mental health settings (Champagne & Stromberg, 2004). *Sensory rooms* use sensorimotor activities that offer a variety of calming and alerting options to promote self-organization and reduce the need for seclusion and restraint (Champagne & Stromberg, 2004). Although initially applied in inpatient psychiatric settings, sensory rooms are now being developed in programs for children. For example, in 2002, most inpatient child and adolescent programs in Massachusetts

Resource 10.4. Avoiding Seclusion and Restraint

- *Tina Champagne, MEd, OTR:* Occupational Therapy Innovation (www.OT-innovations.com)
- *Restraint/Seclusion Reduction Initiative:* The Massachusetts Department of Mental Health developed this initiative to reduce and ultimately eliminate the use of restraint and seclusion in all child and adolescent inpatient and intensive residential treatment facilities in the state. Learn how to create sensory safe environments with The Safety Zone Tool–Adolescents version and the Safety Tool Kids (www.mass.gov/Eeohhs2/docs/dmh/rsri/safety_zone_tool.pdf).

began to develop sensory rooms in response to an initiative led by the Commonwealth of Massachusetts Department of Mental Health aimed at preventing the use of seclusion and restraint (LeBel et al., 2004). Occupational therapy consultants helped develop sensory spaces for children and adolescents, giving the rooms names such as the Zen Room, Cool Room, and Chillville. Resource 10.4 suggests additional sources of information on how to avoid the use of seclusion and restraint.

Summary

Children and youth with SED have severe behavioral problems that directly limit their participation in school and community occupations. They are frequently placed in alternative educational environments requiring the close collaboration of a team of professionals, including occupational therapists. This chapter provided information on how occupational therapy services can promote the reduction of problem behaviors and the development of competencies by applying a variety of approaches, including occupation-based, behavioral, social and emotional, and sensory-based approaches.

References

Abt Associates. (2008). *Characteristics of residential treatment for children and youth with serious emotional disturbances.* Cambridge, MA: Author. Retrieved August 13, 2010, from www.naphs.org/documents/AbtFINALReport.8.4.08_000.pdf

American Occupational Therapy Association. (2006). *Transforming caseload to workload in school-based and early intervention occupational therapy services.* Retrieved July 14, 2009, from www.aota.org/Practitioners/Resources/Docs/FactSheets.aspx

American Occupational Therapy Association. (2008a). *FAQ on school mental health.* Retrieved November 19, 2009, from www.aota.org/Practitioners/PracticeAreas/Pediatrics/Browse/School.aspx

American Occupational Therapy Association. (2008b). Occupational therapy practice framework: Domain and process (2nd ed.). *American Journal of Occupational Therapy, 62,* 625–683.

American Psychiatric Association. (2000). *Diagnostic and statistical manual of mental disorders* (4th ed., text rev.). Arlington, VA: Author.

Amish, P., Gesen, E., Smith, J., Clark, H., & Stake, C. (1988). Social problem-solving training for severely emotionally and behaviorally disturbed children. *Behavioral Disorders, 13,* 175–186.

Attwood, T. (2004). *Exploring feelings: Cognitive–behavior therapy to manage anger.* Arlington, TX: Future Horizons.

Barnes, K., Beck, A., Vogel, K., Grice, K., & Murphy, D. (2003). Perceptions regarding school based occupational therapy for children with emotional disturbances. *American Journal of Occupational Therapy, 57,* 337–341.

Barnes, K., Vogel, K., Beck, A., Schoenfeld, H., & Owen, S. (2008). Self-regulation strategies of children with emotional disturbance. *Physical and Occupational Therapy in Pediatrics, 28*(4), 367–385.

Bazyk, S. (2006). Creating occupation-based social skills groups in after-school care. *OT Practice, 11*(7), 13–18.

Bazyk, S. (2007). Addressing the mental health needs of children in schools. In L. Jackson (Ed.), *Occupational therapy services for children and youth under IDEA* (3rd ed., pp. 145–166). Bethesda, MD: AOTA Press.

Beck, A., Barnes, K., Vogel, K., & Grice, K. (2006). The dilemma of psychosocial occupational therapy in public schools: The therapist' perceptions. *Occupational Therapy in Mental Health, 22*(1), 1–17.

Black, M. (1976). Adolescent Role Assessment. *American Journal of Occupational Therapy, 30,* 73–79.

Cantrell, R. P., & Cantrell, M. L. (2007). *Helping troubled children and youth: Continuing evidence for the Re–ED approach.* Westerville, OH: American Re–ED Association.

Carrey, N., & Gregson, J. (2008). A context for classification in child psychiatry. *Journal of Canadian Academic Child and Adolescent Psychiatry, 17*(2), 50–57.

Case-Smith, J., & Archer, L. (2008). School-based services for students with emotional disturbance: Findings and recommendations. *OT Practice, 13*(1), 17–21.

Center for Effective Collaboration and Practice. (2010). *Students with emotional disturbance: Eligibility and characteristics.* Retrieved August 12, 2010, from http://cecp.air.org/resources/20th/eligchar.asp

Champagne, T., & Stromberg, N. (2004). Sensory approaches in inpatient psychiatric settings: Innovative alternatives to seclusion and restraint. *Journal of Psychosocial Nursing and Mental Health Services, 42*(9), 35–43.

Cheney, D., Flower, A., & Templeton, T. (2008). Applying response to intervention metrics in the social domain for students at risk of developing emotional or behavioral disorders. *Journal of Special Education, 42*(2), 108–126.

Cmiel, C., Karr, D., Gasser, D., Oliphant, L., & Neveau, A. (2004). Noise control: A nursing team's approach to noise control. *American Journal of Nursing, 104*(2), 40–48.

Collaborative for Academic, Social, and Emotional Learning. (2008). *What is SEL: Skills and competencies.* Retrieved August 12, 2010, from http://casel.org/basics/skills.php

Cook, C., Gresham, F., Kern, L., Barreras, R., Thorton, S., & Crews, S. (2008). Social skills training for secondary students with emotional and/or behavioral disorders. *Journal of Emotional and Behavioral Disorders, 16*(3), 131–144.

Coster, W., Deeney, T., Haltiwanger, J., & Haley, S. (1998). *School Function Assessment (SFA).* San Antonio, TX: Harcourt Assessment.

Council for Exceptional Children. (2009). *CEC adopts new policy on physical restraint and seclusion.* Retrieved August 13, 2010, from www.cec.sped.org/AM/Template.cfm?Section=Search&TEMPLATE=/CM/HTMLDisplay.cfm&CONTENTID=12996

Dirette, D., & Kolak, L. (2004). Brief Report—Occupational performance needs of adolescents in alternative education programs. *American Journal of Occupational Therapy, 58,* 337–341.

Dodge, N., Keenan, S., & Lattanzi, T. (2002). Strengthening the capacity of schools and communities to serve students with serious emotional disturbance. *Journal of Child and Family Studies, 11*(1), 23–34.

Dunn, W. (1999). *Sensory Profile.* San Antonio, TX: Psychological Corporation.

Dwyer, K. (2002). Mental health in the schools. *Journal of Child and Family Studies, 11*(1), 101–111.

Fecser, F. A. (2003). Positive Education Program's day treatment centers. *Reclaiming Children and Youth, 12,* 108–112.

Foley, R., & Pang, L. (2006). Alternative education programs: Program and student characteristics. *High School Journal, 89*(3), 10–21.

Ganz, J. (2008). Self-monitoring across age and ability levels: Teaching students to implement their own positive behavioral interventions. *Preventing School Failure, 53*(1), 39–48.

Gioia, G., Espy, K., & Isquith, P. (2003). *Behavior Rating Inventory of Executive Functioning–Preschool Version (BRIEF–P).* Lutz, FL: Psychological Assessment Resources.

Gresham, F. M., Cook, C. R., & Crews, D. (2004). Social skills training for children and youth with emotional and behavioral disorders: Validity consideration and future directions. *Behavioral Disorders, 30*(1), 32–46.

Gresham, F., & Elliott, S. (1990). *Social Skills Rating System.* Circle Pines, MN: American Guidance Center.

Heathfield, L. T., & Clark, E. (2004). Shifting from categories to services: Comprehensive school-based mental health for children with emotional disturbance and social maladjustment. *Psychology in the Schools, 41*(8), 911–920.

Hobbs, N. (1966). Helping disturbed children: Psychological and ecological strategies. *American Psychologist, 21,* 1105–1115.

Ikiugu, M. (2007). *Psychosocial conceptual practice models in occupational therapy: Building adaptive capability.* St. Louis, MO: Mosby.

Individuals With Disabilities Education Improvement Act of 2004, Pub. L. 108–446, 20 U.S.C. § 1400 *et seq.*

Jackson, L., & Arbesman, M. (2005). *Occupational therapy practice guidelines for children with behavioral and psychosocial needs.* Bethesda, MD: AOTA Press.

Keller, J., Kafkes, A., Basu, S., Federico, J., & Kielhofner, G. (2004). *The Child Occupational Self-Assessment (COSA)* (Version 2.0). Chicago: Model of Human Occupation Clearinghouse.

Keller, T. E., Bost, N. S., Lock, E. D., & Marcenko, M. O. (2005). Factors associated with participation of children with mental health problems in structured youth development programs. *Journal of Emotional and Behavioral Disorders, 13*(3), 141–151.

Kellner, M. H., & Bry, B. H. (1999). The effects of anger management groups in a day school for emotionally disturbed adolescents. *Adolescence, 34*(136), 645–651.

King, G., Law, M., King, S., Hurley, P., Rosenbaum, P., Hanna, S., et al. (2004). *Children's Assessment of Participation and Enjoyment (CAPE).* San Antonio, TX: Harcourt Assessment.

Kleiner, B., Porch, R., & Farris, E. (2002). *Public alternative schools and programs for students at risk of education failure: 2000–01* (NCES 2002–004). Washington, DC: National Center for Education Statistics.

Koller, J. R., & Bertel, J. M. (2006). Responding to today's mental health needs of children, families, and schools: Revisiting the preservice and training and preparation of school-based personnel. *Education and Treatment of Children, 29,* 197–217.

Kunz, K., & Brayman. S. (1999). The Comprehensive Occupational Therapy Evaluation. In B. Hemphill (Ed.), *Assessments in occupational therapy mental health: An integrative approach* (pp. 259–274). Thorofare, NJ: Slack.

LeBel, J., Stromberg, N., Duckworth, K., Kerzner, J., Goldstein, R., Weeks, M., et al. (2004). Child and adolescent inpatient restraint reduction: A state initiative to promote strength-based care. *Journal of the American Academy of Child and Adolescent Psychiatry, 43,* 37–45.

Lee, D., & Axelrod, S. (2005). *Behavior modification: Basic principles* (3rd ed.). Austin, TX: Pro-Ed.

Lehr, C. A., Lanners, E. J., & Lange, C. M. (2003). *Alternative schools: Policy and legislation across the United States.* Minneapolis: University of Minnesota, Institute on Community Integration.

Lehr, C., Tan, C., & Ysseldyke, J. (2009). Alternative schools: A synthesis of state-level policy and research. *Remedial and Special Education, 30*(1), 19–32.

Leone, P., & McLaughlin, J. (1995). Appropriate placement of students with emotional and behavioral disorders: Emerging policy options. In J. M. Kauffman, J. Lloyd, & T. Astuto (Eds.), *Issues in the educational placement of pupils with emotional and behavioral disorders* (pp. 335–362). Hillsdale, NJ: Lawrence Erlbaum.

Maas, C., Mason, R., & Candler, C. (2008). "When I get mad. . . ." *OT Practice, 13*(9), 9–14.

Mahoney, J. L., Eccles, J. S., & Larson, R. W. (2004). Processes of adjustment in organized out-of-school activities: Opportunities and risks. *New Directions for Youth Development,* pp. 115–144.

Missiuna, C., Pollock, N., & Law, M. (2004). *Perceived efficacy and goal setting system.* San Antonio, TX: Harcourt Assessment.

Mori, A. B., & Piantanida, D. B. (2007). *Every child wants to play: Simple and effective strategies for teaching social skills.* Torrance, CA: Pediatric Therapy Network.

Murray-Slutsky, C., & Paris, B. A. (2005). *Is it sensory or is it behavior? Behavior problem identification, assessment, and intervention.* Austin, TX: Hammill Institute on Disabilities.

National Center for Education Statistics. (2002). *Characteristics of the 100 largest public elementary and secondary school districts in the United States: 2000–01* (NCES 2002–351). Washington, DC: Author.

National Center for Education Statistics. (2006). *Digest of education statistics.* Retrieved August 13, 2010, from http://nces.ed.gov/programs/digest/d05/tables/dt05_051.asp

Narrow, W. E., Reiger, D. A., Goodman, S. H., Rae, D. S., Roper, M. T., Bourdon, K. H., et al. (1998). A comparison of federal definitions of severe mental illness among children and adolescents in four communities. *Psychiatric Services, 49*(12), 1601–1608.

Olson, L., Colangelo, C., & Shaw, M. (2009, April). *Addressing children's social participation.* Presentation at the 89th AOTA Annual Conference & Expo, Houston, TX.

Positive Education Program. (2008). [Home page]. Retrieved November 23, 2010, from http://www.pepcleve.org/

Reddy, L. (2001). Serious emotional disturbance in children and adolescents: Current status and future directions. *Behavior Therapy, 32,* 667–691.

Reddy, L. A., De Thomas, C. A., Newman, E., & Chun, V. (2009). School-based prevention and intervention programs for children with emotional disturbance: A review of treatment components and methodology. *Psychology in the Schools, 46*(2), 132–153.

Repie, M. S. (2005). A school mental health issues survey from the perspective of regular and special education teachers, school counselors, and school psychologists. *Education and Treatment of Children, 28*(3), 279–298.

Roberts, M. (2008). Life skills. In J. Creek & L. Lougher (Eds.), *Occupational therapy and mental health* (4th ed., pp. 359–379). Edinburgh: Elsevier.

Silver, S. E., Duchnowski, A. J., Kutash, K., Friedman, R. M., Eisen, M., Prange, M. E., et al. (1992). A comparison of children with serious emotional disturbance served in residential and school settings. *Journal of Child and Family Studies, 1*(1), 43–59.

Simpson, G. A., Bloom, B., Cohen, R. A., & Blumberg, S. (2005). *U.S. children with emotional and behavioral difficulties: Data from the 2001, 2002, and 2003 National Health Interview Surveys* (Advance Data From Vital and Health Statistics No. 360). Hyattsville, MD: National Center for Health Statistics. Retrieved August 13, 2010, from www.cdc.gov/nchs/products/ad.htm

Stemmac, L., & Josefowits, N. (1985). A board game for teaching social skills to institutionalized adolescents. *Journal of Child Care, 2,* 31–37.

Trott, M. C. (2002). *Oh behave! Sensory processing and behavioral strategies: A practical guide for clinicians, teachers, and parents.* San Antonio, TX: Psychological Corporation.

U.S. Department of Health and Human Services. (2000). *Report of the Surgeon General's Conference on Children's Mental Health: A national action agenda.* Washington, DC: Author.

Vernberg, E. M., Roberts, M. C., & Nyre, J. E. (2008). The intensive mental health program: Development and structures of the model of intervention for children with serious emotional disturbances. *Journal of Child and Family Studies, 17,* 169–177.

Whitehouse, E., & Pudney, W. (1996). *Volcano in my tummy: Helping children to handle anger.* Gabriola Island, BC: New Society.

Williams, M., & Shellenberger, S. (1996). *How does your engine run? A leader's guide to the Alert Program for self-regulation.* Albuquerque, NM: Therapy Works.

Williamson, G. G., & Dorman, W. J. (2002). *Promoting social competence.* San Antonio, TX: Therapy Skill Builders.

World Health Organization. (2008). *The international statistical classification of diseases and health-related problems.* Geneva: Author.

Zeitlin, S., & Williamson, G. (1985). *Coping Inventory.* Bensenville, IL: Scholastic Testing Service.

Zigmond, N. (2006). Twenty-four months after high school: Paths taken by youth diagnosed with severe emotional and behavioral disorders. *Journal of Emotional and Behavioral Disorders, 14*(2), 99–107.

CHAPTER 11

Children With Attention Deficit Hyperactivity Disorder, Developmental Coordination Disorder, and Learning Disabilities

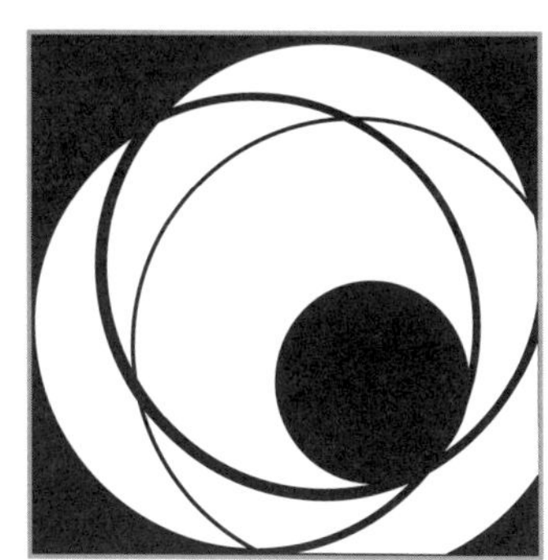

Anne A. Poulsen, PhD

Learning Objectives

After reading this material and completing the examination, readers will be able to

- Recognize the shared features and commonalities experienced by children with attention deficit hyperactivity disorder, developmental coordination disorder, and learning disabilities;
- Determine the impact of these conditions on children's mental health and social participation;
- Identify how fulfilling needs for relatedness, competence, and autonomy influences positive mental health in this population; and
- Identify occupation-focused strategies to enhance social participation and promote mental health within a three-tiered approach (universal, targeted, intensive).

Attention deficit hyperactivity disorder (ADHD), developmental coordination disorder (DCD), and learning disabilities (LD) have many links and overlaps in terms of shared occupational performance difficulties and similar confusion over management and service access. These conditions can affect up to 3 children in a classroom of 30, and significantly more boys than girls are referred for therapy services (Barkley, 2006; Cermak & Larkin, 2002). Only a small proportion of children, however, actually receive intervention. Parents are typically confronted with long waiting lists for occupational therapy services (Green et al., 2005), and receiving a runaround in obtaining accurate diagnosis and service provision is common (Rodger & Mandich, 2005). Many children simply slip between the cracks in service provision and receive no early intervention to prevent lifelong struggles with everyday tasks that others master with ease.

Historically, the three conditions have received several labels. Consensus on appropriate terminology and diagnostic criteria is poor, and some confusion exists on the matter (Missiuna & Polatajko, 1995). Has labeling been constructive in terms of helping to direct services to these populations? Or have the various labels been ineffective or, at worst, destructive for these children's mental health and social participation? The pragmatic considerations for accuracy in terms of diagnosis and symptom description must be carefully weighed alongside the risks of stigmatization, social exclusion, and participation restrictions that can occur whenever any labels are applied to children.

For children with ADHD, DCD, and LD, it is imperative that occupational therapists act early to identify individual vulnerabilities while supporting whole-school and population-based strategies to enhance strengths, prevent ill health, and help children develop their full potential. The key aim of occupational therapy services is to facilitate occupational performance role fulfillment through an optimal person–environment–occupation fit (Law et al., 1996). This fit underpins occupational flourishing, which occurs when there is a full discovery of life's possibilities in everyday activities.

This chapter first describes how to recognize the unique and overlapping characteristics of the "alphabet buddies"—ADHD, DCD, and LD—as described in the *Diagnostic and Statistical Manual of Mental Disorders* (4th ed., text rev.; *DSM–IV–TR;* American Psychiatric Association [APA], 2000) and the proposed revisions in the *DSM–V* (APA, 2010). It identifies the shared features and commonalities experienced by children with these disorders and outlines the need for supportive services to improve mental health outcomes and social participation for people with these disorders throughout their lives.

Second, the chapter outlines how to be aware of the mental health and social participation needs of people with these conditions. It aims to answer the following questions:

- What is the potential lifelong impact of these conditions on mental health?
- What is the impact in and out of school on social participation?
- What are the benefits and disadvantages of labeling?

Third, the chapter delineates the key aims of occupational therapy service provision to improve mental health and social participation for children with ADHD, DCD, and LD. It presents examples of how these aims are met using the Synthesis of Child, Occupational Performance, and Environment–In Time (SCOPE–IT) Model and Self-Determination Theory (Deci & Ryan, 2000) so that readers can understand how fulfilling the three basic psychological needs for relatedness, competence, and autonomy influences positive mental health in this population.

Finally, the chapter uses an expanded occupational lens to describe occupation-focused strategies aimed at enhancing social participation and promoting mental health, using a three-tiered approach. The aim is for readers to be able to delineate strategies at Tier 1 (promoting mental health and social participation at a universal level), Tier 2 (small-group or targeted interventions for at-risk children), and Tier 3 (intensive one-on-one assessments and interventions for high-risk children).

Overview of the Alphabet Buddies: ADHD, DCD, and LD

The specific criteria used to diagnose ADHD, DCD, and LD according to the *DSM–IV–TR* (APA, 2000) are presented in Tables 11.1, 11.2, and 11.3. However, heterogeneity in symptom presentation and functional impact is common. Children who have any of these conditions can experience serious restrictions in social participation, a problem that has implications for mental health. Building up a picture of each child's unidentified and identified abilities and contextualizing those strengths within the unique physical and social ecology of everyday activities make it possible to open doors to healthy participation and functioning. For example, part of the occupational therapy perspective is understanding that a boy with DCD who spends his spare time in his bedroom on the computer or watching television for long periods has strengths in playing electronic games with cyber-friends but would also like to join the soccer team with his classmates and needs

Table 11.1. Definition of ADHD

Terminology	Description
Examples of other terms used to describe ADHD	• Attention deficit disorder • Hyperkinetic disorder.
Subtypes	• ADHD, combined type • ADHD, predominantly inattentive type • ADHD, predominantly hyperactive–impulsive type.
APA (2000) criteria. Proposed revisions to the classification of ADHD in the *DSM–V* are currently under consideration; changes to all criteria are debated (APA, 2010).	
Criterion A	Six or more symptoms of inattention and/or hyperactivity–impulsivity (as listed in the *DSM–IV–TR;* APA, 2000) have persisted for at least 6 months or to a degree that is maladaptive and inconsistent with developmental level.
Criterion B	Age of onset is before age 7. Some symptoms that interfered with everyday functioning were present before age 7. *Note:* The proposed revisions for the *DSM–V* suggest that this age limit will be increased to age 12 (APA, 2010).
Criterion C	Some impairment from symptoms is observed in at least two settings, e.g., at school and at home.
Criterion D	Clinically significant evidence of impaired functioning in social, academic, or occupational functioning must be clearly evident.
Criterion E	*Exclusion criteria:* A diagnosis of ADHD is excluded if people have been diagnosed as having schizophrenia or other psychotic disorder, pervasive developmental disorder, mood or anxiety disorder, dissociative or personality disorder.
Other descriptive information	
Gender ratio	Male:female ratio is 4:1 (Gaub & Carlson, 1997).
Prevalence	3%–5% for children ages 5–11 (APA, 2000)

Note. APA = American Psychiatric Association; ADHD = attention deficit hyperactivity disorder; *DSM = Diagnostic and Statistical Manual of Mental Disorders; DSM–IV–TR = DSM,* 4th edition, text revision; *DSM–V = DSM,* 5th edition.

Source. APA (2000).

Table 11.2. Definition of DCD

Terminology	Description
Examples of other terms used to describe DCD	• In the United Kingdom, the commonly used term is developmental dyspraxia. • Historical terms include minimal cerebral dysfunction, congenital maladroitness, and clumsy child syndrome. • Term used in the EHA, as amended by IDEA, is *learning disability–minimal brain dysfunction.*
APA (2010) criteria	
Criterion A	Motor performance is substantially below levels that would be expected for chronological age and past skill acquisition opportunities. This poor motor performance can be manifested as coordination difficulties and clumsiness, poor balance, dropping or bumping into things, marked delay in achieving developmental milestones (e.g., sitting, crawling, and walking), or in the acquisition of basic motor skills (e.g., cutting, coloring, printing, writing, catching, throwing, kicking, running, jumping, and hopping).
Criterion B	The disturbance in Criterion A, without accommodations, significantly interferes with academic achievement or activities of daily living.
Criterion C	*Exclusion criteria:* The disturbance is not the result of a general medical condition, such as cerebral palsy, hemiplegia, or muscular dystrophy.
Criterion D (has been omitted in the proposed *DSM–V* revisions)	The *DSM–IV–TR* (APA, 2000) stated that "if Mental Retardation is present, the motor difficulties are in excess of those usually associated with it." Sugden (2006) interpreted this to mean children with scores <70 on a standardized test of intelligence were not considered to have DCD.
Other descriptive information	
Gender ratio	Male:female ratio varies from 1.3:1 (Martin, Pick, & Hay, 2006) to 3:1 (Missiuna, Pollock, et al., 2008).
Prevalence	6% for children ages 5–11 (APA, 2000)

Note. APA = American Psychiatric Association; DCD = developmental coordination disorder; *DSM = Diagnostic and Statistical Manual of Mental Disorders; DSM–IV–TR = DSM,* 4th edition, text revision; *DSM–V = DSM,* 5th edition; EHA = Education for All Handicapped Children Act of 1975; IDEA = Individuals With Disabilities Education Act of 1990.

Source. APA (2010).

some support (and organizational change) to realize that goal. This viewpoint forms the basis for planning to expand every child's capacity so that full participation in meaningful everyday activities is possible, whether on the sports field, in the classroom, or at home.

Key occupational performance challenges facing children with ADHD, DCD, and LD are presented in Tables 11.4, 11.5, and 11.6. Briefly,

- Children with ADHD have persistent patterns of inattention, hyperactivity–impulsivity, or both that interfere with functioning in at least two areas of living.
- DCD is a condition that is diagnosed when children have significant motor impairments that are incommensurate with chronological age and measured intelligence and are not the result of a medical condition, such

Table 11.3. Definition of LD

Terminology	Description
Examples of other terms used to describe LD	• Academic skills disorder • Specific learning disabilities.
Subtypes	• Subtypes listed in *DSM–V* proposed revisions (APA, 2010) include dyslexia (reading disorder) and dsycalculia (mathematics disorder). Dysgraphia and learning disorder not otherwise specified have been omitted. • Historical terms include academic skills disorder.
APA (2010) criteria	
Criterion A	Difficulties in (1) accuracy or fluency of reading (for dyslexia) or (2) production or comprehension of quantities, numerical symbols, or basic arithmetic operations that are not consistent with the person's chronological age, educational opportunities, or intellectual abilities. Multiple sources of information are to be used to assess these abilities, one of which must be an individually administered, culturally appropriate, psychometrically sound standardized measure of these skills.
Criterion B	Academic achievement, activities of daily living, or both that require these specific abilities (i.e., reading, mathematics) are functionally impaired, without accommodations, because of deficits identified in Criterion A.
Other descriptive information	
Gender ratio	Variable male:female ratios have been reported, ranging from 2:1 to 5:1, with more males affected. However, for dyslexia a more equivalent gender ratio, 1.6:1, is now reported (Chan, Ho, Tsang, Lee, & Chung, 2007).
Prevalence	3%–5% for children ages 5–11 (APA, 2000), although some estimates are as high as 1 in 10 or 1 in 15 (Hendrikson et al., 2007).

Note. APA = American Psychiatric Association; *DSM–V* = *Diagnostic and Statistical Manual of Mental Disorders,* 5th edition; LD = learning disabilities.

Source. APA (2010).

as cerebral palsy. These motor difficulties significantly interfere with performance in daily activities in the classroom, playground, sporting field, workplace, or home environment.

- The principal occupational performance area in which children with LD experience functional difficulties is the academic realm. Having difficulties with reading, mathematics, or written expression has potential repercussions across many occupational performance areas beyond schoolwork alone.

Shared Features and Commonalities Experienced by Children With These Conditions

The overlap among ADHD, DCD, and LD is well recognized (Spencer, Biederman, & Mick, 2007; Visser, 2003). Children with these conditions often share similarities in basic neurobiological background, or "hard wiring." Historically, biologically,

Table 11.4. Impact of ADHD on Occupational Performance

Skill Issue	Examples
Process skills for pacing, attending, and completing tasks	• *At school:* Work output uneven and messy, frequent shifts from one unfinished activity to another, failure to pay close attention to details, careless errors, low persistence in independent work, fidgets or squirms in seat, motor restlessness • *Basic ADLs:* Forgets or is inconsistent in washing body parts; wiping self; flushing toilet; personal care tasks unfinished or messy; lids of toothpaste, toilet, and other grooming items left off; buttons and zippers not fully fastened or irregularly fixed; clothes untucked; belts not threaded through loops • *IADLs:* Leaves table before end of meal, homework incomplete, low persistence with effortful tasks or chores • *Leisure:* Performance erratic, steps not performed in sequence recommended by instructor or instruction manual, attends to other features of the environment rather than leisure task, excessive running or climbing when not appropriate, difficulty playing quietly
Process skills for organization of space, objects, and time	• *At school:* Difficulties with searching, locating, and organizing materials in lockers, desks, and bags; forgets to bring homework, lunch, and appropriate clothing to school; pencils, papers, and books misplaced, lost, and scattered; damage to property occurs through spilling, dropping, and mishandling • *At home (basic ADLs):* Messy eating and drinking patterns and use of utensils, restless sleep patterns and irregular breathing interrupt night time sleeping, incomplete recall of personal care routines • *At home (IADLs):* Untidy, disorganized bedroom and study desktops, inconsistent putting away toys, keeping cupboards organized • *Leisure:* Forgets to bring sports equipment and clothing to matches, forgets timing of practices and matches or performances
Communication skills for maintaining relationships and performing tasks	• *Across domains:* Appears to not be listening, particularly in busy environments; frequent shifts in attention during a conversation; mind appears to be on other tasks—does not hear instructions, cannot block out trivial noises or background conversations so that an activity cannot be completed without interruption; blurting out answers inappropriately • *Leisure:* Inattention to instructions of adult or peer leaders; does not appear to listen to adult leader's advice, game tips, or feedback; cannot block out spectators' behavior or external stimuli irrelevant to game
Maintaining attention throughout a task; difficulties are associated with adverse emotional reactions	• *Across domains:* Strong dislike or avoidance of challenging academic tasks that require sustained mental effort and self-application, adverse emotional reactions to activities with high organizational demands • *At home:* Frustration and anger in response to effortful and complex dressing tasks involving multiple items, layers, difficult fasteners, etc.; low perceived competence in getting ready on time • *Leisure:* Strong emotional reactions—anxiety, anger, fear, and avoidance—directed toward tasks or toward the physical and social environment
Impulsivity	• *Across domains:* Difficulty delaying responses, impatience, interrupting, restlessness, noncompliant, off task, may respond aggressively to frustrations, reduced awareness of danger • *Leisure:* Difficulty waiting for turn, grabs objects from others, clowns around, touches objects and people inappropriately, bangs into others, takes risks • *At home (IADLs):* Difficulty maintaining and acquiring a driver's license

Note. ADHD = attention deficit hyperactivity disorder; ADLs = activities of daily living; IADLs = instrumental activities of daily living.

and functionally, the conditions have many commonalities. It is not unusual for a child with any one condition to exhibit signs of other conditions. Co-occurring symptoms may represent a risk of double or triple jeopardy with respect to potentially adverse social participation and mental health outcomes. Not only do ADHD, DCD, and LD co-occur, but they may overlap with other conditions, such as autism

Table 11.5. Impact of DCD on Occupational Performance

Skill Issue	Examples
Process skills for pacing, attending, and completing tasks	• *At school/college:* Slower learning motor tasks, quicker using a computer than writing by hand (as college student), difficulty organizing thoughts while doing written classwork • *At home (basic ADLs):* Slow learning to tie shoes • *At home (IADLs):* Slow learning to drive a car • *Leisure:* Slow learning to ride a bicycle, difficulty understanding how to do activities because they may not be able to follow instructions
Process skills for sequencing and performing motor tasks fluently	• *At school:* Difficulty negotiating way around desks, playgrounds, without bumping into others; copying from a board when multiple sequences of looking up and down while writing and perhaps listening at the same time are required. • *Basic ADLs:* Dressing difficulties (e.g., tying shoelaces, putting clothes on in the right order); getting ready for school or changing clothes for physical education classes in a timely fashion is problematic • *IADLs:* Difficulty walking alongside parent in shopping center without bumping into parent or other people • *Leisure:* Forgets to bring sports equipment and clothing to matches, forgets timing of practices and matches or performances
Difficulties with performance of motor tasks; relate to avoidance, conflict, or low self-esteem	• *At school:* Avoidance of written tasks, refusal or reluctance to participate in school physical education classes and sports days, low self-esteem, anxiety, exhaustion after lengthy sessions of handwriting, dissatisfaction and disappointment with messy or untidy written work, slumps over desk or rocks on chair while performing writing or cutting • *At home:* Conflict over homework completion; either avoids or covers up problems when possible; difficulty getting ready on time, knocking over cups, difficulty pouring from jugs, etc., can be stressful • *Leisure:* Low persistence in socially evaluative physical activities and social loafing or making less effort to achieve a goal when in a group situation, anxiety about balance or climbing activities
Peer relationships	• *School:* Vulnerable to bullying and teasing, being laughed at and ridiculed for poor motor performance or letting the team down • *Leisure:* Few invitations to play after school or attend other children's birthday parties, low motivation to participate in team sports and competitive physical activities

Note. ADLs = activities of daily living; IADLs = instrumental activities of daily living; DCD = developmental coordination disorder.

spectrum disorder (Green et al., 2009); speech and language impairment (Rechetinikov & Maitrat, 2009); Tourette's syndrome (Keen, 2005); sensory impairments such as retinopathy of prematurity (Goyen & Lui, 2009) or hearing impairments (Engel-Yeger & Weissman, 2009); sleep, depression, and anxiety disorders (Bart et al., 2009); and overweight and obesity (Cairney, Hay, Faught, & Hawes, 2005). More than half the children diagnosed with ADHD also exhibit behavior characteristics of oppositional defiant disorder (ODD; Barkley, 2006). An example of a child diagnosed with several disorders is presented in Box 11.1.

Rates of overlap among children with ADHD, DCD, and LD are difficult to determine. Diagnostic criteria recommended by the Ontario and Leeds summits (Polatajko, Fox, & Missiuna, 1995; Sugden, 2006) have not been widely adopted, which has hampered collection of reliable data on incidence or prevalence. Unknown or imprecise rates of occurrence for secondary and co-occurring disorders

Table 11.6. Impact of LD on Occupational Performance

Skill Issue	Examples
Cognitive processing across one or more domains	• *At school:* Underlying disabilities in visual perception, poor short- and long-term memory, auditory processing, difficulties with organization of ideas, objects, and time; may affect classroom performance throughout the day • *Leisure:* May forget to bring sports equipment and clothing to matches, forgets timing of practices and matches or performances
Social relations	• *Across domains:* LD may affect behavior in social situations across the lifespan, but this is not always the case (e.g., children may be less popular with their peers, remain loners in a group), inappropriate social responses to adults, difficulty with sharing • *Communication:* May be slow to process language, may be able to decode but struggle with comprehension, may have poor sequencing of instructions, may have poor understanding of pragmatics of language, which influences social participation, choice of hobbies, and vocations
Variable emotional reactions	• Not all children with LD exhibit behavioral problems that affect occupational performance. However, perhaps as many as 30% of children with LD will have emotional or behavioral disorders, including both internalizing and externalizing problems that are long term and influence decisions to participate in social activities and to engage in and persist with academic studies, vocations, and leisure pursuits (Hallahan, Lloyd, Kauffman, Weiss, & Martinez, 2005) • May have good days and bad days—variability in performance is observed • At risk for developing secondary problems such as depression, anxiety, and substance abuse, which have significant lifelong occupational performance implications

Note. LD = learning disabilities.

have contributed to inadequate reporting of statistics to estimate future service provision requirements.

New diagnostic categories and labels have been adopted in some countries to account for the overlap among conditions. For example, the estimate that approximately half of all children with DCD also have attention deficit disorder (Fox & Lent, 1996) has led to the development of a new diagnostic category called *deficits in attention and motor processing,* or DAMP (Gillberg, 2003; Stein & Chowdhury, 2006). Other labels proposed to account for the nonspecific and heterogeneous nature of these conditions include *atypical brain development* (Kaplan, Wilson, Dewey, & Crawford, 1998) and *specific developmental disorder* (Rispens & van Yperen, 1997).

Providing Supportive Services

Specialist services to support these children are limited. A case can be made for providing more direct services within schools or communities and indirect services through consultation and advocacy at a population level, an approach that would ensure that children with ADHD, DCD, and LD can benefit from broad changes to learning and performance climates in which the emphasis is on positive activity engagement and mental well-being.

The key goals of occupational therapy service provision aimed at improving mental health outcomes and social participation for children with ADHD, DCD, and LD are presented in Table 11.7. Achieving health for all children through full participation in occupations and activities in their home, school, and community

Box 11.1. Case Example: Aaron

Aaron was a bright 6-year-old whose high-achieving father was the principal of the school Aaron attended. Aaron was initially referred because of handwriting difficulties, problems with attention in class, and social skills deficits. His teacher described him as a "happy little boy for most of the time but as stubborn as can be when asked to participate in sports—refusing to take his shoes off and join in with his classmates and being generally disruptive when forced to participate." Clinical examination revealed that Aaron's poor gross and fine motor performance on the Movement Assessment Battery for Children–2 (Henderson, Sugden, & Barnett, 2007) was below the 5th percentile for his age. His functional difficulties with handwriting, shoelace tying, and sports meant that he met the criteria for a diagnosis of DCD. Aaron's father appeared relieved when told the results of the motor assessment because it helped explain why Aaron was experiencing troubles in the classroom. His father further investigated Aaron's difficulties, taking him to a child psychologist and a speech–language pathologist.

Aaron's father used the term *alphabet kid* to describe his child. He explained that his son had now acquired a long list of labels, including ADHD, DCD, ODD, and LD. He commented,

> I now understand some of the problems Aaron is experiencing. He's an alphabet kid, and I don't want that to be a cop-out. But maybe it will convince the classroom teacher that Aaron needs help. I think she believes he is simply not trying his hardest and plays up because he's the principal's son.

is consistent with the World Health Organization's (2001) biopsychosocial view of health and functioning. Promoting well-being through participation in meaningful activities may also prevent some of the secondary emotional and behavioral disturbances seen in these children (Missiuna, Moll, King, Stewart, & Macdonald, 2008). Having a holistic, preventive focus aimed at all children and their families also meets concerns about low generalization of treatment effects across settings over time, specifically for populations such as those with ADHD (Abikoff, 2009).

An interdisciplinary professional approach centered on child and family needs is the gold standard for the care of children with ADHD, DCD, and LD (Salmon & Kirby, 2008) because most of them have multiple diagnoses and difficulties across many domains (Hendriksen et al., 2007). Occupational therapy models of practice, such as Engaging and Coaching for Health–Child (EACH–Child; Ziviani, Poulsen, & Hansen, 2009) and Occupational Performance Coaching (OPC; Graham, Rodger, & Ziviani, 2009), are examples of recent, holistic, occupation-based approaches with an ecological focus. Older models, such as the Model of Social Interaction (Doble & Maggill-Evans, 1992), focus on a person's social enactment skills within the context of occupational performance, and less attention is paid to environmental influences.

Models such as EACH–Child are based on person–environment–occupation (PEO) principles (Law et al., 1996). One PEO framework developed for children with DCD but applicable to all populations described in this chapter is the SCOPE–IT model (Poulsen & Ziviani, 2004a, 2004b; Haertl, 2009). At the heart of the SCOPE–IT model (Figure 11.1) are three clock hands that represent quantity of time (hour hand), choice in how time is allocated (minute hand), and quality of time and effort (minute hand) spent in four key occupational performance areas. The occupational performance areas are (1) work (obligatory activities, such as chores, schoolwork, and structured out-of-school time); (2) leisure and play; (3) activities of daily living (ADLs), both instrumental and basic; and (4) rest. Motivation to spend time in different activities activates the hands of the SCOPE–IT clock. Self-Determination Theory (Deci & Ryan, 2000, 2008) helps explain how motivation to engage in

Table 11.7. Key Aims of Occupational Therapy Service Provision to Improve Mental Health Outcomes and Social Participation for Children With ADHD, DCD, and LD

Aims	Means of Achieving Aims
To help children fulfill their basic psychological needs for autonomy, competence, and relatedness	Through engagement in personally meaningful activities that meet these psychological needs (Deci & Ryan, 2000)
To identify and maintain occupational balance	By ensuring that children have healthful and moderate balanced time use among the occupations of work, play, rest, and sleep (see Ziviani, Desha, & Rodger, 2006)
To encourage and support healthy community participation in physical, social, cultural, service, and skill-based activities	By adopting a coaching approach, such as the–EACH–Child model (Ziviani et al., 2009)
To ensure that there is a good fit or match among child capabilities, ecological assets, and occupational performance	By using a frame of reference, such as the Person–Environment–Occupation model (Law et al., 1996) or SCOPE–IT (Poulsen & Ziviani, 2004a, 2004b)
To adopt a client- or family-centered approach in which collaborative goal setting guides practice	Through the use of principles about guiding clients to set their own goals for occupational performance, e.g., OPC (Graham, Rodger, & Ziviani, 2009)

Note. ADHD = attention deficit hyperactivity disorder; DCD = developmental coordination disorder; EACH–Child = Engaging and Coaching for Health–Child; LD = learning disabilities; OPC = Occupational Performance Coaching; SCOPE–IT = Synthesis of Child, Occupational Performance and Environment–In Time.

personally meaningful occupations is fueled by a drive to satisfy basic psychological needs. When psychological needs are satisfied, the foundations for flourishing occupational performance and optimal mental health are created.

For children with ADHD, nurturing the fulfillment of occupational performance roles might be seen when classrooms are organized to support attention, home spaces are designed to enable self-regulation during homework tasks, and preparation for joining in valued activities is facilitated by the occupational therapist. *Occupational jeopardy,* which occurs when basic psychological needs are not met in everyday activities, can be seen in the case of a child such as Aaron, who was reluctant to participate in sports because he had low actual and perceived motor ability (i.e., unmet competence needs); who tried to control his environment by refusing to participate but was forced to join in by his teacher (i.e., low autonomy); and whose disruptive behavior placed him at risk of being avoided or rejected by his peers (i.e., unmet relatedness needs).

Literature Review of Mental Health and Social Participation Needs of Children With ADHD, DCD, and LD

Small initial differences in the neurodevelopment and genetic makeup of children with ADHD, DCD, and LD, when combined with supportive or adverse environmental conditions, contribute to significantly divergent life courses throughout school and later life (Cantell, Smyth, & Ahonen, 2003). For some children, identifying the initial core problems behind an unfolding life course of low social participation and poor mental well-being can be difficult. Secondary emotional disturbance

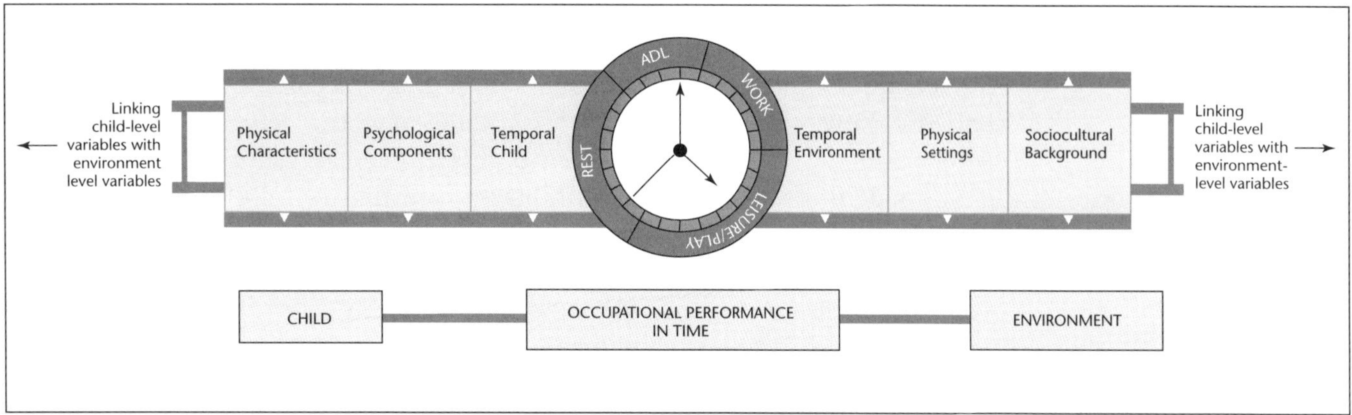

Figure 11.1. Synthesis of Child, Occupational Performance, and Environment–In Time (SCOPE–IT) model.

Note. ADL = activities of daily living.

Source. Poulsen and Ziviani (2004b).

and occupational performance difficulties in key areas such as academics, ADLs, and leisure affect a child's mental health and social participation. Frustration and confusion on the part of parents, teachers, and other community members who observe a downward spiral when performance difficulties interfere with functioning may also occur (Missiuna, Moll, King, King, & Law, 2007).

Some members of the wider community and, indeed, many health professionals and teachers, believe that subtle initial difficulties are transitory and that children will just outgrow early problems. Negative labels inferring lack of effort, such as *lazy,* may be applied, reflecting a lack of understanding and knowledge about these children's unique and persistent difficulties (Hallahan et al., 2005). It is now well recognized that the behavior, motor, and academic difficulties experienced by children with ADHD, DCD, and LD can continue to have an impact on full participation in daily activities throughout the lifespan (Cantell, Smith, & Ahonen, 2003). It has even been argued that conditions such as DCD could be considered social disorders because of their impact on social participation (Kirby, 2004). Problems with peer relationships and peer relation self-concept not only persist into adulthood but may increase for some people, such as those with ADHD or combined ADHD and DCD (Bagwell, Brooke, Pelham, & Hoza, 2001; Rasmussen & Gillberg, 2000). A widespread need for public and professional education about these conditions exists (Fox & Lent, 1996).

Impact on Child Mental Health

Children with ADHD, DCD, and LD can experience acute and chronic mental anguish at any time in their lives (e.g., Cantell et al., 2003; Rasmussen & Gillberg, 2000). Low self-esteem, social exclusion, reduced employment prospects, and increased chances of offending can influence mental health (Kaufmann, 2005). For children with DCD, anxiety and depression may emerge by early adolescence (Piek, Dworcan, Barrett, & Coleman, 2000). Extreme variability is common, however, and mental health outcomes are individually determined.

Evidence has shown that accumulative risks associated with having multiple coexisting conditions are particularly adverse for mental health (Gregg, 2009). If children are not provided with adequate support and accommodations, their generalized negative self-perceptions can contribute to global feelings of learned helplessness and negative expectations of success. Adolescents and adults with these "childhood" disorders fall into a no-man's land between child and adolescent psychiatry and receive few support services (Kirby, Sugden, Beveridge, & Edwards, 2008). The importance of increasing public and professional awareness, without overtly medicalizing these conditions, cannot be overly stressed. The factors affecting mental health for these children are summarized in Table 11.8.

Box 11.2 presents a case example of a 12-year-old girl, Mia, who had learning and motor coordination difficulties and was referred to the KOALA program (Kinder, for children and families; Overweight, for *overcoming and being OK!;* Activity, for a*n active mind and an active body;* Lifestyle, for *a living, life-giving diet;* Actions, for *all together and ahead we look*) at the Mater Children's Hospital, South Brisbane, Queensland, Australia. Mia's story highlights some of the mental health and social issues faced by children with LD and DCD.

Impact on Social Participation

Children with ADHD, DCD, and LD report peer rejection and fewer friendships than their age-related peers without these difficulties (Bagwell et al., 2001; Missiuna et al.,

Table 11.8. Factors Contributing to Mental Health Issues for Children With ADHD, DCD, and LD

Factors	Actions
Quality evidence of pathophysiology or etiology and life course for each of these conditions is insufficient and still emerging.	Research and education campaigns need to continue to inform teachers, practitioners, and policymakers.
Occupational performance difficulties are first identified in childhood but continue to present challenges throughout life.	People with these conditions need awareness and support throughout the lifespan.
A gender imbalance exists, with more boys than girls affected.	The most vulnerable within each society need to be supported, but minority subgroups, such as girls with these conditions, need to be recognized.
The disorders often cluster in families.	All family members' mental, social, and physical health needs must be considered.
Prolonged occupational performance difficulties across a range of contexts have implications for mental health.	Early intervention is needed before primary problems contribute to secondary issues.
No "gold standard" intervention program exists for any of these conditions, although an increasing body of evidence is accumulating about effective strategies aimed at improving occupational performance (e.g., Polatajko & Mandich, 2004). Many children with ADHD, DCD, and LD do not receive or are ineligible for publicly funded interventions.	Ongoing research is needed on effectiveness of interventions and strategies. Population-based preventive programs addressing social and physical activity participation needs have mental and physical health implications for all children and may therefore be considered a priority over one-on-one intensive interventions.

Note. ADHD = attention deficit hyperactivity disorder; DCD = developmental coordination disorder; LD = learning disabilities.

Box 11.2. Case Example: Mia

Mia first saw an occupational therapist when she was referred to the KOALA (*K*inder, *O*verweight, *A*ctivity, *L*ifestyle, *A*ctions) program. Although her family was concerned about her steady weight gain, sedentary lifestyle, and poor coordination, Mia was more worried about the fact that no one would play with her at school. She reported having no friends to talk to or sit with during breaks and nobody to play with after school or on weekends. Her favorite pastimes included watching television and reading in her bedroom. Cooking and eating pasta with her large family was an activity she enjoyed on the weekends.

As part of the KOALA program, Mia and her family attended three specially targeted weekend camps run by the SCOUTS Australia program. The focus was on family participation in fun, noncompetitive physical activities and healthy nutritional experiences. During the camp, Mia had difficulties with all the gross motor activities and was a reluctant starter on the hikes.

At the occupational therapy clinic between camps, she was assessed on the Bruininks–Oseretsky Test of Motor Proficiency–2 (Bruininks & Bruininks, 2005), and her performance was well below average for her age and measured intelligence. Her scores on the Self-Description Questionnaire–I (SDQI; Marsh, 1990) revealed low peer relations and general self-concept. Scores on both the Physical Ability and Physical Appearance self-concept subscales were well below age norms. While completing the SDQI, she described being bullied on the playground and being called names. During this session, Mia listed some leisure and social performance goals that she would like to achieve. With her mother present, Mia explored physical and social leisure time activity options that might help her reach these goals.

By the second and third camps, Mia's persistence in tackling increasingly challenging tasks alongside the other children was noticeable. Her parents noted that Mia's improving confidence during group activities in the camp environment seemed to have an effect at school as well, where she reported a tentative friendship with a classmate. Mia decided to continue with the SCOUTS experience and enrolled in her local SCOUT group.

2007; Wong & Donahue, 2002). Limited participation in community activities, such as team sports, has been reported for children with ADHD or DCD (Harvey & Reid, 1997; Poulsen, Ziviani, Cuskelly, & Smith, 2007). Less exposure to the associated social worlds surrounding these pursuits can mean that concepts, ideas, skills, and attitudes acquired in these contexts are limited (Vygotsky, 1978).

Restricted social participation can be experienced throughout life, particularly in the leisure domain, in which decisions to join and continue attending sports practices or classes are more likely to be optional. Teasing and stigmatization can contribute to dropout and avoidance of social and physical activities. Secondary emotional health issues (Missiuna et al., 2007) have been reported, including anxiety (Bart et al., 2009) and depression (Piek, Barrett, Allen, Jones, & Louise, 2005). Retrospective accounts by adults who described themselves as being physically awkward during their school years recount the humiliation associated with public exposure of poor physical coordination on the sports fields (Fitzpatrick & Watkinson, 2003).

Attention difficulties and impulsivity influence the ability of children with ADHD to listen to and follow instructions, which can be problematic in out-of-school activities in which volunteers with limited experiences in managing large groups of children are required to teach complex or new skills. Children with ADHD may experience aggression, emotional reactivity, difficulty waiting for turns, rowdiness, and physical injury when playing team sports (Johnson, 2000). Inattention and misinterpretation of key social cues and having an intrusive response style and poor conversational peer-entry abilities can make it difficult for children with ADHD to move into social settings with ease.

Boys with DCD in the upper years of primary or elementary school are particularly at risk of having low self-perceptions of physical ability, physical appearance, and peer relations if they are unable to participate in popular extracurricular activities, such as team sports (Poulsen et al., 2007). To be part of a team or group that accomplishes something is to be part of a social whole. Performance competency plays an important part in being accepted by peers and being able to be a member of a group (Mandich, Polatajko, & Rodger, 2003). Children who do not have the prerequisite strengths or abilities can miss out on these important group experiences. According to Aristotle, "the whole is more than the sum of its parts."

To flourish is to enable others to flourish as well. Co-flourishing helps children meet their potential by using individual strengths to partake more fully in social contexts. Adult leaders can help children with ADHD, DCD, and LD identify their unique contributions and become part of the social whole. More often, children with these conditions have been found to be at increased risk of victimization, bullying, and social rejection than children without these disorders (Piek et al., 2005). During adolescence, greater social isolation may occur, particularly for boys, if the school culture is biased toward physical elitism and prowess in organized or formally structured power sports (Endresen & Olweus, 2005). On the playground, poor gross motor coordination can also affect selection in informal teams that are not organized by adults.

Low participation in social and physical activities during early adolescence has been reported as spreading to low participation in all social activities, whether physical or nonphysical, as youth with DCD grow older (Cantell et al., 1994). This pattern raises concerns about the poverty of some children's leisure participation when they experience reduced exposure to a range of social and physical informal and formal pursuits.

Young adults (ages 18–25) with DCD are significantly more likely to be living at home with their parents than are those of the same age with LD such as dyslexia (Kirby et al., 2008). Ongoing difficulties with ADLs and a need for continuing parental support have been suggested as contributing to delay in leaving the family home and increased social isolation with age for young adults with DCD. In contrast, young adults with ADHD are more likely than those without ADHD to leave their homes and families at younger ages, enter romantic and sexual relationships earlier (and experience more breakdowns of those relationships), be involved in crime, and have poorer early work histories and higher rates of unemployment (Schachar & Tannock, 2002). The combination of DCD and ADHD is associated with poorer outcomes than either disorder alone. Of a sample of young adults with both disorders, 80% had ongoing problems with alcohol and drug abuse, mental health difficulties, and higher rates of breaking the law compared with 13% in a comparison group with ADHD alone (Rasmussen & Gillberg, 2000).

Benefits and Disadvantages of Labels: First Do No Harm

Sugden (2006) argued that international consensus regarding diagnostic features, familial patterns, course and specific culture, age, and gender features is necessary to build knowledge about prevalence, associated features, and evidence-based service provision. The benefits and disadvantages of labeling have been vigorously debated by researchers and clinicians working with children with ADHD, DCD, and LD. The arguments are outlined in Table 11.9.

Labels are only beneficial when they can serve as springboards to build and strengthen capacity in vulnerable people. They can be seen as flags to identify areas of need and to alert communities to provide support for people at risk. Ensuring that a child's health and well-being are optimized rather than jeopardized by the use of disease reference points and labels is a key consideration. An example of the referral runaround and poor labeling that contribute to slow understanding of the occupational performance needs and mental health issues for a child with DCD can be seen in the description of Phillip, an 11-year-old boy with DCD (Box 11.3).

Table 11.9. Benefits and Disadvantages of Labels for Children With ADHD, DCD, and LD

Benefits	Rationale
Authenticity	The levels of confusion over terminology, combined with uncertainty about how to describe the core characteristics of these disorders, have contributed to questioning of the authenticity of these conditions by some health practitioners and members of the public. For example, DCD has been considered an invisible or hidden disorder of childhood (Lingam, Hunt, Golding, Jongmans, & Emond, 2009).
Service provision	Service provision is positively affected by accurate labeling, both for preventive services—broad community strategies to promote health and well-being—and for intervention development and delivery.
Medical rebate	Medical rebate and funding for further research and resource provision are more likely if there is an agreed-on label and clear diagnostic criteria.
Knowledge	Further refinement in understanding the unique characteristics and needs of children is facilitated by well-defined criteria for each diagnostic label.
Research	Not having clear diagnostic criteria and labeling affects international scientific research endeavors to collate and compare evidence globally.
Nonemotive terminology	Informed labeling may be less detrimental than use of common or slang terms used to describe these conditions. There is more likely to be sensitive consideration and debate over officially accepted terminology.
Screening	Screening of children for these conditions cannot occur without clear diagnostic criteria and labeling.
Disadvantages	**Rationale**
Stigma	Labels may be associated with negative views about poor coordination, inattention, hyperactivity, and learning difficulties that are debilitating for children and their family members.
Burden	Physicians and teachers may be reluctant to identify conditions or difficulties that they perceive to be minor. There is a view that labeling will burden parents and their children needlessly (Missiuna, Moll, et al., 2008).
Impact of multiple labels	There may be too many boxes to tick for these children. The heterogeneous nature of these conditions and the fact that disorders co-occur may mean that children do not fit neatly into discrete boxes, which can be disadvantageous in terms of directing service provision because some students with overlapping presentation may miss out on support because of mild symptoms across a range of disorders and, therefore, not meeting the criteria for any one defined category (Kirby et al., 2008).
Bullying	External characteristics or identifying features, such as wearing glasses, having red hair, having speech difficulties, speaking with a dialect, being from a different ethnic background, and having a diagnostic label, are associated with an increased tendency to be bullied (Olweus, 2010).
Medicalization	Applying a label might be considered to be a medicalization of a personal characteristic or ability that is at the extreme end of a developmental spectrum. At worst, this can mean that children and their families adopt a sick role requiring medical treatment. Is it possible to change labels to reflect a more positive outlook, e.g., making LD stand for "learns differently" rather than "learning disabled"?

Note. ADHD = attention deficit hyperactivity disorder; DCD = developmental coordination disorder; LD = learning disabilities.

Box 11.3. Case Example: Phillip

Phillip's family had been seeking answers to questions about his occupational performance difficulties since he turned 4 years old. His first teacher noted Phil's reluctance to join in physical games with his peers and his fear of climbing on the playground apparatus. He preferred solitary fantasy play and was described as a loner.

Phil's parents were worried that Phil had no friends. His dad enrolled him in a soccer club because Phil expressed a desire to try this activity. He might even get a few invitations to play after school, something that had never happened before. Instead, it seemed to make things worse. Phil's coach singled him out to work on his skills, saying that he needed to play "like a Phillip, not a Phillippa." Phil became a reluctant starter and then refused to go to training. Phil's coach put more effort into getting Phil to join in and kept working on Phil's weaknesses. Admittedly, Phil wasn't a star participant. He had difficulty following instructions and couldn't catch the ball. He tended to prance up and down the side of the field at a safe distance from the main action. Phil begged to give up.

His parents didn't know what to do and turned for help to the local doctor, who assured them that Phil would soon outgrow his problems. So they encouraged him to join in and offered rewards if he put more effort into the matches. But Phil had developed a new approach to the game. He would spend his time on the field sitting at the end of the field picking dandelions during the game. The roar from disappointed spectators and his teammates when he failed to join in the action was deafening. His parents couldn't bear to watch their son's failure. His father recalled similar experiences from his own childhood and decided to avoid watching the games, leaving it up to the experts. Perhaps the coach could motivate Phil to join in the action. Instead, his teammates derided him, and his coach became exasperated at his behavior and his parents' apparent lack of support. Phil's wishes to be left alone were totally fulfilled. His parents didn't know what to do or where to go.

At school, Phil's social isolation increased. He was never picked by other boys for recess games, and he never received those valued invitations to play after school. He was labeled a *klutz* by his classmates. He had feelings of sadness, considered himself stupid, and felt guilty and confused about why he hated the physical activities his classmates enjoyed. To Phil, it was all pain and humiliation. His teacher noticed that he was increasingly quiet in class and slow to finish his written work. But because he was really no problem, especially when there were children in the class with much more severe learning and behavior difficulties, she left him alone, sad and quiet, at the back of the class. The teacher would have liked to refer him for help, but the waiting lists were long, and besides, she couldn't quite put her finger on what was actually wrong.

It turned out that Phil never outgrew his problems. He was teased and later bullied throughout his school life. At first, he withdrew from physical activity participation at school. Then he stopped participating in all leisure activities with peers and family members. His recollections of school physical education are colored by terms such as "torture" and "agony." He was called "doughnut" as he grew older and became overweight and physically unfit. Perhaps a more accurate description or label, along with informed understanding and support at an early stage, would have helped. How could flourishing rather than languishing have been promoted for Phil?

Evidence for Flourishing and Resilience

May the hand of a friend always be near you,
May successes help you grow,
May you realize your dreams one step at a time.

—Traditional Irish friendship wish

Researchers have identified in longitudinal and retrospective studies a subgroup of people with ADHD, DCD, and LD who display characteristics of resilience, including persistence, determination, and positive views of self (Cantell et al., 1994, 2003; Fitzpatrick & Watkinson, 2003). These studies have provided insights into various individual or ecological factors that positively influence life pathways (Missiuna, Moll, et al., 2008). Unfortunately, the literature focusing on flourishing and

Box 11.4. Case Example: Sam

Sam's parents coached and managed the under-12 basketball team. Sam was a keen, enthusiastic player who regularly practiced at home. Not only was his grandfather a founding member of the basketball association, but his uncle had played on an Olympic basketball team. This boy had early and repeated exposure to excellent coaching both on the court and at home, in which every minute out of school was spent practicing and having fun with his family around the hoop. His cousins played on his team, his mother was the team manager, and his dad was the assistant coach. He lived and breathed basketball. Additionally, he was very tall for his age and was focused on improving his game. He had a deep sense of connection with the basketball community (meeting needs for relatedness); he felt competent (through repeated opportunities to acquire skills); and he had his own personal goals for improvement (autonomy). His basic psychological needs for well-being and flourishing in this leisure pursuit were met at this point in time. His family background provided strong social capital to support ongoing participation even though Sam had been diagnosed as having DCD at the early age of 4.

resilience is less prolific than are studies reporting mental illness and other adverse long-term outcomes.

Evidence has increased that children with ADHD, DCD, and LD flourish when there is a good fit among child skills and attributes, environmental factors, and the activities selected by the child or adult (e.g., Kirby et al., 2008; Miller, 2002). It is important to look closely at whether a child is able to participate in a range of activities that promote flourishing through psychological need fulfillment. It is also important to investigate social and physical environmental factors, such as the contribution of social capital to activity participation. *Social capital* is defined as the social connections, norms, and trust formed by participating in community activities (Putnam, 2000). The potential benefits for children who may be on the fringe of fitting into and fully participating in a leisure pursuit are considerable. Increasing social capital can strengthen interpersonal ties, offer opportunities for power or positions of responsibility, and provide a means of acquiring skills and knowledge. The example of Sam, a 10-year-old boy with DCD whose family had high social capital within the leisure pursuit of basketball, is presented in Box 11.4.

According to Self-Determination Theory (Deci & Ryan, 2008), the three basic psychological needs that must be satisfied for effective functioning and optimal mental health are (1) relatedness, (2) autonomy, and (3) competence. When relatedness needs are fulfilled, autonomy is facilitated, and strengths and talents are nurtured to ensure competent participation in desired occupations, broad health benefits result not only for the target children but for all children, their families, and the wider community.

Psychological Need 1: Relatedness

> Don't walk in front of me; I may not follow. Don't walk behind me; I may not lead. Just walk beside me and be my friend.
>
> —Albert Camus (as cited in Parker, 2008, p. 2)

Having a positive relationship with a significant adult—usually a parent but sometimes a teacher, grandparent, or trusted family friend—contributes to resilience in children with ADHD (Weiss, Hechtman, Perlman, Hopkins, & Wener, 1979). Being able to identify people who can provide support in difficult times increases resilience for people with LD (Al-Yagon & Mikulincer, 2004; Miller, 2002). For young adults with DCD, the ability to relate well to others, meet new people, and communicate with others has been associated with resilience (Kirby et al., 2008).

Another characteristic that has been associated with higher self-perceptions of social confidence is a sense of humor, or viewing oneself as a fun person to be with (Fitzpatrick & Watkinson, 2003; Kirby et al., 2008). Persistence in staying involved in team sports has also been described as a positive force for participants who manage to endure the agony of these challenging activities (Cantell et al., 1994). As Cantell et al. noted, some players with DCD showed fortitude and were intrinsically motivated to persist even when they were physically injured. Resource 11.1 presents an example of resilience in a young man with DCD who has received awards for his Internet sites that are dedicated to supporting others with motor coordination difficulties.

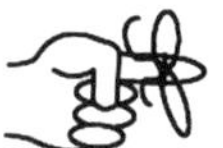

Remember this. . . .
Self-Determination Theory identifies three basic psychological needs:

1. ***Relatedness,*** **which refers to interconnectedness or a sense of being cared for;**
2. ***Competence,*** **or the need to feel a sense of mastery of the environment; and**
3. ***Autonomy,*** **which means volition through self-organized experiences and determining one's own behavior without external interference.**

Psychological Need 2: Competence

> And will you succeed? Yes indeed, yes indeed! Ninety-eight and three-quarters percent guaranteed.
>
> —Dr. Seuss (Geisel, 1990, p. 42)

Resilient people with LD have described how being able to identify successful experiences and reflect on positive abilities that outshine deficits in other areas enhances confidence (Miller, 2002). Being well coordinated and having clear memories of specific events and times that were positive motivators during stressful periods have been described as being protective. Knowledge of one's own strengths in good times and bad is also protective (Peterson & Seligman, 2004). In a study of healthy people with LD (Lackaye, Margalit, Ziv, & Ziman, 2006), participants who were found to have positive views of their self-worth and competence and a clear understanding of their strengths in specific domains were resilient. In addition, they viewed their problems as setbacks that were controllable and modifiable rather than pervasive and permanent. Resource 11.2 presents tools for identifying individual strengths.

Opportunities to develop new skills outside school in structured extracurricular activities (SEAs) are associated with personal development, exploration and identity work, emotional self-regulation, teamwork, and the development of social and work skills (Bazyk, 2005). Improved cognitive and emotional development (Hofferth & Sandberg, 2001), better academic attitudes and emotional development (Cooper, Valentine, Nye, & Lindsay, 1999), and higher educational aspirations (Marsh, 1992) are associated with youth involvement in SEAs. Time spent in such activities is also related to increased high social status (Gilman, 2001), increased life chances and resilience (Masten & Coatsworth, 1998), and initiative (Larson, 2000).

Resource 11.1. Matt's Hideout

Matt's Hideout (www.matts-hideout.co.uk) was developed to inform and educate the wider public about the daily experiences and hassles of living with severe coordination difficulties. More than an educational site about difficulties, Matt's Hideout tells a positive story of resilience in the face of some teachers' and school principals' construal of episodes of poor coordination and bumping into others on the playground as deliberate misbehaviors that merited punishment.

Matt has opened another site called "Dyspraxic Teens" (www.dyspraxicteens.org.uk), in which people with DCD share stories about their life experiences and concerns. It is an enlightening site for anyone involved in the care of people with these conditions and their families.

Finally, youth who are involved in SEAs have higher scores on the Five Cs of positive youth development: *c*ompetence, *c*onfidence, *c*onnection, *c*haracter, and *c*aring–compassion (Lerner et al., 2005).

To date, few studies have explored associations between participation in SEAs and resilience or flourishing of children with ADHD, DCD, and LD. Further research is warranted because these developmentally beneficial activities extend children's competencies, provide socialization experiences, and are autonomy enhancing, thus meeting basic psychological needs and theoretically contributing to optimal growth and flourishing (Larson, 2000). A well-established body of evidence has described the positive psychosocial outcomes for children who participate in activities that emphasize fun and enjoyment, personal achievement of self-referenced goals, goal-referenced and situation-specific feedback, and focus on process rather than performance outcomes (Kingston & Wilson, 2008).

Resource 11.2. Values in Action Surveys for Youth and Adults

The Values in Action (VIA) Youth Survey for 10- to 17-year-olds and the adult version, the VIA Inventory of Strengths, are freely available at www.viacharacter.org/VIASurvey/tabid/55/Default.aspx. These instruments are foundation tools used in positive education classrooms and allow children and adults to identify and reflect on character strengths.

Psychological Need 3: Autonomy

You have brains in your head.
You have feet in your shoes.
You can steer yourself in any direction you choose.

—Dr. Seuss (Geisel, 1990, p. 2)

According to Hope Theory (Snyder, 2000), people who demonstrate perseverance in reaching self-determined goals (e.g., "I meet the goals that I set for myself," an example of *agentic thinking*) and who also believe that they can work out ways of achieving these goals (e.g., "I can think of many ways to get what I want", an example of *pathways thinking*) are likely to be resilient. Adoption of these two types of hopeful thinking help fulfill psychological needs for autonomy and competence. Agentic and pathway thinking are positively associated with physical health, psychological adjustment, and performance in school and sport (Snyder, 2000).

Higher levels of self-determination and internal regulation occur when children are more autonomous in thinking about how to set achievable goals. The ability to take ownership and control of personally meaningful goals is seen in decision making, self-management, self-advocacy, and problem solving. For people with LD, social skills development and self-determined behavior are closely related (Pierson, Carter, Lane, & Glaeser, 2008).

Adopting an Occupational Lens to Describe Occupational Therapy's Role With These Populations at Three Levels

What actions can occupational therapists take to raise awareness and ensure that all children can fully participate in a range of developmentally fulfilling occupations that meet the three basic psychological needs for relatedness, competence, and autonomy? How can they best adopt an occupational lens to protect the more vulnerable members of the community, such as children with ADHD, DCD, or LD, from occupational deprivation? Flow-on effects are generated for all community participants if occupational flourishing is the collective aim. The unique occupational therapy perspective and strong professional values mean that occupational therapists are well positioned to provide multitiered intervention and prevention strategies and programs to promote mental health and social participation for these children.

Tier 1: Promoting Mental Health and Social Participation at a Community Level

> Education is the most powerful weapon which you can use to change the world.
>
> —Nelson Mandela (2003)

To combat the bullying, social exclusion, and low participation in valued leisure pursuits experienced by many children with ADHD, DCD, and LD, a new prototype of socially responsible and humanistic action focused on ensuring that all children have optimal mental health and social participation is essential. This approach requires advocating for social justice through education programs and policies aimed at increasing children's mental health at a population level. For example, with children who are less physically capable, it means ensuring that people in positions of authority, who may prioritize funding and resources for elite athletes over less talented athletes, are encouraged to adopt a broader view of physical activity participation for all members of the community. The following sections describe levels of influence that need to be targeted.

Government

At the government level, policy and funding priorities can do much to improve the chances of children with ADHD, DCD, or LD having optimal mental health and social participation:

- *Equality of opportunity:* Policies require ongoing development to ensure that all children are able to access affordable physical activity options for lifelong physical and social fitness.
- *Internet forums and education:* A growing number of Web sites have advocated for the benefits of physical activity engagement throughout life. Contributions from occupational therapists will enrich these sites.
- *Mental health promotion for children through full social and physical activity participation in SEAs:* Participation in meaningful and varied SEAs is associated with enhanced resilience when psychological needs are met. Ensuring that these activity contexts have positive motivational climates focused on mastery, learning, and self-paced goal achievement rather than on social comparison and individual competition with others is required.
- *Interdisciplinary collaborations:* Developing health promotion programs through interdisciplinary collaborations is necessary because the solutions to these myriad health challenges are complex, and there is no single solution.

- *Health messages:* These messages must be examined for unintended negative outcomes or inadvertent transference of stereotypes and misinformation. Ideally, messages on health information regarding activity participation for children with ADHD, DCD, and LD need to be carefully designed and pretested on target audiences.

Schools

At the school level, several approaches can help enhance the outlook for the children who are the subject of this chapter:

- *Advocacy for mental health programs:* Advocacy needs to be embedded in all classrooms. An increasing body of scientific evidence has demonstrated the need to introduce social–emotional learning to promote development of social and emotional skills for all students in the classroom (Payton et al., 2008).
- *Support school-based programs aimed at targeting bullying:* Such programs include the Olweus Bullying Prevention Program (Olweus, 2010) and the Australian Bounce Back program (McGrath & Noble, 2006).
- *Promote play opportunities during recess:* School policies that restrict children's play by removing playground equipment from school grounds and limiting recess time have been criticized by Bundy et al. (2008) for restricting playfulness opportunities. Playfulness on adapted playgrounds increases creativity, decreases a focus on physical prowess, and increases opportunities for leadership for children with poor motor coordination. Occupational therapists are well positioned to provide input into playground design (Bundy et al., 2008).
- *Responsible television advertising and programming:* Television advertising and programming can help develop healthy habits in all children (e.g., promoting television-free family mealtimes, physical activity routines for all family members, pet ownership, recreational opportunities for families during school time and vacations).
- *Recess planning:* Occupational therapists can help identify and expand activity options during recess (e.g., cultural pursuits, clubs, noncompetitive physical activities, relaxation and mindfulness training, martial arts, service activities). Recognizing recess as an opportunity for introducing youth to a range of skills, noncompetitive physical activity options, clubs and service activities, and lifelong leisure pursuits has long-term benefits associated with positive youth development (Lerner et al., 2005).
- *After-school programs:* Conversations between occupational therapists and personnel involved in developing and implementing after-school programs need to be strengthened to address the occupational needs of children with ADHD, DCD, and LD in these settings. These contexts offer opportunities for children who are further disadvantaged by low socioeconomic circumstances to benefit from SEA involvement (Vandell, 2000).
- *Safe sports:* Occupational therapists' work in physical rehabilitation settings with young adults who have experienced spinal and head injuries

associated with trauma and physical injury on the sporting fields means that they are well informed to advocate for safe sports. In addition, pediatric therapists have developmental and behavioral knowledge to contribute to policy about characteristics, such as age and maturity, that underpins healthy involvement in a range of sports.

- *Driving:* Occupational therapists have an established role in working with older people and those with physical and mental impairments on driving. Older adolescents and young adults with ADHD, DCD, and LD also need support in the acquisition of driving skills.
- *Vacation programs and use of school facilities over long vacation periods:* Underused physical facilities and resources in schools can be considered for occupational therapy programs to support children with ADHD, DCD, and LD.

Communities and Community Organizations

At the community level, occupational therapists' values and beliefs about democratic inclusion, coupled with professional knowledge and understanding of the personal attributes of children and the environments in which different occupations are performed, offer multiple entry points for assisting participation in community activities.

- *Youth information networks:* To assist children and their families in identifying realistic, affordable, and interest-linked activities, updated information on current recreational options within the local community should be readily accessible.
- *Activity portfolio balancing:* Occupational therapists have the necessary skills to provide expert consultation in activity portfolio balancing in programs such as the Duke of Edinburgh program (www.dukeofed.org.au/), which exists in 120 countries around the world.
- *Public recreational opportunities:* Evidence has shown that youth who have low participation in structured extracurricular activities, including sports and community service activities, may participate in more gang activity and drug use and report higher levels of boredom (Davis & Jones, 1996). Town plans should consider the importance of having outdoor natural spaces with rugged and hilly terrain to encourage walking, which is considered a lifestyle physical activity (Ziviani et al., 2008).
- *Physical activities for nonelite athletes:* Encouraging communities and schools to adopt models such as the "sports for peace" approach in which affiliation and learning processes are emphasized (Ennis et al., 1999) or the *T*asks, *A*uthority, *R*ecognition, *G*rouping, *E*valuation, and *T*ime (TARGET) model, an applied coaching program based on the principles of achievement goal theory (Epstein, 1989), has the potential to increase participants' enjoyment, persistence, and involvement in team sports. Such programs will have an impact on all children's participation levels, particularly for nonelite athletes.
- *Active transport:* Occupational therapists have been called on (Ziviani et al., 2008) to work with town planners, politicians, and health economists to enrich everyday physical activity options for all children by ensuring that

safe, accessible, and affordable public transport, sporting amenities, walkways and dedicated bicycle paths, and community spaces are available in communities.

Families

At the family level, many opportunities exist to link families with existing school and community programs and support exploration, choice, and sustained participation in a range of activities.

- *Parenting skills programs:* Occupational therapists can provide input into these programs in relation to occupational performance and supported self-regulation.
- *Education programs:* Occupational therapists are encouraged to expand these programs to increase parental awareness of the benefits of structured extracurricular activities, daily routines, readiness for school, sleep patterns, and occupational performance that underpin healthy lifestyles.
- *Leisure opportunities:* Information can be provided to update parents about leisure opportunities in their area and include parents in social groups to exchange information about possible community resources to support children's interests and developmental stage.
- *Family routines and holidays:* Practitioners can advocate for television-free family mealtimes; physical activity and relaxation routines embedded in everyday family time; caring for pets; and importance of outdoor adventure activities and lifelong pursuits, such as walking.
- *Social connectivity using the Internet and Internet technology domain:* It remains a challenge for occupational therapists to facilitate social participation beyond the Internet, to expand online chat rooms to the real world.

Professionals

For all practitioners, a professional need for currency in lifelong learning exists as well as a professional responsibility to increase awareness and knowledge about legislation, practice changes, and advances that relate to children with ADHD, DCD, and LD.

- *Professional self-development:* An important foundation stone for all positive occupational therapy programs is to persuade the professionals who work with children with ADHD, DCD, and LD of the need to adopt a positive science stance in their own professional lives (Csikzentmihalyi & Csikzentmihalyi, 2006) and to pursue educational opportunities to acquire skills in whole-school approaches, such as social and emotional learning programs (see, e.g., www.casel.org).
- *Advocacy:* All therapists need to be aware of current legislation and advocate through their professional organizations for removal of societal barriers or potential restrictions on full activity participation for children with ADHD, DCD, and LD.
- *Education about ADHD, DCD, and LD:* To address limited community and professional knowledge about some of these disorders, information needs

Resource 11.3. CanChild

The CanChild Web site (http://dcd.canchild.ca/en/ourresearch/dcdeducationalmaterialshome.asp) includes practical flyers to distribute to physicians, classroom teachers, and parents. Take particular note of the teaching case report and attached video of a child with DCD, published in the *Canadian Medical Association Journal* in August 2006, called "Why Every Office Needs a Tennis Ball," which can be found in the section devoted to resources for physicians or www.cmaj.ca/cgi/content/full/175/5/471.

to be provided to therapists about readily available resources to enable early recognition and remediation. Flyers and other materials are available on Web sites (Resource 11.3).

Tier 2: Small-Group Interventions

Small-group interventions for youth at risk of mental ill health or social exclusion include recess, classroom, and out-of-school groups.

Leisure Coaching Model Using EACH–Child

EACH–Child (Ziviani et al., 2009) is an occupation-based coaching model that has been used to promote physical activity participation with children with movement skill difficulties. It is a tailored coaching program that can be used with small groups of children to scaffold their participation in local community activities, and it is a framework for supporting graduated occupational engagement that is appropriate for children with ADHD, DCD, and LD. The EACH–Child process has three steps: (1) engaging the child in motivating physical activity options that are congruent with the child's needs, interests, and abilities and are context sensitive; (2) coaching the child to facilitate activity participation using self-referenced goals, rather than age-related standards, and teaming with community specialists; and (3) scaffolding transitions into appropriate community organizations. These stages are presented in Figure 11.2.

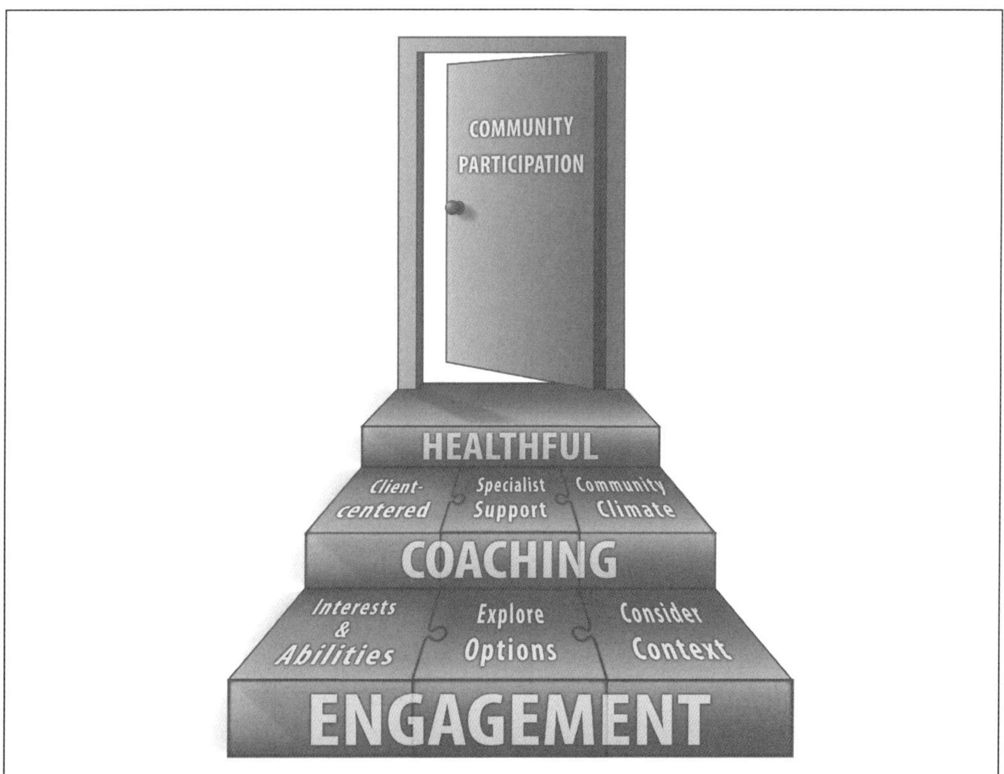

Figure 11.2. Engaging and Coaching for Health (EACH)–Child model.

Source. Ziviani et al. (2009).

The intention of the EACH–Child approach is for the therapist to provide graduated support to allow children to have successful and ongoing participation in leisure pursuits in the communities in which they live. In the EACH–Child model of practice, the therapist is envisaged as a "guide on the side" rather than a "sage on the stage" (Miller & Rollnick, 2002). The emphasis is on collaborative problem solving to identify and implement solutions to occupational performance difficulties. The skillful therapist facilitates change by shadowing the client's journey to healthy participation, assisting in the discovery of how to open doors to community participation.

Self-Determination Theory (Deci & Ryan, 2000, 2008) helps explain how self-directed activity engagement allows children to satisfy basic psychological needs in supportive environments. The occupational therapist acts as a coach or mentor, facilitating a child's participation in valued everyday activities so that these needs are met, which means providing consultative skills and support to children, their families, and activity leaders to enable optimal ongoing engagement. The motivational climate focuses on mastery and learning and achieving self-referenced, rather than other-referenced, goals. Changes in activity participation can be measured using the Measure of Processes of Care–20 (King, King, & Rosenbaum, 2004) or the Reliable Change Index (Chu & Reynolds, 2007).

Whole-School Approaches and Small-Group Programs

Examples of whole-school approaches and small-group programs to enhance the mental health and social participation of children with ADHD, DCD, and LD are presented in Table 11.10. Many of these interventions can also be used in one-on-one contexts. This list is not comprehensive; it does not enumerate the myriad approaches that can be used to address both social participation and mental health needs of children with ADHD, DCD, and LD. Current and emerging approaches and strategies are briefly described.

Tier 3: Intensive One-on-One Assessments and Interventions

More intensive one-on-one interventions require a detailed workup to analyze PEO fit for each child. The use of SCOPE–IT blends well with whole-school approaches but represents a more exhaustive analysis of PEO fit. Data synthesis occurs using a top-down approach in which intrinsic and extrinsic factors restricting full participation in age-appropriate activities are evaluated. The process is health and growth oriented, and the evaluation process is not adverse or disempowering, disability focused, or centered on identification of weaknesses and problems that are within the child. In-depth evaluations can be organized using the SCOPE–IT framework.

S = Synthesis

A global picture of each child's strengths and tapped and untapped potential is formed so that goodness of fit among child, activity, and environment can be analyzed from SCOPE–IT evaluations. The emphasis is on describing functional and healthy synthesis and to identify pathways for growth when there is poor "fit" among these elements (Law et al., 1996). Goodness of fit is determined based on the gradings used in Hemmingsson, Egilson, Hoffman, and Kielhofner's (2005) School Setting Interview from 1 to 4.

Table 11.10. Examples of Interventions to Enhance Mental Health and Social Participation of Children With ADHD, DCD, and LD

Intervention	Description
Social and emotional learning (SEL)	A whole-school approach such as SEL has more potential than social skills training for children with ADHD, DCD, and LD. SEL has a mental health focus, and increasing evidence has been found for its effectiveness in fostering stronger school communities and in academic performance, positive social behavior, and reducing conduct problems and emotional distress (Payton et al., 2008). See www.casel.org.
Positivity portfolio	The positivity portfolio is an approach that has received little research attention from occupational therapists but is more widely used in educational contexts in which positive psychology principles are embedded within the curriculum. The potential to apply these principles to out-of-school time use and to integrate these techniques within daily habits is encouraging. Useful Web sites include www.positivepsychology.org and www.authentichappiness.sas.upenn.edu/Default.aspx. The VIA strengths questionnaires for youth ages 10–17 provide children with the language to evaluate their personal strengths: www.viacharacter.org/VIASurvey/tabid/55/Default.aspx
Cognitive-based interventions	These interventions aim to improve occupational performance in areas self-determined by the child but with some family-centered negotiation of additional goals using an approach called CO-OP (Polatajko & Mandich, 2004). CO-OP can be implemented using occupational performance coaching (Graham et al., 2009). This intervention is a promising one-on-one intervention for use with families of children with ADHD, DCD, or LD.
Positive behavioral interventions and supports (PBIS)	PBIS is a decision-making framework that is implemented at a whole-school level with a focus on addressing problem behaviors. See www.pbis.org
Social skills training	Scant evidence exists that explicit social skills training programs are effective for children with ADHD, DCD, and LD (Hallahan et al., 2005). However, the limited success of many of these programs may be linked to issues such as insufficient program duration and lack of embedded practice in real life.
Environmental supports and coaching	Morning routines and homework are particularly problematic for children with ADHD, and it has been suggested that occupations and routines be brought to the foreground of occupational therapists' approach to these children and their families (Segal, 1998). Programs that enhance resilience and social connectedness in children with ADHD, DCD, and LD are more likely to be sustainable because they are ecologically sensitive than are clinic-based approaches in which environmental supports are not considered. (See Graham et al., 2009, and Lim & Rodger, 2008.)
Mindfulness training	An increasing body of evidence supports the use of yoga, meditation, and mindfulness training on emotional, social, and behavioral outcomes for children with ADHD (Singh et al., 2010). Occupational therapists can include these approaches in a balanced daily activity routine.

Note. ADHD = attention deficit hyperactivity disorder; CO–OP = Cognitive Orientation to Occupational Performance; DCD = developmental coordination disorder; LD = learning disabilities.

- 4 = an *ideal fit,* where no adjustments need to be made to the environment.
- 3 = a *good fit,* in which adjustments have been made to meet the child's needs and there is satisfactory child, environment, occupation fit.
- 2 = a *partial fit,* in which some changes have been made but further changes are required to enhance the fit.
- 1 = *unfit,* meaning that no changes have been made to improve fit to date.

Table 11.11. Child-Level Assessment Tools

Dimensions	Measures
Physical characteristics	• Evaluations of physical ability include the Movement ABC–2 (Henderson et al., 2007) and the Bruininks–Oseretsky Test of Motor Proficiency–2 (Bruininks & Bruninks, 2005). • Evaluations of sensory processing can also be grouped in this section and include the Sensory Profile (Dunn, 1999).
Psychological components	• For evaluating self-concept perceptions, therapists might select from any of the self-description questionnaires, which span the age range from preschool to adulthood (Marsh, 1990) and can be downloaded from the University of Oxford SELF Centre at www.self.ox.ac.uk/. • Occupational therapists wishing to measure psychological needs for self-determined activity engagement are directed to http://psych.rochester.edu/SDT/measure/index.html for a range of assessments for children and youth. The scales for children with LD are for academic performance rather than other occupational performance areas. • Social skills rating scales are comprehensively reviewed and detailed for occupational therapists by Merrell (1993). • Examples of social skills rating scales developed by occupational therapists for children with social skills difficulties, such as seen in target groups, include the ACIS (Forsyth, Li, & Kielhofner, 1999), the Social Profile (Donohue, 2007), and the ESI (Fisher & Griswold, 2008).
Temporal dimensions	• Recognizing the changing pattern of interests, abilities, and capabilities according to the child's chronological age and developmental status but also acknowledging state and trait variability and the influence of context on responses at any point in time.

Note. ACIS = Assessment of Communication and Interaction Skills; ESI = Evaluations of Social Interaction; Movement–ABC = Movement Assessment Battery for Children.

C = Child-Level Data

Examples of assessments of current skills and abilities of children with ADHD, DCD, and LD to provide data about the intrinsic factors affecting a child's occupational performance are presented in Table 11.11; these represent only a few of the child-level assessments available to practitioners.

OP = Occupational Performance

An increasing number of measures are available to therapists to evaluate a child's occupational performance interests and experiences (Table 11.12). Subjective and objective ratings of what children with ADHD, DCD, and LD currently "do" and also what they "can do" provide activity-based data to help a child form occupation-centered goals (Hammel et al., 2008). Where possible, triangulation of data using other data sources (e.g., questionnaires or scales, parent and teacher reports, self-recording or monitoring information using electronic diaries; e.g., Whalen et al., 2006) is recommended. Adoption of intervention approaches, such as Cognitive Orientation to Occupational Performance (CO–OP; Polatajko & Mandich, 2004), which was historically developed to enhance occupational performance of children with DCD, has been expanded to address the occupational performance difficulties of children with other conditions. The OPC Model (Graham et al., 2009) provides a framework for

Table 11.12. Occupational Perfomance (OP)–Level Assessment Tools

OP–Level Dimensions	Measures
Interests	• Pediatric Interest Profiles (Henry, 2000) • Assessment of Ludic Behaviors (Ferland, 1997) • Pediatric Card Sort (Mandich, Polatajko, Miller, & Baum, 2004) • Personal Projects Analysis (Christiansen, Little, & Backman, 1998) • Personal Projects Analysis–for Children (Poulsen, Barker, & Ziviani, 2010)
Ratings of current participation	• Pediatric Volitional Questionnaire (Version 2.1; Basu, Kafkes, Schatz, Kiraly, & Kielhofner, 2008) • Short Child Occupational Profile (Bowyer, Ross, Schwartz, Kielhofner, & Kramer, 2005) • Child Occupational Self-Assessment (Keller, Kafkes, Basu, Federico, & Kielhofner, 2005) • Children's Assessment of Participation and Enjoyment (King, Law, & Rosenbaum, 2004) • Leisure Diagnostic Battery (Witt & Ellis, 1989) • Assessment of Life Habits for Children (Fougeyrollas et al., 1998) • Child and Adolescent Scale of Participation (Bedell, 2004) • Canadian Occupational Performance Measure (Law et al., 1998) • Peer Interactive Play Scales (Fantuzzo, Mendez, & Tigher, 1998) • Play Assessment in Group Setting (Lautamo, Kottorp, & Salminen, 2005)
Observation of current participation	• Peer Social Behavior Code, part of the Systematic Screening for Behavior Disorders (Walker & Severson, 1992) • Direct observation during activities provides objective data that can be replicated by independent observers or at another point in time if criteria are met for (1) use of previously designated codes and categories, (2) use of same procedure, (3) use of clearly specified rules and procedure, and (4) recording of biases or reactivity on part of child or other people present

using approaches that are cognitive based and occupational performance focused (see Resource 11.4 for a creative approach to using the CO–OP and OPC models). Both CO–OP and OPC use collaborative goal setting and are child centered.

E = Environment

Extrinsic elements that are assessed under this category include contextual factors associated with a child's participation in a range of occupations. Although both the physical and the social environments may be evaluated separately, most assessments comprehensively address both the social and the physical worlds of the child or adolescent. Examples of assessments to evaluate the environment include the Test of Environmental Supportiveness (Bundy, 1999) and the widely used Home Observation (HOME) tools for measurement of the environment. The HOME tools are applicable across a wide range of age groups, including infants and toddlers, early childhood, middle childhood, and early adolescence (Bradley & Caldwell, 1979; Bradley et al., 1989; Caldwell & Bradley, 1984). In addition, context- and activity-specific environmental assessment tools are available, such

Resource 11.4. CO–OP + OPC

Combining the CO–OP with the OPC Model provides a practical child- or family-centered approach to working with children who have occupational performance difficulties. See Polatajko and Mandich (2004) and Graham et al. (2009) for more practical information and evidence of effectiveness of this approach with children who have DCD.

as the Children's Perceptions of Physical and Social Environments, which support physical activity participation at home and in the wider neighborhood (Hume, Ball, & Salmon, 2006). School–environment fit is assessed with the School Setting Interview (Hemmingsson et al., 2005). The impact of environment on occupational participation is one component of the SCOPE–IT measure (Bowyer et al., 2005).

IT = In Time

A review of the many types of time-use methodologies, including reliability and validity data for child populations, is presented in Juster's seminal and subsequent work (Juster, 1985; Juster, Ono, & Stafford, 2003). The advantages of always incorporating an interview to gain an overview of time use are as follows:

- Parents and children can provide a truly child- or parent-centered view of their lives as their personal stories of everyday living unfold.
- Family routines and habits can be described as part of a guided journey of self-reflection with no prejudicial questions or judgments from the interviewer. For example, exploration of family time use can be conducted using the ecocultural family interview (www.npi.ucla.edu/iweisner/index.htm).
- Information about activities that might be overlooked (e.g., sleep routines, social companions) can be gathered; it provides another avenue or area to consider in developing comprehensive strategies to enhance activity participation.

Time-use inventories are a low-cost, convenient means of acquiring detailed information about daily activity participation and, as such, should be a cornerstone of occupational therapy assessments for children with ADHD, DCD, and LD.

Summary

Children with ADHD, DCD, and LD are at risk of low social and physical participation in meaningful occupations at school, at home, and in the community. To ensure flourishing and well-being, it is essential that their basic psychological needs for autonomy, competence, and relatedness are met. This need fulfillment occurs when occupational therapists support full participation in personally valued activities that are child identified but ecologically sustainable. The EACH–Child model describes the steps leading to full and satisfying participation in personally meaningful activities for children with these conditions. EACH–Child uses a coaching process based on exploration and identification of interests, abilities, and support options within the child's social and physical environment to facilitate progression toward community participation.

Evaluation of the child–occupational performance–environment fit precedes identification of child-centered coaching goals. Understanding the factors that enable full participation and optimal fit among child, activity, and environment has physical, cognitive, social, and emotional benefits. A three-tiered occupational therapy approach to achieve those benefits has a multilayered, comprehensive impact. Tier 1 strategies emphasizing advocacy for social justice help ensure that healthy communities are primed to support children's participation in valued pursuits. Tier

2 and 3 interventions will always have their place alongside Tier 1 strategies, providing more in-depth support for children who are particularly vulnerable.

Although a holistic emphasis on mental health promotion for all children is a preferred strategy to prevent adverse mental health and social participation outcomes for vulnerable groups such as children with ADHD, DCD, and LD, this utopia cannot always be realized. However, if occupational justice aimed at ensuring full participation for all children is the desired endpoint, it requires committed action by occupational therapists.

References

Abikoff, H. (2009). ADHD psychosocial treatments: Generalization reconsidered. *Journal of Attention Disorders, 13,* 207–210.

Al-Yagon, M., & Mikulincer, M. (2004). Patterns of close relationships and socio-emotional and academic adjustment among school-age children with learning disability. *Learning Disabilities Research and Practice, 19,* 12–19.

American Psychiatric Association. (2000). *Diagnostic and statistical manual of mental disorders* (4th ed., text rev.). Washington, DC: Author.

American Psychiatric Association. (2010). *Proposed draft revisions to DSM disorders and criteria.* Retrieved March 28, 2010, from www.dsm5.org/Pages/Default.aspx

Bagwell, C., Brooke, M., Pelham, W., & Hoza, B. (2001). Attention-deficit hyperactivity disorder and problems in peer relations: Predictions from childhood to adolescence. *Journal of the American Academy of Child and Adolescent Psychiatry, 40,* 1285–1292.

Barkley, R. A. (2006). *Attention deficit hyperactivity disorder: A handbook for diagnosis and treatment* (3rd ed.). New York: Guilford Press.

Bart, O., Bar-Haim, Y., Weizman, E., Levin, M., Sadeh, A., & Mintz, M. (2009). Balance treatment ameliorates anxiety and increases self-esteem in children with comorbid anxiety and balance disorder. *Research in Developmental Disabilities, 30,* 486–495.

Basu, S., Kafkes, A., Schatz, R., Kiraly, A., & Kielhofner, G. (2008). *The Pediatric Volitional Questionnaire* (Version 2.1). Chicago: Model of Human Occupation Clearinghouse, University of Illinois at Chicago.

Bazyk, S. (2005). Exploring the development of meaningful work for children and youth in Western contexts. *WORK: A Journal of Prevention, Assessment, and Rehabilitation, 24,* 11–20.

Bedell, G. M. (2004). Developing a follow-up survey focused on participation of children and youth with acquired brain injuries after discharge from inpatient rehabilitation. *NeuroRehabilitation, 19,* 191–205.

Bowyer, P., Ross, M., Schwartz, O., Kielhofner, G., & Kramer, J. (2005). *The Short Child Occupational Profile (SCOPE)* (version 2.1). Chicago: Model of Occupational Clearinghouse.

Bradley, R. H., & Caldwell, B. M. (1979). Home observation for measurement of the environment: A revision of the preschool scale. *American Journal of Mental Deficiency, 84,* 235–244.

Bradley, R. H., Caldwell, B. M., Rock, S. L., Barnard, K. E., Gray, C., Hammond, M. A., et al. (1989). Home environment and cognitive development in the first 3 years of life: A collaborative study involving six sites and three ethnic groups in North America. *Developmental Psychology, 25,* 217–235.

Bruininks, R. H., & Bruininks, B. D. (2005). *Bruininks–Oseretsky Test of Motor Proficiency, Second Edition.* Circle Pines, MN: American Guidance Service.

Bundy, A. (1999). *Test of Environmental Supportiveness.* Ft. Collins: Colorado State University.

Bundy, A., Luckett, T., Naughton, G. A., Tranter, P. J., Wyer, S. R., Ragen, J., et al. (2008). Playful interaction: Occupational therapy for all children on the school playground. *American Journal of Occupational Therapy, 62,* 522–527.

Cairney, J., Hay, J. A., Faught, B. E., & Hawes, R. (2005). Developmental coordination disorder and overweight and obesity in children aged 9–14 years. *International Journal of Obesity, 29,* 369–372.

Caldwell, B. M., & Bradley, C. B. (1984). *Home observation for the measurement of the environment.* Little Rock: University of Arkansas, College of Education.

Cantell, M. H., Smyth, M. M., & Ahonen, T. P. (1994). Clumsiness in adolescence: Educational, motor, and social outcomes of motor delay detected at 5 years. *Adapted Physical Activity Quarterly, 11,* 115–129.

Cantell, M. H., Smyth, M. M., & Ahonen, T. P. (2003). Two distinct pathways for developmental coordination disorder: Persistence and resolution. *Human Movement Science, 22,* 413–431.

Cermak, S. A., & Larkin, D. (2002). *Developmental coordination disorder.* Albany, NY: Delmar.

Chan, D. W., Ho, C., Tsang, S.-M., Lee, S.-H., & Chung, K. K.-H. (2007). Prevalence, gender ratio, and gender differences in reading-related cognitive abilities among Chinese children with dyslexia in Hong Kong. *Education Studies, 33,* 249–265.

Christiansen, A. S., Little, B. R., & Backman, C. (1998). Personal projects: A useful approach to the study of occupation. *American Journal of Occupational Therapy, 52,* 439–446.

Chu, S., & Reynolds, F. (2007). Occupational therapy for children with attention deficit hyperactivity disorder (ADHD), Part 2: A multicentre evaluation of an assessment and treatment package. *British Journal of Occupational Therapy, 70,* 439–448.

Cooper, H., Valentine, J. C., Nye, B., & Lindsay, J. J. (1999). Relationships between five after-school activities and academic achievement. *Journal of Educational Psychology, 91,* 369–378.

Csikszentmihalyi, M., & Csikszentmihalyi, I. S. (2006). *A life worth living: Contributions to positive psychology.* New York: Oxford University Press.

Davis, A., & Jones, L. J. (1996). Children in the urban environment: An issue for the new public health agenda. *Health and Place, 2,* 107–113.

Deci, E. L., & Ryan, R. M. (2000). The "what" and "why" of goal pursuits: Human needs and the self-determination of behavior. *Psychological Inquiry, 11,* 227–268.

Deci, E. L., & Ryan, R. M. (2008). Self-determination theory: A macrotheory of human motivation, development, and health. *Canadian Psychology, 49,* 182–185.

Doble, S. E., & Maggill-Evans, J. (1992). A model of social interaction to guide occupational therapy practice. *Canadian Journal of Occupational Therapy, 59,* 141–150.

Donohue, M. V. (2007). *Social Profile manual.* Retrieved March 15, 2010, from www.social-profile.com/index.html

Dunn, W. (1999). *Sensory Profile—User's manual.* San Antonio, TX: Psychological Corporation.

Education for All Handicapped Children Act of 1975, Pub. L. 94–142, 20 U.S.C. § 1400 *et seq.*

Endresen, I. M., & Olweus, D. (2005). Participation in power sports and antisocial involvement in preadolescent and adolescent boys. *Journal of Child Psychology and Psychiatry, 46,* 468–478.

Engel-Yeger, B., & Weissman, D. (2009). A comparison of motor abilities and perceived self-efficacy between children with hearing impairments and normal hearing children. *Disability and Rehabilitation, 31,* 352–358.

Ennis, C. D., Solmon, M. A., Satina, B., Loftus, S. J., Mensch, J., & McCauley, M. T. (1999). Creating a sense of family in urban schools using the "Sport for Peace" curriculum. *Research Quarterly for Exercise and Sport, 70,* 273–285.

Epstein, J. (1989). Family structures and student motivation: A developmental perspective. In C. Ames & R. Ames (Eds.), *Research on motivation in education. Vol. 3: Goals and cognitions* (pp. 259–295). New York: Academic Press.

Fantuzzo, J., Mendez, J., & Tigher, E. (1998). Parental assessment of peer play: Development and validation of the parent version of the Penn Interactive Peer Play Scale. *Early Childhood Research Quarterly, 13,* 659–676.

Ferland, F. (1997). *Play, children, and physical disabilities and occupational therapy.* Ottawa: University of Ottawa.

Fisher, A. G., & Griswold, L. A. (2008). *Evaluation of social interaction: Research edition IV.* Retrieved March 15, 2010, from www.social-interaction.com/

Fitzpatrick, D. A., & Watkinson, E. J. (2003). The lived experience of physical awkwardness: Adults' retrospective views. *Adapted Physical Activity Quarterly, 20,* 279–297.

Forsyth, K., Li, K., & Kielhofner, G. (1999). The Assessment of Communication and Interaction Skills (ACIS): Measurement properties. *British Journal of Occupational Therapy, 62,* 69–74.

Fougeyrollas, P., Noreau, L., Berferon, H., Cloutier, R., Dion, S., & St.-Michel, G. (1998). Social consequences of long-term impairments and disabilities: Conceptual approach and assessment of handicap. *International Journal of Rehabilitation Research, 21,* 127–141.

Fox, A. M., & Lent, B. (1996). Clumsy children—Primer on developmental coordination disorder. *Canadian Family Physician, 42,* 1965–1971.

Gaub, M., & Carlson, C. (1997). Gender differences in ADHD: A meta-analysis and critical review. *Journal of the American Academy of Child and Adolescent Psychiatry, 36,* 1036–1047.

Geisel, T. [Dr. Seuss]. (1990). *Oh, the places you'll go!* London: Harper Collins.

Gillberg, C. (2003). Deficits in attention, motor control, and perception: A brief review. *Archives of Disease in Childhood, 88,* 904–910.

Gilman, R. (2001). The relationship between life satisfaction, social interest, and frequency of extracurricular activities among adolescent students. *Journal of Youth and Adolescence, 30,* 749–767.

Goyen, T. A., & Lui, K. (2009). Developmental coordination disorder in "apparently normal" schoolchildren born extremely preterm. *Archives of Disease in Childhood, 94,* 298–302.

Graham, F., Rodger, S., & Ziviani, J. (2009). Coaching parents to enable children's participation: An approach for working with parents and their children. *Australian Occupational Therapy Journal, 56,* 16–23.

Green, D., Bishop, T., Wilson, B. N., Crawford, S. G., Hooper, R., Kaplan, B. J., et al. (2005). Is questionnaire-based screening part of the solution to waiting lists for children with developmental coordination disorder? *British Journal of Occupational Therapy, 68,* 2–10.

Green, D., Charman, T., Pickles, A., Chandler, S., Loucas, T., Simonoff, E., et al. (2009). Impairment in movement skills of children with autistic spectrum disorders. *Developmental Medicine and Child Neurology, 51,* 311–316.

Gregg, N. (2009). *Adolescents and adults with learning disabilities and ADHD: Assessments and accommodation.* New York: Guilford Press.

Haertl, K. (2009). A frame of reference to enhance childhood occupations: SCOPE–IT. In P. Kramer & J. Hinjosa (Eds.), *Frames of reference for pediatric occupational therapy* (3rd ed., pp. 266–305). Baltimore: Lippincott Williams & Wilkins.

Hallahan, D. P., Lloyd, J. W., Kauffman, J. M., Weiss, M. R., & Martinez, E. A. (2005). *Learning disabilities: Foundations, characteristics, and effective teaching* (3rd ed.). Boston: Pearson Education.

Hammel, J., Magasi, S., Heinemann, A., Whiteneck, G., Bogner, J., & Rodriguez, E. (2008). What does participation mean? An insider perspective from people with disabilities. *Disabilities and Rehabilitation, 30,* 1445–1460.

Harvey, W., & Reid, G. (1997). Motor performance of children with attention-deficit hyperactivity disorder: A preliminary investigation. *Adapted Physical Activity Quarterly, 14,* 189–202.

Hemmingsson, H., Egilson, S., Hoffman, O., & Kielhofner, G. (2005). *The School Setting Interview* (Version 3.0). Chicago: Swedish Association of Occupational Therapists.

Henderson, S. E., Sugden, D. A., & Barnett, A. L. (2007). *Movement Assessment Battery for Children—Second edition (Movement ABC–2).* London: Psychological Corporation.

Hendriksen, J. G. M., Keulers, A. H. H., Feron, F. J. M., Wassenberg, R., Jolles, J., & Vles, J. S. H. (2007). Subtypes of learning disabilities: Neuropsychological and behavioural functioning of 495 children referred for multidisciplinary assessment. *European Child and Adolescent Psychiatry, 16,* 517–524.

Henry, A. D. (2000). *Pediatric interest profiles: Surveys of Play for Children and Adolescents, Kid Play Profile, Preteen Play Profile, Adolescent Interest Profile.* San Antonio, TX: Therapy Skill Builders.

Hofferth, S. L., & Sandberg, J. F. (2001). How American children spend their time. *Journal of Marriage and Family, 63,* 295–308.

Hume, C., Ball, K. K., & Salmon, J. (2006). Development and reliability of a self-report questionnaire to examine children's perceptions of the physical environment at home and in the neighbourhood. *International Journal of Behavioral Nutrition and Physical Activity, 3,* 3–16.

Individuals With Disabilities Education Act of 1990, Pub. L. 101–476, 20 U.S.C., Ch 33.

Johnson, R. C. (2000). Sports behavior of ADHD children. *Journal of Attention Disorders, 4,* 150–160.

Juster, F. T. (1985). Conceptual and methodological issues involved in the measurement of time use. In F. T. Juster & F. P. Stafford (Eds.), *Time, goods, and well-being* (pp. 19–62). Ann Arbor: University of Michigan, Institute for Social Research.

Juster, F. T., Ono, H., & Stafford, F. P. (2003). An assessment of alternative measures of time use. *Sociological Methodology, 33,* 19–54.

Kaplan, B. J., Wilson, B. N., Dewey, D., & Crawford, S. G. (1998). DCD may not be a discrete disorder. *Human Movement Science, 17,* 471–490.

Kaufmann, J. M. (2005). *Characteristics of emotional and behavioral disorders of children and youth* (8th ed.). Upper Saddle River, NJ: Prentice Hall.

Keen, D. V. (2005). ADHD and the paediatrician: A guide to management. *Current Paediatrics, 15,* 133–142.

Keller, J., Kafkes, A., Basu, S., Federico, J., & Kielhofner, G. (2005). *The Child Occupational Self-Assessment* (Version 2.1). Chicago: Model of Occupational Therapy Clearinghouse.

King, G., Law, M., & Rosenbaum, P. (2004). *Children's Assessment of Participation and Enjoyment (CAPE) and Preferences for Activities of Children (PAC).* San Antonio, TX: Harcourt Assessment.

King, S., King, G., & Rosenbaum, P. (2004). Evaluating health service delivery to children with chronic conditions and their families: Development of a refined Measure of Processes of Care (MPOC–20). *Children's Health Care, 33,* 35–57.

Kingston, K. M., & Wilson, K. M. (2008). The application of goal setting in sport. In S. D. Mellalieu & S. Hanton (Eds.), *Advances in applied sport psychology* (pp. 75–123). New York: Routledge.

Kirby, A. (2004). Is dyspraxia a medical condition or a social disorder? *British Journal of General Practice, 54,* 6–8.

Kirby, A., Sugden, D., Beveridge, S. K., & Edwards, L. (2008). Developmental coordination disorders (DCD) in adolescents and adults in further and higher education. *Journal of Research in Special Educational Needs, 8,* 120–131.

Lackaye, T., Margalit, M., Ziv, O., & Ziman, T. (2006). Comparisons of self-efficacy, mood, effort, and hope between students with learning disabilities and their non-LD-matched peers. *Learning Disabilities Research and Practice, 21,* 111–121.

Larson, R. W. (2000). Toward a psychology of positive youth development. *American Psychologist, 55,* 170–183.

Lautamo, T., Kottorp, A., & Salminen, A. C. (2005). Play assessment for group settings: A pilot study to construct an assessment tool. *Scandinavian Journal of Occupational Therapy, 12,* 136–144.

Law, M., Baptiste, S., Carswell, A., McColl, M. A., Polatajko, H., & Pollock, M. A. (1998). *Canadian Occupational Performance Measure* (2nd ed., rev.). Ottawa: CAOT Publications.

Law, M., Cooper, B., Strong, S., Stewart, D., Rigby, P., & Letts, L. (1996). The Person–Environment–Occupation Model: A transactive approach to occupational performance. *Canadian Journal of Occupational Therapy, 63,* 9–23.

Lerner, R. M., Lerner, J. V., Almerigi, J. B., Theokas, C., Phelps, E., Gestsdottir, S., et al. (2005). Positive youth development, participation in community youth development programs, and community contributions of fifth-grade adolescents: Findings from the first wave of the 4–H study of positive youth development. *Journal of Early Adolescence, 25,* 17–71.

Lim, S. M., & Rodger, S. (2008). An occupational perspective on assessment of social competence in children. *British Journal of Occupational Therapy, 71,* 469–481.

Lingam, R., Hunt, L., Golding, J., Jongmans, M., & Emond, A. (2009). Prevalence of developmental coordination disorder using the *DSM–IV* at 7 years of age: A UK population-based study. *Pediatrics, 123,* e693–e700.

Mandela, N. R. (2003, July 16). *Lighting your way to a better future.* [Speech delivered at the launch of the Mindset Network]. Retrieved August 10, 2010, from www.nelsonmandela.org

Mandich, A. D., Polatajko, H. J., Miller, L., & Baum, C. (2004). *The Paediatric Activity Card Sort.* Ottawa: CAOT Publications.

Mandich, A. D., Polatajko, H. J., & Rodger, S. (2003). Rites of passage: Understanding participation of children with developmental coordination disorder. *Human Movement Science, 22,* 583–595.

Marsh, H. W. (1990). *Self Description Questionnaire–I: Manual.* Campbelltown, New South Wales, Australia: University of Western Sydney, Publication Unit.

Marsh, H. W. (1992). Extracurricular activities: Beneficial extension of the traditional curriculum or subversion of academic goals. *Journal of Educational Psychology, 84,* 553–562.

Martin, N. C., Piek, J. P., & Hay, D. (2006). DCD and ADHD: A genetic study of their shared aetiology. *Human Movement Sciences, 25,* 110–124.

Masten, A. S., & Coatsworth, J. D. (1998). The development of competence in favorable and unfavorable environments. *American Psychologist, 53,* 205–220.

McGrath, A., & Noble, T. (2006). *Evidence-based approaches to bullying in Australian schools.* Frenchs Forest, New South Wales, Australia: Pearson Education.

Merrell, K. W. (1993). Using behavior rating scales to assess social skills and antisocial behavior in school settings: Development of the School Social Behavior Scales. *School Psychology Review, 22,* 115–133.

Miller, M. (2002). Resilience elements in students with learning disabilities. *Journal of Clinical Psychology, 58,* 291–198.

Miller, W. R., & Rollnick, S. (2002). *Motivational interviewing: Preparing people for change.* New York: Guilford Press.

Missiuna, C., Moll, S., King, A. C., King, G., & Law, M. (2007). A trajectory of troubles: Parents' impressions of the impact of developmental coordination disorder. *Physical and Occupational Therapy in Pediatrics, 27,* 81–101.

Missiuna, C., Moll, S., King, G., Stewart, D., & Macdonald, K. (2008). Life experiences of young adults who have coordination difficulties. *Canadian Journal of Occupational Therapy, 75,* 157–166.

Missiuna, C., & Polatajko, H. J. (1995). Developmental dyspraxia by any other name: Are they all just clumsy children? *American Journal of Occupational Therapy, 49,* 619–627.

Missiuna, C., Pollock, M. A., Egan, M., Delaat, D., Gaines, R., & Soucie, H. (2008). Enabling occupation through facilitating the diagnosis of developmental coordination disorder. *Canadian Journal of Occupational Therapy, 75,* 26–34.

Olweus, D. (2010). *Olweus Bullying Prevention Program.* Retrieved August 10, 2010, from www.olweus.org/public/index.page

Parker, P. M. (2008). *Parading: Webster's quotations, facts, and phrases* (p. 2). San Diego, CA: ICON Group International.

Payton, J., Weissberg, R. P., Durlak, J. A., Dymnicki, A. B., Taylor, R. D., Schellinger, K. B., et al. (2008). *The positive impact of social and emotional learning for K–8 students: Finding from three scientific reviews.* Chicago: Collaborative for Academic, Social, and Emotional Learning. Retrieved June 10, 2009, from www.lpfch.org/sel

Peterson, C., & Seligman, M. E. P. (2004). *Character strengths and virtues: A handbook and classification.* Washington, DC: Oxford University Press.

Piek, J. P., Barrett, N. C., Allen, L. S. R., Jones, A., & Louise, M. (2005). The relationship between bullying and self-worth in children with movement coordination disorders. *British Journal of Educational Psychology, 75,* 453–463.

Piek, J. P., Dworcan, M., Barrett, N. C., & Coleman, R. (2000). Determinants of self-worth in children with and without developmental coordination disorder. *International Journal of Disability, Development and Education, 47,* 259–272.

Pierson, M. R., Carter, E. W., Lane, K. L., & Glaeser, B. C. (2008). Factors influencing the self-determination of transition-age youth with high-incidence disabilities. *Career Development for Exceptional Individuals, 31,* 115–125.

Polatajko, H. J., Fox, A. M., & Missiuna, C. (1995). An international consensus on children with developmental coordination disorder. *Canadian Journal of Occupational Therapy, 62,* 4–6.

Polatajko, H., & Mandich, A. (2004). *Enabling occupation in children: The Cognitive Orientation to Daily Occupational Performance (CO–OP) approach.* Ottawa: CAOT Publications.

Poulsen, A. A., Barker, F., & Ziviani, J. (2010). Personal projects of boys with developmental coordination disorder. *OTJR: Occupation, Participation and Health.* Advance online publication. doi:10.3928/15394492-20100722-02

Poulsen, A. A., & Ziviani, J. M. (2004a). Can I play too? Physical activity engagement patterns of children with developmental coordination disorders. *Canadian Journal of Occupational Therapy, 71,* 100–107.

Poulsen, A. A., & Ziviani, J. M. (2004b). Health-enhancing physical activity: Factors influencing engagement patterns in children. *Australian Occupational Therapy Journal, 51,* 69–79.

Poulsen, A. A., Ziviani, J., Cuskelly, M., & Smith, R. (2007). Boys with developmental coordination disorder: Loneliness and team sport participation. *American Journal of Occupational Therapy, 61,* 463–474.

Putnam, R. D. (2000). *Bowling alone: The collapse and revival of American community.* New York: Touchstone.

Rasmussen, P., & Gillberg, C. (2000). Natural outcome of ADHD with developmental coordination disorder at age 22 years: A controlled, longitudinal, community-based study. *Journal of the American Academy of Child and Adolescent Psychiatry, 39,* 1424–1431.

Rechetinikov, R. P., & Maitrat, K. (2009). Motor impairments in children associated with impairments of speech or language: A meta-analytic review of research literature. *American Journal of Occupational Therapy, 63,* 255–263.

Rispens, J., & van Yperen, T. A. (1997). How specific are "specific developmental disorders"? The relevance of the concept of specific developmental disorders for the classification of childhood developmental disorders. *Journal of Child Psychology and Psychiatry, 38,* 351–362.

Rodger, S., & Mandich, A. (2005). Getting the run around: Accessing services for children with developmental coordination disorder. *Child: Care, Health and Development, 31,* 449–457.

Salmon, G., & Kirby, A. (2008). Schools: Central to providing comprehensive CAMH services in the future? *Child and Adolescent Mental Health, 13,* 107–114.

Schachar, R., & Tannock, R. (2002). Syndromes of hyperactivity and attention deficit. In M. Rutter & E. Taylor (Eds.), *Child and adolescent psychiatry* (4th ed., pp. 399–418). Oxford, England: Blackwell Science.

Segal, R. (1998). The construction of family occupations: A study of families with children who have attention deficit/hyperactivity disorder. *Canadian Journal of Occupational Therapy, 65,* 286–292.

Singh, N. N., Singh, A. N., Lancioni, G. E., Singh, J. E., Winton, A. S. W., & Adkins, A. D. (2010). Mindfulness training for parents and their children with ADHD increases the children's compliance. *Journal of Child and Family Studies, 19,* 1062–1024.

Snyder, C. R. (2000). *Handbook of hope: Theory, measures, and applications.* New York: Academic Press.

Spencer, T. J., Biederman, J., & Mick, E. (2007). Attention deficit/hyperactivity disorder: Diagnosis, lifespan, comorbidities, and neurobiology. *Ambulatory Pediatrics, 7,* 73–81.

Stein, S. M., & Chowdhury, U. (2006). *Disorganized children: A guide for parents and professionals.* London: Jessica Kingsley.

Sugden, D. A. (2006). *Devlopmental coordination disorder as a specific learning difficulty: Leeds consensus statement.* Leeds, England: Economic and Social Research Council.

Vandell, D. L. (2000). Parents, peer groups, and other socializing influences. *Developmental Psychology, 36,* 699–710.

Visser, J. (2003). Developmental coordination disorder: A review of research on subtypes and comorbidities. *Human Movement Science, 22,* 479–493.

Vygotsky, L. S. (1978). *Mind in society: The development of higher psychological process.* Cambridge, MA: Harvard University Press.

Walker, H. M., & Seversen, H. H. (1992). *Systematic screening for behaviour disorders.* Longmont, CO: Sopris West.

Weiss, G., Hechtman, L., Perlman, T., Hopkins, J., & Wener, A. (1979). Hyperactives as young adults: A controlled prospective ten-year follow-up of 75 children. *Archives of General Psychiatry, 36,* 675–681.

Whalen, C. K., Henker, B., Jamner, L. D., Ishikawa, S. S., Floro, J. N., & Swindle, R. (2006). Toward mapping daily challenges of living with ADHD: Maternal and child perspectives using electronic diaries. *Journal of Abnormal Child Psychology, 34,* 115–130.

Witt, P. A., &. Ellis, G. D. (1989). *The Leisure Diagnostic Battery.* State College, PA: Venture.

Wong, B. Y. L., & Donahue, M. (2002). *The social dimensions of learning disabilities: Essays in honor of Tanis Bryan.* Mahwah, NJ: Lawrence Erlbaum.

World Health Organization. (2001). *International classification of functioning, disability and health.* Geneva: Author.

Ziviani, J., Desha, L., & Rodger, S. (2006). Children's occupational time use. In S. Rodger & J. Ziviani (Eds.), *Occupational therapy with children: Understanding children's occupations and enabling participation* (pp. 91–112). Oxford, England: Blackwell.

Ziviani, J., Poulsen, A. A., & Hansen, C. (2009). Movement skills proficiency and physical activity in 6- to 12-year-old children: A case for Engaging and Coaching for Health (EACH–Child). *Australian Occupational Therapy Journal, 56,* 259–265.

Ziviani, J., Wadley, D., Ward, H., Macdonald, D., Jenkins, D., & Rodger, S. (2008). A place to play: Socioeconomic and spatial factors in children's physical activity. *Australian Occupational Therapy Journal, 55,* 2–11.

CHAPTER 12

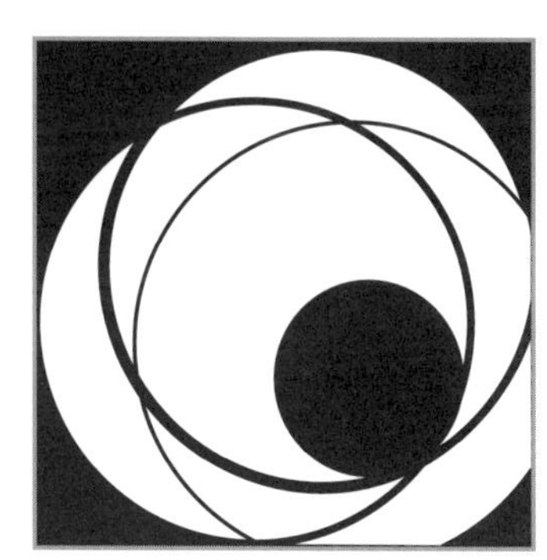

Begin With the End in Mind: Promoting Mental Health, Social Participation, and Self-Determination in the Transition From School to Adult Life

Lisa Crabtree, PhD, OTR/L, and
Andrea B. Sherwin, PhD, OTR/L

Learning Objectives

After reading this material and completing the examination, readers will be able to

- Delineate the importance of considering a vision for the future, inclusive experiences, and person-centered planning during the transition planning process;
- Identify the role of occupational therapists in promoting the successful transition of youth (including those with and without disabilities and mental health challenges) into adulthood;
- Identify key components of self-determination that influence positive outcomes for children and youth;
- Identify the role of occupational therapists in the development of self-determination and empowerment of youth that support positive outcomes; and
- Delineate strategies that occupational therapists can use within a three-tiered approach to foster positive mental health, social participation in school and community activities, and the development of self-determination skills for transitional youth.

> If you don't make a conscious effort to visualize who you are and what you want in life, then you empower other people and circumstances to shape you and your life by default.
>
> —Covey (2010)

This chapter presents information about the process of transition from the school-age years into adulthood, with a focus on supporting positive mental health and social participation and promoting self-determined behaviors throughout the process. Youth who experience a successful transition process have increased positive outcomes in work, relationships, and independent living as adults. Occupational therapists, as related service providers under the Individuals With Disabilities Education Improvement Act of 2004 (IDEA), have a significant role in promoting such transitions for children and youth with mental health challenges or disabilities and supporting best practices for the successful transition of all youth into adulthood.

Transition and Self-Determination

Transition to adulthood is a longitudinal process rather than a predetermined occurrence at one point in time. The process includes a vision for the future; inclusive experiences; and a "blueprint for navigating the waters of the community, workplace, finances, personal life, and home" (Wehman, 2006, p. 10). Person-centered planning is critical to successful transitions. Recognizing these basic constructs offers a more complete understanding of how to plan interventions more effectively and support people throughout the transition process.

Outcomes

Despite more than 30 years of mandated educational and related services for youth with disabilities, outcomes remain poor for their transition into competent adulthood. Indeed, dropout rates, unemployment rates, and arrest records among youth with disabilities are higher than those in a comparable typical population (Clark, Koroloff, Geller, & Sondheimer, 2008; Haber, Karpur, Deschenes, & Clark, 2008; Howlin, Goode, Hutton, & Rutter, 2004; Wehmeyer & Schwartz, 1997). Youth with serious mental illness have the highest unemployment rate of any disability group and have significantly lower rates of high school completion (National Collaborative on Workforce and Disability, 2009). The dropout rate for people with disabilities is approximately 11%. Students with emotional disorders, behavioral disorders, or both have a dropout rate of 50% to 59%, and students with learning disabilities have a dropout rate of 32% to 36% (Kemp, 2006). Additionally, reduced access to social networks and support services further limits the resources for transitional youth with mental health needs (Davis & Sondheimer, 2005).

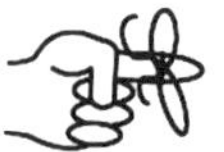

Remember this. . . .
The dropout rate for people with disabilities is approximately 11%. Students with emotional disorders, behavioral disorders, or both have a dropout rate of 50% to 59%, and students with learning disabilities have a dropout rate of 32% to 36%.

These bleak projections are significant, considering that positive adult outcomes in employment, community living, and community interaction are causally linked to self-determined behaviors and seamless transition from secondary school (Wehman, 2006). Despite legislation designed to improve employment outcomes and provide a variety of transitional employment services for people with disabilities, including the Rehabilitation Act of 1973, the Ticket to Work and Work Incentives Improvement Act of 1999, and the Workforce Investment Act of 1998, "systemic barriers . . . lack of consistency in service provision . . . as well as barriers in coordination and collaboration with other workforce development systems" continue to exist (Muthumbi, 2008, p. 102). For youth with serious mental health needs, the challenges are even more significant because it is difficult to find support services to address their mental health treatment, housing, and employment needs (National Collaborative on Workforce and Disability, 2009). Differences in eligibility criteria among child and adult service agencies frequently create challenges in navigating multiple services and programs that are often not coordinated with one another. The need for multidimensional, integrated services among agencies serving transitional youth is critical.

In addition to addressing needs related to independent living, encouraging social networks and participation of transitioning youth can have a significant impact on life satisfaction, peer interaction, and employment. Through the promotion of positive mental health, social participation in school and community activities, and development of self-determination skills, occupational therapists, in collaboration with team members and outside agencies, can positively affect all students' outcomes.

Role of Occupational Therapy

The American Occupational Therapy Association (AOTA; 2008) has described the overarching domain of the occupational therapy profession as "supporting health and participation in life through engagement in occupation" (p. 626). In collaboration with team members, occupational therapists can support children, youth, and their families through the transition process by considering individual client factors, performance skills and patterns, activity demands, and context and environment (see the resources listed in Box 12.1). By focusing on long-term outcomes and goals throughout the evaluation and intervention process, occupational therapists facilitate development of social and employability skills in preparation for community participation as adults. For example, enabling a preschooler to engage in a classroom job such as watering plants, subsequently integrating the child's abilities and interests related to horticulture during occupational therapy interventions in the elementary school years, and then encouraging his or her participation in a career interest inventory during middle school could lead to volunteer or work experiences related to those horticultural interests when he or she is in high school. By fostering interests, self-knowledge, control over environment, and choice-making skills throughout the school-age years, occupational therapists promote self-determined behaviors that lead to more self-satisfied adults.

A growing body of literature offers various strategies to support successful transitions for children and youth at the individual (Wehman, 2006) and systems level (National Collaborative on Workforce and Disability for Youth, 2010). Better outcomes can be achieved if youth have access to support services and accommodations, positive relationships, collaborative teams, supported employment, safe places to interact with peers, and an inclusive process that supports self-determined behaviors (National Collaborative on Workforce and Disability, 2009).

Occupational therapists have the capacity to be instrumental in promoting positive transitions that incorporate these factors by using their expertise in promoting social participation, independent skills, and work behaviors. Well-structured and timely supports transform the transition process from stressful to successful. Caring relationships, high expectations, and greater opportunities for participation have been shown to be protective factors for transitioning youth (Benard & Marshall,

Box 12.1. Transition Resources on the Internet

- *The 411 on Disability Disclosure: A Workbook for Youth With Disabilities (www.ncwd-youth.info/resources_&_Publications/411.html):* This resource is designed to help youth and the adults working with them learn how to make informed decisions about disclosing their disability and understand how that decision might affect their education, employment, and social lives.
- *American Occupational Therapy Association (www.aota.org/Practitioners/ProfDev/CE/Aota/CEonCD/Transition.aspx):* Visit the "Professional Development" section of AOTA's Web site for a continuing education course on occupational therapy and transition (Conaboy, Nochajski, Schefkind, & Schoonover, n.d.). Consumers can visit www.aota.org/Consumers/Work/Job.aspx for Tip Sheets on work transition for people who are newly unemployed or returning to work (AOTA, 2004).
- *Disability Law Lowdown (http://english.disabilitylawlowdown.com/showlist.php):* This Web site provides podcasts in English, Spanish, and American Sign Language on a variety of subjects related to disability laws and disability rights, including one titled *Self-Advocacy for High School Students With Disabilities.*
- *Division on Career Development and Transition (DCDT; www.dcdt.org/index.cfm):* DCDT's mission is to promote national and international efforts to improve the quality of and access to career and vocational and transition services, increase the participation of education in career development and transition goals, and influence policies affecting career development and transition services for people with disabilities.
- *Medical Home Portal (www.medicalhomeportal.org/):* This site provides information for families and professionals on topics such as self-advocacy and transition issues.
- *National Center on Secondary Education and Transition (NCSET; www.ncset.org/default.asp):* The center coordinates national resources, offers technical assistance, and disseminates information related to secondary education and transition for youth with disabilities to create opportunities for youth to achieve successful futures.
- *National Collaborative on Workforce and Disability/Youth (www.ncwd-youth.info/):* This Web site provides many resources for addressing the transition of youth to work settings, including *Guideposts for Success for Youth With Mental Health Needs,* available in English and Spanish (www.ncwd-youth.info/topic/mental-health).
- *National Standards and Quality Indicators: Transition Toolkit for Systems Improvement (www.nasetalliance.org):* Developed by the National Alliance for Secondary Education and Transition, this toolkit contains information and tools to provide a common and shared framework for helping school systems and communities identify what youth need to achieve successful participation in postsecondary education and training, civic engagement, meaningful employment, and adult life.
- *Ohio Center for Autism and Low Incidence (OCALI; www.ocali.org/_archive/pdf_trans_guide/Trans_Guide_1.pdf):* This Web site provides archived Webcasts related to transition to adulthood and a resource titled *Transition to Adulthood Guidelines for Individuals With Autism Spectrum Disorders (ASD)* that identifies 13 steps to incorporate into the transition-planning process.
- *Partnerships for Youth Transition (PYT; http://ntacyt.fmhi.usf.edu):* PYT is an initiative of the Substance Abuse and Mental Health Services Administration focusing on developing transition service systems for youth with behavioral or emotional difficulties. The National Technical Assistance Center for Youth Transition at the University of South Florida coordinates PYT Project activities and evaluation. This Web site includes an extensive collection of Web links, e-newsletters, and other publications.
- *TransCen, Inc. (www.transcen.org/):* TransCen is a nonprofit organization dedicated to improving educational and employment outcomes for people with disabilities by developing, implementing, and researching innovations regarding school-to-adult life transition and career development for people with disabilities.
- *Transition to Independence Process (TIP; http://tip.trustedts.com/Home.aspx):* The mission of the TIP system is to assist young people with emotional or behavioral difficulties in making a successful transition into adulthood, with all youth achieving, within their potential, their goals in the transition domains of employment, education, living situation, and community life.
- *Wright's Law (http://wrightslaw.com/info/iep.index.htm):* Wright's Law contains articles, regulations, and helpful tips about getting transition services into a child's individualized education program.
- *Youthhood.org (www.youthhood.org):* This Web site provides opportunities for youth to interact with adults and discuss topics such as employment, independent living, health, and other issues related to a transition to adult life. Adults can create activities for youth to work on when they log on to the site, including journaling, a life map, and a class notebook.

2001), allowing them to develop necessary skills to prevent high-risk behaviors from affecting emotional and physical health. Also, problem solving, decision making, and goal setting all contribute to the development of positive self-concept and more self-determined behaviors. Caring and nurturing relationships, in particular, offer a sense of connection to the community (Jivanjee, Kruzich, & Gordon, 2008). Providing opportunities to master and apply skills, including leadership and personal relationship skills, may significantly contribute to resiliency and success in the transition to adulthood. These opportunities can be incorporated into a variety of peer play or social opportunities supported by occupational therapists throughout the elementary, middle, and high school years. Inclusive intervention strategies, games, social clubs, and after-school programming are all experiences that foster a range of interaction skills that concurrently lead to a positive sense of self-worth and self-determined behaviors over the span of years.

Self-Determination

The concept of *self-determination,* a term used originally in political science to conceptualize internally determined human behaviors, emphasizes that one determines "one's own fate or course of action without compulsion" (Wehmeyer, Palmer, Agran, Mithaug, & Martin, 2000, p. 107). Seemingly a logical connection to individual rights, it was not linked to people with disabilities until the 1970s with the introduction of the normalization movement (Cobb, 1973) promoting self-governance, self-advocacy, community involvement and, above all, respect for people with intellectual disabilities (previously referred to as *mental retardation;* Wehmeyer et al., 2000). This elemental principle later burgeoned into the Independent Living, Self-Advocacy, and Disability Rights Movements (Shapiro, 1993; Ward & Meyer, 1999). At the crux of each of these movements is the core concept that people have the right to control their own lives.

Self-Determination and Education

Principles of self-determination are incorporated into a variety of models of educational curricula for people with disabilities (Carter, Lane, Pierson, & Stang, 2008; Martin, Dycke, D'Ottavio, & Nickerson, 2007; Sands & Doll, 1996; Wehmeyer & Schwartz, 1997). Doing so is considered best practice in working with youth with disabilities because IDEA mandates increased student involvement in transition planning (Wehmeyer, 2002). The concept and application of self-determination principles within education exist because of two major initiatives: The U.S. Department of Education launched a research initiative in the early 1990s, and the Robert Wood Johnson Foundation funded a second wave of research in the mid-1990s. These proactive investigative agendas brought the concept and language of self-determination to the forefront of educational curricula and programming for people with disabilities and thereby offered a powerful voice to people seeking greater independence and control (Hoffman, 2003; Wehmeyer & Schwartz, 1997).

Such in-depth research in education has yielded a growing body of literature on outcomes and strategies for promoting self-determination in curricular instruction. Martin et al. (2007) described their Student-Directed Summary of Performance tool as a "summative repository of crucial information that students with disabilities need to know when they leave school" on which one can "record and report the results of ongoing, student-directed transition assessment" (p. 16). Such an instrument enables students to become more involved in the transition process.

Another example is the Self-Determined Learning Model of Instruction, developed by Wehmeyer, Palmer, et al. (2000). This model uses a "three-phase instructional process" that enables teachers to empower students to become greater self-advocates and become "a causal agent in one's life" (Wehmeyer, Palmer, et al., 2000, p. 441). The three phases of this mode are as follows: (1) Set a goal, (2) take action, and (3) adjust goal or plan. These phases are further broken down into specific guiding questions that teachers can use to allow students to make decisions and solve problems for themselves with guidance from adults, rather than follow through with directions from adults in their lives who problem solve for them. Thus, it is the individual who causes things to happen in his or her life.

This construct of *causal agency,* which is the basis of empowerment, self-advocacy, and self-efficacy, offers people with disabilities the language to speak out on their own behalf. Although these constructs and related interventions, outcomes, and applications are prevalent in the educational realm, self-determination is an emergent concept in the profession of occupational therapy. As presented in this chapter, however, self-determination is integral to the transition process and occupational therapy practice. Occupational therapists focus on quality of life, client-centered practice, and promoting positive self-worth and independence, all of which are essential aspects of self-determined behavior, as they support people across the lifespan (Box 12.2).

Self-Determination and Transition

Wehmeyer, Kelchner, and Richards (1996) wrote that *self-determined behaviors* are "acting as the primary causal agent in one's life and making choices and decisions

Box 12.2. Component Elements of Self-Determined Behavior

- Choice-making skills
- Decision-making skills
- Problem-solving skills
- Goal-setting and attainment skills
- Independence, risk-taking, and safety skills
- Self-observation, evaluation, and reinforcement skills
- Self-instruction skills
- Self-advocacy and leadership skills
- Internal locus of control
- Positive attributions of efficacy and outcome expectancy
- Self-awareness
- Self-knowledge.

Source. Wehmeyer, Gragoudas, and Shogren (2006, p. 43).

regarding one's quality of life free from undue external influence or interference" (p. 632). This definition encapsulates the concepts of personal choice, participation, and quality of life, concepts that are associated with empowerment and self-efficacy and with advocacy behaviors. Self-determined behaviors have four essential characteristics: (1) the person acts autonomously, (2) behaviors are self-regulated, (3) the person is psychologically empowered, and (4) the person acts in a self-realizing manner (Wehmeyer et al., 1996). The transitional process, as described previously in this chapter, necessitates all of these skills. At each critical transition point throughout the educational process—a move from one grade level to the next, a change in schools, or graduation from postsecondary school—self-determined behaviors are fundamental. Consequently, an occupational therapist helping people increase awareness of their personal preferences, interests, strengths, and limitations provides an indispensable resource supporting the transitional process.

The concept of self-determination encompasses the notion that people are "causal agents . . . and must make things happen in their lives" (Wehmeyer, Palmer, et al., 2000, p. 440). Also, as a self-determined person, one takes responsibility for and control over one's actions using strategies and problem-solving approaches to goal-directed actions (Mithaug, 1996). The outcome is that people with disabilities "have opportunities to exert control in their lives and are provided supports that enable them to take advantage of such opportunities in ways that respect their values, beliefs, and customs" (Wehmeyer, 2004, p. 338).

To achieve such outcomes, the transition process must be inclusive at each stage (Sands & Doll, 1996) and consistently encourage and support self-determined behaviors throughout the educational process (Wehmeyer, Bersani, & Gagne, 2000). As Brotherson, Cook, Erwin, and Weigel (2008) noted, the home environment is the primary learning atmosphere; therefore, to support a participatory process at this stage, families must be at the center of the discussion regarding any transition. Erwin et al. (2009) explored this idea further and delineated strategies to support family-directed transitions, identifying questions that therapists may ask of families to promote culturally sensitive involvement. For example, during early childhood transitions, in which family members participate, occupational therapists may actively engage the child's parents in the planning process by asking them questions, providing suggestions for facilitating engagement in outdoor family leisure activities, and offering online and printed reading material about family support groups or other areas of need (Erwin et al., 2009). Similar supports may be used with older students, as asking youth about preferences and engaging them in the discussion of choice foster problem solving and decision making, which are essential life skills that promote self-determined behaviors. For people with intellectual disabilities or emotional disturbance, these core skills become more challenging.

Under these circumstances, promoting communication to be able to become aware of choices and options and to self-evaluate decisions is essential (Wehmeyer & Gragoudas, 2004). One study examining youth and employment noted that a disproportionate number of self-determined students were likely to remain in their jobs at the time of follow-up compared with students without these skills (Wehmeyer & Gragoudas, 2004).

Promoting Self-Determination

Promoting self-determined behaviors in children, youth, and their families also necessitates an approach toward positive perception and expectation. Recognizing that students and their families are capable of making their own decisions and choices about what is best and how they choose to spend their time in the community is critical to successful long-term outcomes. The unsubstantiated perception of professionals that students with disabilities are incapable of making their own decisions propagates a lack of opportunities for students to practice self-determined behaviors. This cycle leads to learned helplessness, decreased motivation, and poor decision-making skills and, over time, sabotages any opportunity for self-determined behaviors at home or in the community. Conversely, choice making is motivating, affirming, and enhances capacity, and a just-right challenge offers the opportunity to expand practical skills in decision making and problem solving (Mithaug, 1993; Wehmeyer, Palmer, et al., 2000).

Meeting with parents and families to initiate or review an individualized education program (IEP) also offers a forum to encourage families to present their children with choices and options. Too often, children and youth with disabilities are denied the choices that typically developing children are expected to and usually do make about various aspects of their lives. All children and youth, independent of their level of cognitive function, are aware of the opportunity of choice, including routine choices about clothing, food, sports, or after-school activities, all of which promote a significantly different perception regarding environmental influence on a person. Some examples of questions parents might ask include "Would you like to do T-ball or soccer after school?" "Would you like to wear the blue shirt or the pink shirt?" Alternatively, such choice options may also be generalized to increase community participation: "Would you like to go to the mall or the library?"

Another important choice for youth with disabilities is how to make decisions about disclosing one's disability. Resources are available to assist in the decision-making process related to disclosure, and occupational therapists can play a significant role in supporting students' awareness of their capacities and challenges and in promoting their decision-making skills. Disclosing one's disability is a personal decision and often is dependent upon contextual factors.

Additionally, it is beneficial when parents can recognize their own capacities and schedule limitations. Offering choices to children and youth that cannot be fulfilled because a parent becomes overwhelmed is counterproductive to promoting self-determined behaviors. Alternatively, a parent asking "Would you like to go the post office or the grocery store first?" presents the child with choice while fully recognizing that the parent must complete both tasks. Additional resources for promoting self-determined behaviors include creating social opportunities for interaction with other peers, allowing for risk taking and exploration, and providing honest feedback with communication (Davis & Wehmeyer, 1991).

Occupational therapists can effectively use the therapeutic setting to encourage choice making as well. Asking children and youth which toy they prefer to play with first or which goal they would like to address first provides a medium for discussion and opportunity. Most important, the therapist and the caregivers should remember that all choices must be acceptable before they are asked or offered. Additionally, friendship choices play an increasingly important role as children age and need to assert their independence. Promoting positive peer relationships, supportive friendships, and collaborative and community experiences, along with demonstrating the ability to share feelings and articulate needs and wants, supports self-determined behaviors (Williams & Heslop, 2006).

In most traditional settings, occupational therapists are considered experts. This mindset, however, leads not to a path that fosters self-determination, choice making, and opportunity but to one that consistently places children and youth with disabilities in a place of inferiority. It leads to the erroneous idea that they should wait for others, sit still, and eat the food that is served to them, without protest. By fostering self-determination skills in children and youth, occupational therapists have the ability to empower them to make choices and to shape their own futures.

Self-Determination and Youth Empowerment

According to Self-Determination Theory, creating opportunities for increased participation and leadership generates greater self-confidence and increases self-concept and a sense of psychological empowerment (Chambers et al., 2007). Nevertheless, youth benefit from support and guidance when making choices about levels of participation. As young people develop, however, they need expanding opportunities to be active decision makers in their own care and in shaping policies and procedures that govern youth in community systems of care. The Youth Empowerment Initiative is one approach based on a youth empowerment model that supports young people in having a voice in all decisions that affect their lives and the lives of their peers and families (Jennings, Parra-Medina, Hilfinger-Messias, & McLoughlin, 2006). As such, self-determination can be viewed as a critical ingredient in promoting youth empowerment (Box 12.3).

Transition

According to IDEA 2004, *transition* is

> a coordinated set of activities for a student that—
>
> > (A) is designed to be within a results-oriented process that is focused on improving the academic and functional achievement of the child with a disability to facilitate the child's movement from school to post-school

Box 12.3. Dimensions of the Youth Empowerment Initiative

- A welcoming and safe environment
- Meaningful participation and engagement
- Equitable power sharing between youth and adults
- Reflection of interpersonal and sociopolitical processes
- Participation in sociopolitical activities to foster change
- Integrating individual- and community-level empowerment.

Source. Jennings et al. (2006).

> activities, including post-secondary education, vocational education, integrated employment (including supported employment), continuing and adult education, adult services, independent living, or community participation.
>
> (B) is based on the individual child's needs, taking into account the child's strengths, preferences, and interests; and
>
> (C) includes instruction, related services, community experiences, the development of employment and other post-school adult living objectives, and when appropriate, acquisition of daily living skills and functional vocational evaluation. (§ 602.34)

This definition of the transition process focuses on achievable outcomes for students with disabilities, although it is based on expectations that families have for all youth as they reach the end of their secondary school experience. The federal law mandates that a transition plan be in place beginning at age 16, although many state laws require teams to address transition issues beginning at age 14. However, by taking a broader view of transition as a process that starts when the child begins school at age 3 and increasing the focus on active student participation and self-determination, successful outcomes can be achieved as youth transition out of the school environment. This broad transition process is illustrated by a schema developed by George Tilson of TransCen, an organization dedicated to assisting youth in the transition to adulthood (Figure 12.1).

Transition Continuum

Occupational therapists can support development of transitional skills throughout the continuum from preschool to after high school. At the preschool level, occupational therapy services can include direct intervention to support independent skills in the classroom and at home in addition to workshops for teachers and parents aimed at developing activities to support community social participation. The transition continuum begins with a child's awareness of self and the community while developing independent skills and positive work habits. Specific attention to the development of positive work attitudes and beliefs should be considered at each stage of development (Box 12.4).

When children are in elementary school, practitioners can provide occupational therapy intervention in group settings that facilitate positive social interactions and assist students in cultivating abilities and interests related to later career development. In addition to direct services, therapists can also support children's social and employability skills through newsletter tips to parents, membership on policy committees that promote community participation, or providing consultation to classroom teachers related to classroom accommodations. In collaboration with team members, occupational therapists work to create inclusive, supportive classroom environments that promote social–emotional health. Early programming that addresses social–emotional needs in elementary school can provide a foundation for developing self-determination skills needed in the transition to adulthood later on.

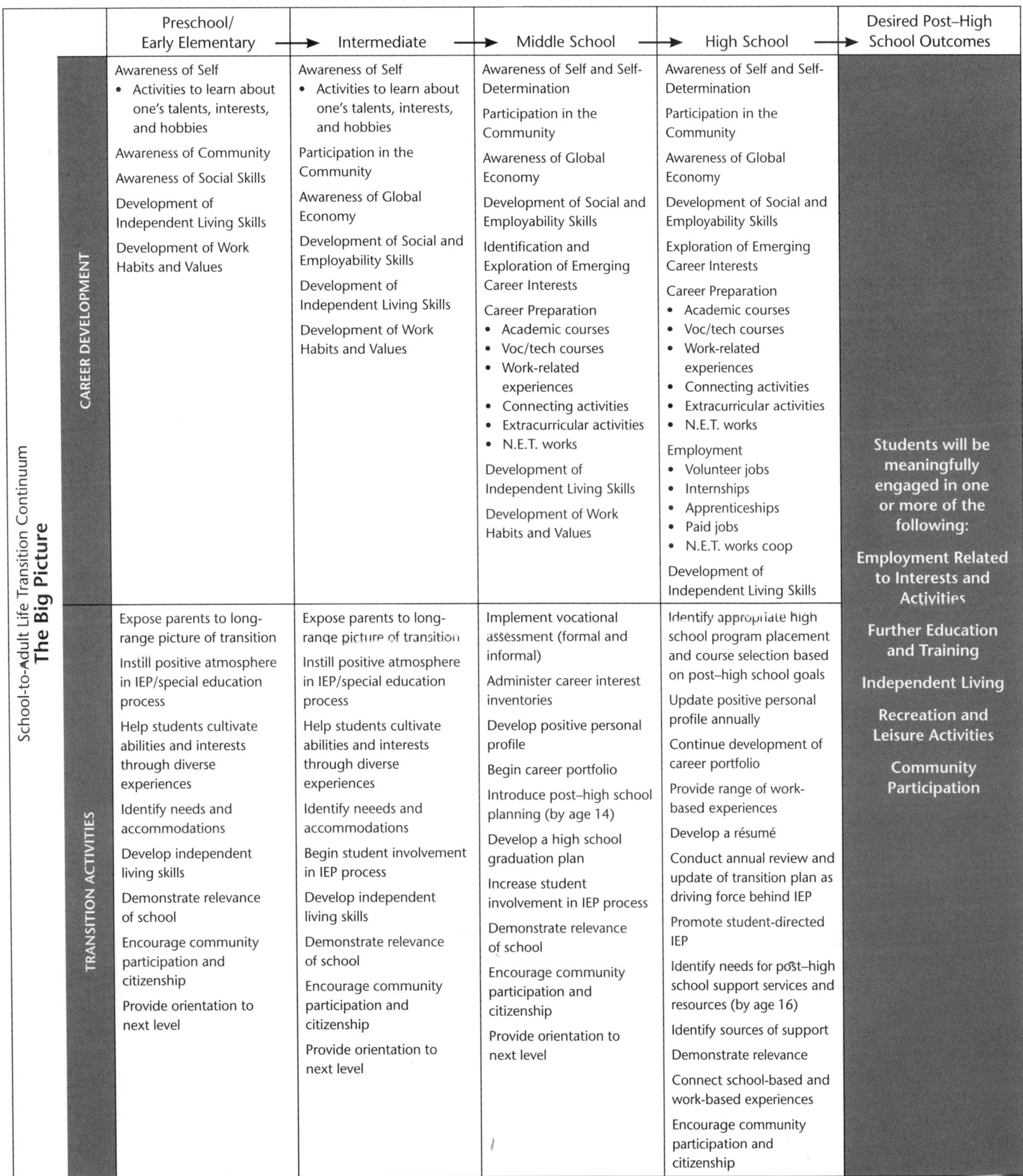

School-to-Adult Life Transition Continuum
The Big Picture

	Preschool/ Early Elementary →	Intermediate →	Middle School →	High School →	Desired Post–High School Outcomes
CAREER DEVELOPMENT	Awareness of Self • Activities to learn about one's talents, interests, and hobbies Awareness of Community Awareness of Social Skills Development of Independent Living Skills Development of Work Habits and Values	Awareness of Self • Activities to learn about one's talents, interests, and hobbies Participation in the Community Awareness of Global Economy Development of Social and Employability Skills Development of Independent Living Skills Development of Work Habits and Values	Awareness of Self and Self-Determination Participation in the Community Awareness of Global Economy Development of Social and Employability Skills Identification and Exploration of Emerging Career Interests Career Preparation • Academic courses • Voc/tech courses • Work-related experiences • Connecting activities • Extracurricular activities • N.E.T. works Development of Independent Living Skills Development of Work Habits and Values	Awareness of Self and Self-Determination Participation in the Community Awareness of Global Economy Development of Social and Employability Skills Exploration of Emerging Career Interests Career Preparation • Academic courses • Voc/tech courses • Work-related experiences • Connecting activities • Extracurricular activities • N.E.T. works Employment • Volunteer jobs • Internships • Apprenticeships • Paid jobs • N.E.T. works coop Development of Independent Living Skills	**Students will be meaningfully engaged in one or more of the following:** **Employment Related to Interests and Activities** **Further Education and Training** **Independent Living** **Recreation and Leisure Activities** **Community Participation**
TRANSITION ACTIVITIES	Expose parents to long-range picture of transition Instill positive atmosphere in IEP/special education process Help students cultivate abilities and interests through diverse experiences Identify needs and accommodations Develop independent living skills Demonstrate relevance of school Encourage community participation and citizenship Provide orientation to next level	Expose parents to long-range picture of transition Instill positive atmosphere in IEP/special education process Help students cultivate abilities and interests through diverse experiences Identify neeeds and accommodations Begin student involvement in IEP process Develop independent living skills Demonstrate relevance of school Encourage community participation and citizenship Provide orientation to next level	Implement vocational assessment (formal and informal) Administer career interest inventories Develop positive personal profile Begin career portfolio Introduce post–high school planning (by age 14) Develop a high school graduation plan Increase student involvement in IEP process Demonstrate relevance of school Encourage community participation and citizenship Provide orientation to next level	Identify appropriate high school program placement and course selection based on post–high school goals Update positive personal profile annually Continue development of career portfolio Provide range of work-based experiences Develop a résumé Conduct annual review and update of transition plan as driving force behind IEP Promote student-directed IEP Identify needs for post–high school support services and resources (by age 16) Identify sources of support Demonstrate relevance Connect school-based and work-based experiences Encourage community participation and citizenship	

Figure 12.1. Transition continuum: The big picture. Taking a broad view of the transition process from preschool through postsecondary school supports successful outcomes in adulthood.

Note. IEP = individualized education plan.

Source. School-to-Adult Life Transition Continuum: The Big Picture, by G. Tilson, 2001, Rockville, MD: TransCen, Inc. Copyright © 2001 by TranCen, Inc. Adapted with permission.

Box 12.4. Seven Strategies for Helping Children and Youth Develop Positive Work Attitudes and Beliefs

1. Provide opportunities to observe positive examples of work from the significant adults in children's lives. Ideally, children need to see adults who value and find meaning in their work. Because adult attitudes about work are often contagious, it is important to frame work as effortful activity that is enjoyed rather than as toil or drudgery that is endured.
2. Give children of all ages opportunities to engage in legitimate work activities at home, day care, school and, eventually, in the community. Work skills develop gradually over time, based on the child's development.
   a. Infants, while perched on the parent's hip or sitting in a high chair, have multiple opportunities to observe adults' work—stirring food cooking in a pot, washing dishes, or folding clothes.
   b. Toddlers not only observe adult work but are eager to contribute to portions of tasks, such as fetching a needed item or stirring a bowl of pudding.
   c. Preschoolers can perform most chores with supervision and are also eager to assist.
   d. School-age children can be expected to be independent in self-care and a broader range of work activities (e.g., simple food preparation, cleaning, yard care).
3. Encourage participation in a range of meaningful work and structured leisure activities to help children and youth develop foundation skills for later work. Work and leisure should not be viewed as separate entities but as part of a continuum in the lives of youth—both contribute to the development of positive work behaviors (e.g., time management, persistence, frustration tolerance).
4. Well-defined goals help children understand the reason why the task should be completed. For example, "wiping the crumbs from the table will prevent your homework papers from getting dirty" or "folding these clothes will help keep them from getting wrinkled." Providing feedback also allows children to make associations between their helpful act and the outcome. "Thank you for helping clear the table. It will take less time to clean up after dinner so that we can go on a walk."
5. Co-participation of children and adults in household tasks tends to enhance meaning while increasing a sense of family or group solidarity.
6. Help children begin to visualize a future that involves meaningful work by encouraging them to talk about their interests, options, and dreams.
7. Foster self-reflection to help youth find their "sweet spot," or area of intense personal interest. Identified talents and interests can help the person eventually seek work that is aligned with his or her authentic self.

Source. Bazyk (2005).

When children enter middle school, initial career preparation activities should be explored and implemented. Using the evaluation process, the occupational therapist can assist middle school children in developing a positive personal profile that includes a list of their strengths and interests, and he or she can use group activities to develop a career portfolio. Encouraging participation in after-school activities related to areas of interest can prepare students for career exploration. By the time youth are transitioning to the high school level, they should have identified realistic post–high school goals. The occupational therapist can work with students individually on prevocational skills or, more broadly, through development of program planning that creates opportunities for career exploration activities. Intervention should occur at all three tiers, depending on the needs of each individual student.

At the high school level, involvement in training job coaches in supportive and adaptive strategies can be a collaborative process with students, one that builds leadership skills and a sense of empowerment that increases motivation and participation. Occupational therapists can also assist youth in developing the independent living skills necessary for planned postschool environments. Volunteer and work-based experiences in community settings, along with participation in community leisure activities, are critical to a successful transition into adult life. Occupational therapists have the background and expertise to work collaboratively with youth, family members, and the high school team to ensure a successful transition. One model of transition to higher education possibilities is the Disabilities, Opportunities, Internetworking, Technology (DO–IT) program developed by Burgstahler, Lopez, and Jirikowic (2007) at the University of Washington (Resource 12.1). With funding from the National Science Foundation, promoters use a variety of programs and projects to develop the skills of youth with disabilities who are in their last 2 years of high school. The focus of summer study programs, work-based learning, and e-mentoring programs is on preparing youth for participation in competitive academic programs and careers. By providing mentorship from adults and DO–IT graduates, supporting electronic communication with peers and mentors, providing assistive technology, and developing self-determination skills, the programs have a positive impact on academic and career outcomes.

Resource 12.1. DO–IT

- The Accommodation Model and Student Abilities Profile of DO–IT (Disabilities, Opportunities, Internetworking, and Technology) are tools that can help professionals work with students to create an optimum learning environment.
- DO–IT serves to increase the successful participation of people with disabilities in challenging academic programs such as those in science, engineering, mathematics, and technology. Primary funding for DO–IT is provided by the National Science Foundation, the State of Washington, and the U.S. Department of Education. Resources to replicate the program, including publications, videos, and training materials, can be accessed on the Web site free of charge (www.washington.edu/doit/Brochures/).

Source. Burgstahler et al. (2007).

Transition Practices

Effective transition practices with youth with mental health challenges or disabilities result in increased graduation rates, employment, and positive school outcomes (Benz, Lindstrom, & Yovanoff, 2000; Carter et al., 2008; Wehmeyer & Palmer, 2003; Wehmeyer & Schwartz, 1997). As children develop into adolescents, it is increasingly important to support self-determination and empowerment by requesting and acknowledging their perspective of their needs and concerns (Carrington, Templeton, & Papinczak, 2003). Additionally, a wide variety of supports and opportunities need to be made available to transitioning youth, and it is critical for service coordination to occur with medical assistance, continuing education, vocational rehabilitation, housing, transportation, and medical services.

Recognizing that transition-age youth with mental health needs have unique challenges, the U.S. Department of Labor's Office of Disability Employment Policy, in collaboration with the National Collaborative on Workforce and Disability for Youth (NCWD/Youth) created a framework to guide policymakers in developing an integrated set of services that support better outcomes. This resource, *Tunnels and Cliffs: A Guide for Workforce Development Practitioners and Policymakers Serving Youth With Mental Health Needs* (Podmostko, 2007), provides guidelines on how to develop and improve systems to meet students' needs. Often, transitioning youth are given few options when transition plans are made and are provided with programs or services that are not tailored to their needs, thereby shunting them through service tunnels of what is usually provided to youth through individual agencies or school programs. Alternatively, when youth age out of systems at age 18 or 22, they may have difficulty accessing appropriate services in the adult system, which often has different terminology, eligibility requirements, and service options, creating "transition cliffs." This process can cause youth to lose benefits and services that were provided while they were in school. *Tunnels and Cliffs* emphasized the importance of interagency collaboration and increased awareness of all services available in communities to avoid these issues. Other reports published by NCWD/Youth have addressed the issues of children and transitional youth with mental health needs and are available on its Web site (Box 12.5). In collaboration with an interdisciplinary team, occupational therapists can use these resources to advocate for youth with mental health needs and can incorporate work-based learning and career preparation activities into intervention planning.

Team planning for transitional youth with mental health needs and behavioral disorders is complex, because the onset of psychiatric symptoms often does not occur until ages 18 to 25 (National Institute of Mental Health, 2002). This transitional time of life involves planning for careers, postsecondary education, and intimate social relationships, all of which become critical issues for youth and young adults challenged with simultaneously managing their disability. The mission of the National Network on Youth Transition for Behavioral Health at the University of South Florida is "to improve practices, systems, and outcomes for transition-age youth and young adults (14–29 years of age) with emotional and/or behavioral difficulties" (National Network on Youth Transition for Behavioral Health, 2010).

In keeping with this mission, and using a mental health recovery model, Clark et al. (2008) developed an evidence-supported system called the Transition to Independence Process (TIP) to improve real-life outcomes for youth and young adults with emotional and behavioral disorders. The system incorporates seven guidelines to support a successful transition system, which are outlined in Box 12.6. Online training modules are available that provide a framework for program development related to these guidelines.

Another successful person-centered model for planning transitions that takes into account the student's dreams for the future is the PATH process (Box 12.7; Bunch, Finnegan, & Pearpoint, 2009). This model considers the vision of the person with a disability and uses visual images to identify the specific goals and actions necessary to achieve those goals. The success of this model depends on collaboration and linking students and their families with community agencies for postsecondary

Box 12.5. National Collaborative on Workforce and Disability for Youth Resources Related to Youth With Mental Health Needs

- *Tunnels and Cliffs: A Guide for Workforce Development Practitioners and Policymakers Serving Youth With Mental Health Needs* (www.ncwd-youth.info/tunnels-and-cliffs)
- *Guideposts for Success for Youth With Mental Health Needs* (www.ncwd-youth.info/guideposts/mental-health)
- *Transitioning Youth With Mental Health Needs to Meaningful Employment and Independent Living* (www.ncwd-youth.info/white-paper/transitioning-youth-with-mental-health-needs)
- *Pioneering Transition Programs: The Establishment of Programs That Span the Ages Served by Child and Adult Mental Health* (www.ncwd-youth.info/partnership-guide/pioneering-transition-programs)
- *Young Adults With Serious Mental Illness: Some States and Federal Agencies Are Taking Steps to Address Their Transition Challenges* (www.gao.gov/new.items/d08678.pdf)

Box 12.6. Transition to Independence Process (TIP) System Guidelines

- Engage young people through relationship development, person-centered planning, and a focus on their futures.
- Tailor services and supports to be accessible, coordinated, appealing, nonstigmatizing, and developmentally appropriate, building on strengths to enable the young people to pursue their goals across relevant transition domains.
- Acknowledge and develop personal choice and social responsibility with young people.
- Ensure that a safety net of support is provided by a young person's parents, family members, and other informal and formal key players.
- Enhance young people's competencies to assist them in achieving greater self-sufficiency and confidence.
- Maintain an outcome focus in the TIP system at the young person, program, and system levels.
- Involve young people, parents, and other community partners in the TIP system at the practice, program, and community levels.

Source. From "Navigating the Obstacle Course: An Evidence-Supported Community Transition System," in *Transition of Youth and Young Adults With Emotional or Behavioral Difficulties: An Evidence-Supported Handbook* (pp. 95–97), by H. B. Clark and D. K. Unruh, 2009, Baltimore: Paul H. Brookes. Copyright © 2009 by Paul H. Brookes. Adapted with permission.

support. This type of transition planning lends itself to interagency collaboration through a systems-of-care approach (Cline, 2007), in which there is full participation of everyone involved with the student. Family members and professionals from schools and community agencies are all active partners with the transitioning youth in designing effective supports and services. With this approach, occupational therapists can use skills in goal setting and a focus on meaningful engagement in occupations to contribute to the transition-planning process.

Social Participation and Structured Leisure Pursuits

Whether students are college bound or transitioning to work or community settings, participation in recreational activities with others is important to develop routines and opportunities for social participation. Without the structure of organized activities such as those that occur within school programs, transitioning youth are at risk for social isolation when they leave the school environment (Hillier, Fish, Cloppert, & Beversdorf, 2007). Participation in community leisure and recreational programs during the middle and high school years provides a way for youth to develop supportive peers and a repertoire of skills for lifelong involvement. Occupational therapists can support participation in leisure activities by working with youth on skill development or by working with a local college or university to incorporate service learning activities into after-school or community activities for high school students.

According to a report from the National Longitudinal Transition Study, a nationally representative sample of almost 12,000 students ages 13 to 16 (Wagner, Cadwallader, Garza, & Cameto, 2004), levels of social participation with friends and extracurricular groups vary among youth with disabilities. For example, group membership across disability categories ranged from 56% to 75% of youth, although youth with mental health diagnoses demonstrated participation at the lower end of

Box 12.7. PATH Process

PATH (formerly called Planning Alternative Tomorrows with Hope) is an eight-step creative planning tool developed by Marsha Forest, Jack Pearpoint, and John O' Brien of the Marsha Forest Centre in Toronto, Canada. The process begins with selecting a dream for the future and planning the possible and positive actions necessary to obtain goals related to that dream by working backwards. PATH uses visual graphics to keep the youth (pathfinder) and his or her supporters focused on the dreams and goals developed through the PATH process. Materials to support use of the PATH process can be ordered at www.inclusion.com/.

Source. Bunch et al. (2009).

the range than students diagnosed with learning disabilities or sensory impairments. Of all youth involved in the study, those diagnosed with autism, multiple disabilities, or deaf–blindness were among the least likely to be actively involved with individual friends. From 27% to 40% of youth in those categories were reported never to see friends outside of the classroom, and about half or more were not invited to social activities. This information has critical implications for how youth will be able to cope with the challenges of participating with others in community or work environments as they age out of the school system. Without experiencing social opportunities with peers in an inclusive school environment, they will not develop the necessary skills to meaningfully engage in adult life and are at risk for long-term dependence on family members.

Summary

Transition to adulthood is inevitable for all children and youth. To support successful transitions, a focus on the longitudinal process and the integration of self-determination and student involvement in the process has become best practice. Students who transition from high school as self-determined youth have more positive outcomes and greater choices for their futures.

This chapter has discussed ways in which occupational therapists can support children and youth in the transition process, empowering them to become competent young adults. Using a three-tiered model, the case study of a 19-year-old youth presented in Box 12.8 provides a specific example of how the constructs described in this chapter can be applied by occupational therapists in the school system and in the community. Although all three tiers of services are described in the case example, note that intervention is initiated at Tier 1. If the supports at Tier 1 successfully address the student's needs, the intervention approaches at Tier 2 and Tier 3 may not be necessary. Alternatively, the school team, in collaboration with the student and his family, may decide to implement one or more of the interventions simultaneously at each level. Therefore, for illustration purposes, interventions at all three levels are described. Finally, additional resources that occupational therapists can use to support students with disabilities in the transition process are provided in Box 12.1.

Although the process of transition is complex, particularly for students with disabilities, it is important to facilitate students' participation in the process to the greatest extent possible. By focusing on a student's dreams and meaningful occupations, the transition from postsecondary school to young adulthood can be a successful, person-centered experience.

Box 12.8. Case Example: Blaise

Occupational Profile

Blaise is the 19-year-old son of Heang and Kevin Thien and lives with his parents, a 17-year-old sister, a 16-year-old brother, and his grandparents. Blaise's family is originally from Vietnam, although he has lived in the United States for the past 15 years. Blaise was diagnosed with attention deficit hyperactivity disorder at age 4 and has had challenges with sensory processing, motor coordination, social interactions, and emotional regulation since infancy. At age 13, he was diagnosed with depression and anxiety disorder after several episodes of bullying during middle school. After each episode, Blaise did not report the incidents to his teachers and confided only in his parents, who were unclear about the process of reporting to school personnel. Since he started high school at age 14, Blaise has been more interested in participating in after-school clubs, but starting that process required completing paperwork and self-advocacy. Blaise has not initiated any actions to participate and is becoming further isolated from peers and others at school.

Blaise is able to use strategies such as headphones, yoga breathing, and walking so that he does not become overwhelmed in different environments. Although he has participated in various social skills groups over the years, he has difficulty interacting with peers and has expressed feelings of isolation. Blaise has difficulty with emotional regulation, making it challenging for him to get along with others. He often expresses anxiety about being bullied, and he keeps a low profile at the high school to avoid being picked on. Although he would like to have friends, especially a girlfriend, he is too inhibited to initiate conversations and becomes anxious in large groups. He has one friend, Jamal, who enjoys playing video games and chess with him, and they usually get together once a week. Blaise has a strong interest in science and would like to work in a research field.

Blaise is currently in a transitional program at the high school and has the goal of entering a community college program at the end of the current school year. He has identified transitional goals of working part time at the family store, increasing social participation with peers in the community, and becoming more self-reliant so that he can eventually live on his own. However, he has not expressed those ideas in his individualized education program (IEP) meeting.

Interventions to Address Development of Self-Determination and Effective Transition Skills

Tier 1. The occupational therapist serves on a district committee to incorporate policies addressing bullying and creating welcoming community environments on school campuses. Information about antibullying practices and developing inclusive environments is sent home to all families in the district. As part of this initiative, the occupational therapist facilitates creation of a student committee to create a positive environment at the high school. Blaise participates in classroom discussions about bullying and learns to whom he should report incidents that occur.

Tier 2. Blaise needs some positive supports and some information about self-advocacy and fostering his sense of control over his environment. To that end, the occupational therapist can work with the after-school coordinator and Blaise to develop a video gaming club to promote social participation. This activity will provide an environment that will enable Blaise to use his strengths to feel empowered and build self-confidence. He can be in charge of planning and organizing club activities, thereby improving his organizational skills. The occupational therapist can be a consultant to address problems with emotional regulation and skills.

The occupational therapist might work with a job counselor from the community college to develop an employment workshop series for youth from the high school who are transitioning to the community college. Skills will address resume development, job interviewing skills, social interaction skills with customers and fellow employees, working with a job coach, and self-advocacy skills. The assistant can conduct the workshop on self-advocacy skills, providing interventions tailored to participants' individual strengths and preferences. Community collaborations with employers and agencies to provide work experiences can be fostered.

Tier 3. In collaboration with other team members, the occupational therapist initiates an individualized cognitive–behavioral intervention with Blaise for management of anxiety and frustration. An important component of the program is practicing skills in a supportive naturalistic environment, and the therapist consults with teachers and a job coach to ensure success.

Instructing Blaise in the elements of self-determination skills is critical. The occupational therapist can directly support Blaise by teaching him how to self-advocate, make choices, and practice problem-solving and decision-making skills that positively affect his environment. Role-playing sessions incorporating speaking to a variety of professionals, making his needs known, and choosing options for social and vocational experiences can be facilitated in individualized or small-group sessions. Use of the PATH process during his IEP meeting can facilitate identification of his goals and the people who can support Blaise in meeting those goals.

References

American Occupational Therapy Association. (2004). *Returning to work.* Retrieved November 12, 2010, from www.aota.org/Consumers/consumers/Work/Job.aspx

American Occupational Therapy Association. (2008). Occupational therapy practice framework: Domain and process (2nd ed.). *American Journal of Occupational Therapy, 62,* 626–688.

Bazyk, S. (2005). Exploring the development of meaningful work for children and youth in Western contexts. *WORK: A Journal of Prevention, Assessment, and Rehabilitation, 24,* 11–20.

Benard, M., & Marshall, K. (2001). *Protective factors in individuals, families, and schools: National longitudinal study on adolescent health findings.* Minneapolis, MN: National Resilience Resource Center.

Benz, M. R., Lindstrom, L., & Yovanoff, P. (2000). Improving graduation and employment outcomes of students with disabilities: Predictive factors and student perspectives. *Exceptional Children, 66,* 509–529.

Brotherson, M. J., Cook, C. C., Erwin, E. J., & Weigel, C. J. (2008). Understanding self-determination and families of young children with disabilities in home environments. *Journal of Early Intervention, 31,* 22–43.

Bunch, G., Finnegan, K., & Pearpoint, J. (2009). *Planning for real life after school: Ways for teachers and families to plan for students experiencing significant challenge.* Toronto: Inclusion Press.

Burgstahler, S., Lopez, S., & Jirikowic, T. (2007). *Creating a transition program for teens: How DO–IT does it, and how you can do it, too.* Seattle: University of Washington.

Carrington, S., Templeton, E., & Papinczak, T. (2003). Adolescents with Asperger syndrome and perceptions of friendship. *Focus on Autism and Other Developmental Disabilities, 18*(4), 211–218.

Carter, E. W., Lane, K. L., Pierson, M. R., & Stang, K. K. (2008). Promoting self-determination for transition-age youth: Views of high school general and special educators. *Exceptional Children, 75*(1), 55–70.

Chambers, C. R., Wehmeyer, M. L., Saito, Y., Lida, K. M., Lee, Y., & Singh, V. (2007). Self-determination: What do we know? Where do we go? *Exceptionality, 15*(1), 3–15.

Clark, H. B., Koroloff, N., Geller, J., & Sondheimer, D. L. (2008). Research on transition to adulthood: Building the evidence base to inform services and supports for youth and young adults with serious mental health disorders. *Journal of Behavioral Health Services and Research, 35*(4), 365–372.

Cline, T. (2007). *A systems of care approach to substance abuse and mental health services: Testimony before Committee on Health, Education, Labor, and Pensions, United States Senate.* Retrieved August 13, 2010, from www.hhs.gov/asl/testify/2007/05/t20070508b.html

Cobb, H. V. (1973). Citizen advocacy and the rights of the handicapped. In W. Wolfensberger & H. Zauha (Eds.), *Citizen advocacy and protective services for the impaired and handicapped* (pp. 148–161). Toronto: National Institute on Mental Retardation.

Conaboy, K. S., Nochajski, S. M., Schefkind, S., & Schoonover, J. (n.d.). *Occupational therapy and transition.* Retrieved August 13, 2010, from www.aota.org/Practitioners/ProfDev/CE/Aota/CEonCD/Transition.aspx

Covey, S. R. (2010). Habit 2: Begin with the end in mind. In *The 7 habits of highly effective people.* Retrieved August 13, 2010, from www.stephencovey.com/7habits/7habits-habit2.php

Davis, M., & Sondheimer, D. L. (2005). State child mental health efforts to support youth in transition to adulthood. *Journal of Behavioral Health Services and Research, 32*(1), 27–32.

Davis, S., & Wehmeyer, M. L. (1991). *Ten steps to independence: Promoting self-determination in the home.* Silver Spring, MD: Arc National Headquarters.

Erwin, E. J., Brotherson, M. J., Palmer, S. B., Cook, C. C., Weigel, C. J., & Summers, J. A. (2009). How to promote self-determination for young children with disabilities: Evidenced-based strategies for early childhood practitioners and families. *Young Exceptional Children, 12*(2), 27–37.

Haber, M. G., Karpur, A., Deschenes, N., & Clark, H. B. (2008). Predicting improvement of transitioning young people in the Partnerships for Youth Transition Initiative: Findings from a multisite demonstration. *Journal of Behavioral Health Services and Research, 35*(4), 488–513.

Hillier, A., Fish, T., Cloppert, P., & Beversdorf, D. Q. (2007). Outcomes of a social and vocational skills support group for adolescents and young adults on the autism spectrum. *Focus on Autism and Other Developmental Disabilities, 22*(2), 107–115.

Hoffman, A. (2003). *Teaching decision making to students with learning disabilities by promoting self-determination* (ERIC Digest No. E647). Retrieved August 13, 2010, from www.eric.ed.gov/ERICDocs/data/ericdocs2sql/content_storage_01/0000019b/80/1b/81/18.pdf

Howlin, P., Goode, S., Hutton, J., & Rutter, M. (2004). Adult outcome for children with autism. *Journal of Child Psychology and Psychiatry, 45*(2), 212–219.

Individuals With Disabilities Education Improvement Act of 2004, Pub. L. 108–446, 20 U.S.C. § 1400 *et seq.*

Jennings, L. B., Parra-Medina, D. M., Hilfinger-Messias, D. K., & McLoughlin, K. (2006). Toward a critical social theory of youth empowerment. *Journal of Community Practice, 14,* 31–55.

Jivanjee, P., Kruzich, J., & Gordon, L. J. (2008). Community integration of transition-age individuals: Views of young adults with mental health disorders. *Journal of Behavioral Health Services and Research, 35*(4), 402–418.

Kemp, S. (2006). Dropout policies and trends for students with and without disabilities. *Adolescence, 41*(162), 235–250.

Martin, J. E., Dycke, J. V., D'Ottavio, M., & Nickerson, K. (2007). The student-directed summary of performance: Increasing student and family involvement in the transition planning process. *Career Development for Exceptional Individuals, 30*(1), 13–26.

Mithaug, D. E. (1993). *Self-regulation theory: How optimal adjustment maximizes gain.* Westport, CT: Praeger.

Mithaug, D. E. (1996). *Equal opportunity theory.* Thousand Oaks, CA: Sage.

Muthumbi, J. W. (2008). Enhancing transition outcomes for youth with disabilities: The partnerships for youth initiative. *Journal of Vocational Rehabilitation, 29,* 93–103.

National Collaborative on Workforce and Disability. (2009). *Supporting transition to adulthood among youth with mental health needs: Action steps for policymakers* (Policy Brief: Issue 2). Retrieved August 13, 1010, from www.ncwd-youth.info/policy-brief-02

National Collaborative on Workforce and Disability for Youth. (2010). *About us.* Retrieved August 13, 2010, from www.ncwd-youth.info/about

National Institute of Mental Health. (2002). *Mental disorders in America* (NIH Publication No. 99–4584). Bethesda, MD: Author.

National Network on Youth Transition for Behavioral Health. (2010). *The mission of the NNYT network.* Retrieved August 13, 2010, from http://nnyt.fmhi.usf.edu/

Podmostko, M. (2007). *Tunnels and cliffs: A guide for workforce development practitioners and policymakers serving youth with mental health needs.* Washington, DC: National Collaborative on Workforce and Disability for Youth, Institute for Educational Leadership.

Rehabilitation Act of 1973, Pub. L. 93–112, 29 U.S.C. § 701 *et seq.*

Sands, D. J., & Doll, B. (1996). Fostering self-determination is a developmental task. *Journal of Special Education, 30*(1), 58.

Shapiro, J. P. (1993). *No pity: People with disabilities forging a new civil rights movement.* New York: Times Books.

Ticket to Work and Work Incentives Improvement Act of 1999, Pub. L. 106–170.

Wagner, M., Cadwallader, T. W., Garza, N., & Cameto, R. (2004). *Social activities of youth with disabilities* (Reports from the National Longitudinal Transition Study). Retrieved January 4, 2010, from http://www.ncset.org/publications/viewdesc.asp?id=1470

Ward, M. J., & Meyer, R. N. (1999). Self-determination for people with developmental disabilities and autism: Two self-advocates' perspectives. *Focus on Autism and Other Developmental Disabilities, 14*(3), 133–139.

Wehman, P. (2006). *Life beyond the classroom: Transition strategies for young people with disabilities* (4th ed.). Baltimore: Paul H. Brookes.

Wehmeyer, M. L. (2002). *Self-determination and the education of students with disabilities* (ERIC Digest No. ED470036). Retrieved August 13, 2010, from www.eric.ed.gov/PDFS/ED470036.pdf

Wehmeyer, M. L. (2004). Beyond self-determination: Causal agency theory. *Journal of Developmental and Physical Disabilities, 16*(4), 337–359.

Wehmeyer, M., Bersani, H., Jr., & Gagne, R. (2000). Riding the third wave: Self-determination and self-advocacy in the 21st century. *Focus on Autism and Other Developmental Disabilities, 15*(2), 106–115.

Wehmeyer, M. L., & Gragoudas, S. (2004). Centers of independent living and transition-age youth: Empowerment and self-determination. *Journal of Vocational Rehabilitation, 20,* 53–58.

Wehmeyer, M. L., Gragoudas, S., & Shogren, K. A. (2006). Self-determination, student involvement, and leadership development. In P. Wehman (Ed.), *Life beyond the classroom: Transition strategies for young people with disabilities* (pp. 41–69). Baltimore: Paul H. Brookes.

Wehmeyer, M. L., Kelchner, K., & Richards, S. (1996). Essential characteristics of self-determined behavior of individuals with mental retardation. *American Journal on Mental Retardation, 100*(6), 632–642.

Wehmeyer, M. L., & Palmer, S. B. (2003). Adult outcomes for students with cognitive disabilities three years after high school: The impact of self-determination. *Education and Training in Developmental Disabilities, 38*(2), 131–144.

Wehmeyer, M. L., Palmer, S. B., Agran, M., Mithaug, D. E., & Martin, J. E. (2000). Promoting causal agency: The self-determined learning model of instruction. *Exceptional Children, 66*(4), 439–453.

Wehmeyer, M. L., & Schwartz, M. (1997). Self-determination and positive adult outcomes: A follow-up study of youth with mental retardation or learning disabilities. *Exceptional Children, 63,* 245–255.

Williams, V., & Heslop, P. (2006). Filling the emotional gap at transition: Young people with learning difficulties and friendship. *Learning Disability Review, 11*(4), 28–37.

Workforce Investment Act of 1998, Pub. L.105–220, U.S.C. §2801 *et seq.*

Subject Index

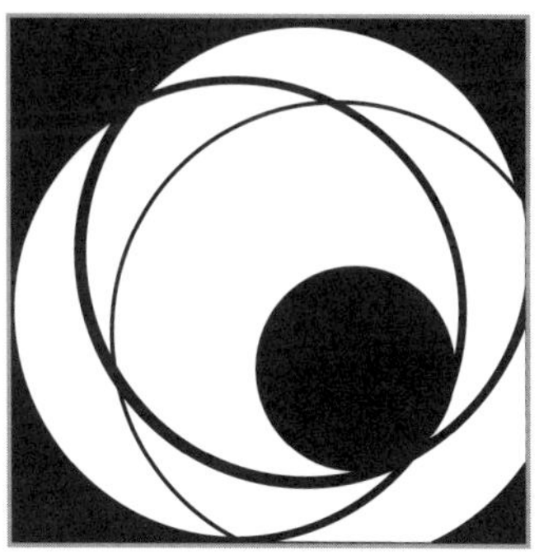

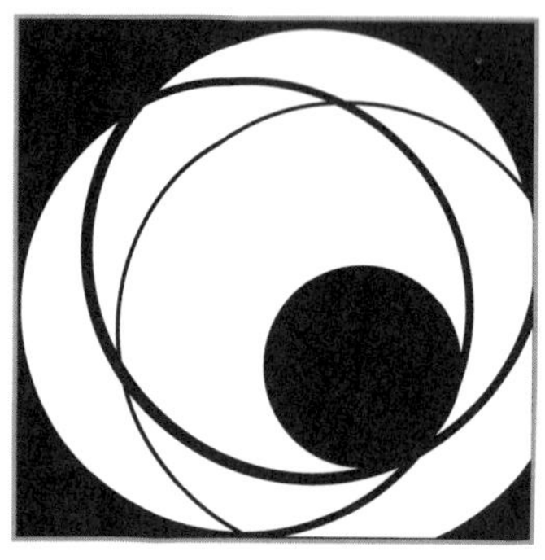

Citation Index

N

O

P

T

U

V

W

Y

Z